10 PRINCIPLES OF RECOVERY
A Positive Psychological Approach to Addiction and Life

By: Trish Barrus, Ph.D. | Jade Ozawa-Kirk, M.Ed.

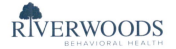

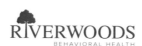

Orem, UT

Copyright © 2021 by Trish Barrus and Jade Ozawa-Kirk

All rights reserved. No part of this book may be reproduced or transmitted in any form or by any means, electronic or mechanical, including photocopying, recording, or any information storage and retrieval system, without permission in writing from Riverwoods Behavioral Health, IP, LLC. P.O. Box 970392 Orem, Utah 84097.

ISBN: 978-0-578-82341-6

Printed in the United States of America   011421

∞This paper meets the requirements of ANSI/NISO Z39.48-1992 (Permanence of Paper)

FOREWORD

In over twenty years of counseling individuals struggling with addiction, I've often heard similar sentiments from both patients and their loved ones: "Why can't I/they just stop?" Addiction recovery has been, and continues to be, a major source of frustration and heartache to all involved, particularly given the frequent lack of lasting outcomes. Studies suggest that over 85 percent of people who engage in treatment for addiction will struggle with significant relapse, having great difficulty maintaining recovery.

No matter the type of addiction (drugs, alcohol, gambling, other), it targets the brain's reward system and changes brain chemistry which can lead to physical symptoms of addiction and withdrawal as well as making it hard for people to think clearly and exercise sound judgment. Treatment for addiction has generally been very negative and highly stigmatizing in its approach. Addiction treatment, perhaps even more so than other mental health treatment, has traditionally focused on what is "wrong" with an individual, perceived "character flaws," and pathology. Though awareness of underlying pathology and motivations for continued use can be valuable, this can also be further damaging and disheartening to the patient and their loved ones. There is great power and benefit in not focusing simply on the problem, but also the solution; on leveraging and building up strengths and highlighting things that are going right, rather than only focusing on the things that are "wrong;" and on promoting self-reliance, increased confidence, and accountability rather than fostering a sense of powerlessness and dependence. In my clinical practice and in my teaching, I have been using a solution-focused, positive approach to managing addiction and promoting recovery and have witnessed so many remarkable transformations and lasting outcomes. I wanted to expand the reach of this work.

In this workbook, I, along with my colleague Jade Ozawa-Kirk, have designed a program that is built on evidence-based positive psychology principles for a strengths-based approach to addiction and recovery. Jade and I agree that the individuals dealing with addiction and recovery are so much more than the negative label of "addict" and we vehemently oppose labeling individuals in this way. That has been a main theme throughout this workbook. We have provided material that is geared towards promoting self-reliance and independence. We focus on hope, optimism and recreating and rebuilding lives through improved self-esteem. We teach about change and how resilience and growth mindset are important in this change. We also explain neuroplasticity and how the brain's main function is to change and adapt. We have created a comprehensive program that provides background, context, and research; examples, anecdotes, and stories from our vast clinical expertise; and importantly, many skills and exercises to help master the concepts and build upon the strength-based principles. Finally, this workbook emphasizes accountability and responsibility for one's life – going forward with courage to change and improve. To be happy, it is imperative to find meaning and purpose, and give back to others some of what is learned through experiences, study, and life's special moments.

Thank you to all who have made this workbook possible–those who have edited, read and re-read, and provided encouragement every step of the way. Thanks to my many patients across the years who have inspired me and trusted me to be part of their treatment and recovery. Thanks to Jade for her insight, wisdom, and collaboration. She started this journey with me years ago as one of my TA's in the Positive Psychology Certificate Program at the University of Utah. Finally, I am so appreciative to my husband and best friend, Lee Barrus, who has tirelessly supported this effort, staying up to wee hours of the morning and providing such relevant insight. The graphic design and layout of this workbook were created and produced by him.

This has been an endeavor of love. Love for those who I have counseled through the years, love for the families who have lost loved ones, and love for those who still struggle with this disease. I hope this workbook is both useful and motivating to those who read and apply its principles. Decide to change and be happy – and pursue that goal with passion and determination! And then pay it forward.

Best wishes to you, wherever you are on your journey.
Trish Barrus, Ph.D.

10 PRINCIPLES OF RECOVERY

PRINCIPLE 1
TAKE ACCOUNTABILITY FOR YOUR LIFE
Examine Yourself with Honesty and Responsibility

PRINCIPLE 2
DISCOVER PURPOSE
Identify what Gives Your Life Meaning

PRINCIPLE 3
CULTIVATE HOPE
Look for Possibilities and Be Optimistic

PRINCIPLE 4
PRACTICE GRATITUDE
Be Aware of Who and What Provides Goodness in Your Life and Show Your Thanks

PRINCIPLE 5
DEFINE & STRENGTHEN YOUR SPIRITUAL SELF
Connect with Your Higher Power

PRINCIPLE 6
FIND YOUR IDENTITY & NURTURE SELF-WORTH
Live from the Inside Out and Not the Outside In

PRINCIPLE 7
CONQUER WITH COURAGE
Use Resilience to Overcome Weaknesses, Setbacks, and Obstacles

PRINCIPLE 8
FORGIVE YOURSELF & OTHERS
Release Yourself from the Past

PRINCIPLE 9
SERVE OTHERS
Enrich Lives with Your Good Works

PRINCIPLE 10
LIVE WITH INTEGRITY
Move Forward with Authenticity and Determination

TABLE OF CONTENTS

Introduction	x
Happiness, Values & the Brain	**1**
What is Happiness	2
The Levels of Happiness	3
The Characteristics of Happy People	4
Values and Happiness	5
The Brain and Addiction	7
Neuroplasticity	11
Labeling and Stigma	13
Emotions	**15**
Types of Emotions	17
The Purpose of Emotion	19
Emotional Numbing	21
How to Treat Emotional Numbing	22
The Process of Change	**25**
The Brain and Change	26
Change	26
Stages of Change	28
Processes of Change	30
Lapses and Relapse	40
Positive Psychology & Addiction	**43**
Gratitude	45
Optimism and Hope	47
Mindfulness and Meditation	49

Savoring	50
Flow	53
Mindset—Fixed versus Growth	55
Resilience	57

Self-Esteem ... 61

What Is Self-Esteem	62
How You Acquire Self-Esteem	63
The Practice of Living Consciously	65
The Practice of Self-Acceptance	67
The Practice of Self-Responsibility	70
The Practice of Self-Assertiveness	71
The Practice of Living Purposefully	73
The Practice of Living with Integrity	74

Self-Compassion, Confidence, & Spirituality ... 77

Confidence versus Self-Doubt	79
Myths about Confidence	79
Doubt	80
The Model of Self-Love	81
Addiction and Spirituality	87

Barriers to Change ... 91

Trauma and Abuse	92
Toxic Relationships	95
Shame and Guilt	97
Forgiveness	99
Self-Defeating Behavior	104
Mental Health Disorders	106

Addictive Thinking ... 109

Self-Deception	112
Denial	113
Rationalization	114

Projection 115
Self-Victimization 116
Manipulating Others 117
Cognitive Distortions (Twisted Thinking) 117
Negative Self-Talk 121

Relationships & Communication **125**
Relationships 126
Attachment 128
Connection, Loneliness, and Addiction 129
Boundaries 133
Codependency 136
Communication 137
Empathy 139
Coping with Difficult People 141
Altruism—Serving Others 144

Living with Integrity **147**
Setting and Achieving Goals 149
Stress Management 151
The Importance of Sleep 156
The Importance of Exercise 157
The Importance of Nutrition 158

Conclusion **161**
Authenticity 161
Honesty 162
Courage 163

Resources **167**
References **179**

INTRODUCTION

We believe that addiction is a disease of the brain—**a curable disease.** You are a person who needs healing, not an addict doomed to a lifetime of recovery. Our unique approach to treating addiction combines science, psychology, and medicine to help you overcome addiction once and for all.

The **Biopsychosocial Model** we use throughout this workbook addresses how recovery is linked to the biological, psychological, and social aspects of a person's life—and how those may need to change to enable recovery.

> "We become slaves of our habits. Happiness occurs when people are most congruent with deeply held values and are holistically or fully engaged."
> —Waterman
>
> "I need to change, and I will change, but to efficiently change you need to do the right things at the right times."
> —Prochaska, Norcross, & DiClemente

Let's look at each of those aspects. The **biological component** of the model looks at how physical and genetic factors can impact recovery from addiction. Those factors include:
- The genetic and inherited factors that may influence drug and/or behavioral addictions.
- The overall health of the body, including the brain, that may impact addiction.
- Changes in diet or nutritional supplements that will increase health and help restore the brain.

The **psychological component** looks at possible psychological causes for addiction. We explore how thoughts lead to emotions and emotions lead to behaviors. For example, negative thought processes, such as "I'm not good enough," cause negative emotions that result in behaviors that can cause or further addiction.
Other psychological factors include:
- Depression
- Abuse/trauma
- Anxiety
- Low self-esteem & lack of self-confidence
- Feelings of unworthiness
- Stress
- Learning disabilities

The **social component** of the model looks at how different social factors—such as education, spirituality, economic factors, legal status, and relationships—might affect or cause addictive behaviors.

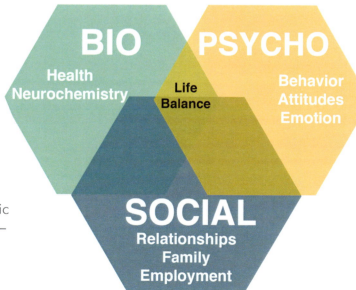

Copyright © 2021 by Trish Barrus and Jade Ozawa-Kirk

All elements of the Biopsychosocial Model are connected, and each one affects the others. Biology can affect a person's psychological state, which can then affect social well-being. Social problems can further affect the biology and the psychological state of a person. It becomes a vicious cycle. Here's an example of how that works: a woman's low hormonal levels (a physical factor) may cause anxiety and depression (psychological factors), which affect self-esteem and confidence (more psychological factors). She then does poorly in her job and her relationships (social factors), which may lead to self-medication and eventual addiction. But it doesn't stop there. As her relationships and job performance worsen, she experiences more anxiety and depression. And those create further physical health problems which continue the cycle.

This model works because linking these related factors taps more effectively into your brain's **neuroplasticity**—its ability to create new thought processes (*neuropathways*) – greatly improving your ability to change your behavior. When this "awakening" or healing of the brain occurs, you'll quickly experience new ways of thinking, feeling, and behaving that can eliminate addiction.

In this workbook, we use both cognitive-behavioral therapy and a positive psychological approach to deal with addiction. **Cognitive therapy** helps you identify faulty self-defeating messages and replace them with positive messages. **Behavioral therapy** teaches strategies that help you regulate emotions and develop the thought processes that will override dysfunctional behaviors of your past.

The **positive psychological approach** helps you capitalize on your strengths rather than be shackled by your weaknesses. Historically, psychology has focused on mental illness and the negatives in human behavior—especially in the addiction world, as evidenced by the label **addict.** In recent years, interest in human potential and well-being has grown, due in part to prominent scholars and psychologists who focused attention on the study of human strengths. These researchers have identified traits and characteristics that most cultures, religions, and philosophies believe contribute to well-being. We will explore these in this workbook.

Scientific interest now looks at how positive emotions sustain mental health. **The positive psychology we use in this workbook focuses more on strengths than on weaknesses, on building the best things in life rather than becoming fixated on the worst, and on those things that contribute to human health rather than take identity from sickness.** Along with these progressive researchers, we believe that people want to lead meaningful and fulfilling lives, to cultivate what is best within themselves, and to enhance their best experiences in love, work, and play.

Our objective for you is to be happy and content with your life, but happiness is a choice. Research shows that happy people process their experiences so that they most often remember their positive experiences. They quickly deal with negative things and push them to the background.

We've identified ten truth-based principles that not only significantly contribute to happiness, but will help you through your recovery. These **10 Principles of Recovery** are emphasized throughout the treatment process and this workbook. With these principles, you'll develop positive, strengths-based ways of thinking that can change your addictive thinking and your life.

1—TAKE ACCOUNTABILITY FOR YOUR LIFE
Examine Yourself with Honesty and Responsibility

2—DISCOVER PURPOSE
Identify What Gives Your Life Meaning

3—CULTIVATE HOPE
Look for Possibilities and Be Optimistic

4—PRACTICE GRATITUDE
Be Aware of Who and What Provides Goodness in Your Life and Show Your Thanks

5—DEFINE & STRENGTHEN YOUR SPIRITUAL SELF
Connect with Your Higher Power

6—FIND YOUR IDENTITY & NURTURE SELF-WORTH
Live from the Inside Out and Not the Outside In

7—CONQUER WITH COURAGE
Use Resilience to Overcome Weaknesses, Setbacks, and Obstacles

8—FORGIVE YOURSELF & OTHERS
Release Yourself from the Past

9—SERVE OTHERS
Enrich Lives with Your Good Works

10—LIVE WITH INTEGRITY
Move Forward with Authenticity and Determination

FLOURISHING

The ultimate goal of our program is to promote living a **flourishing** life that is meaningful and in which you function well (psychologically and socially) and feel good (experience positive emotions). This goes beyond traditional ideas of happiness and well-being. A flourishing life is not without hardship or pain, but it incorporates the perspective that the good outweighs the bad.

Positive psychologist Martin E.P. Seligman identifies five areas crucial to "the good life" (flourishing) and uses the acronym PERMA:
- Positive emotions—seeking out and creating opportunity for more positive emotions
- Engagement—actively engaging in your work and the world

- Relationships—cultivating meaningful relationships with family, friends, and community
- Meaning—finding a sense of meaning and purpose
- Accomplishment—striving to achieve goals

We believe that everyone can live "the good life," and we show you how in this workbook. You can change and grow—and the journey you're about to undertake will help you create your best life.

> "Reliving the states that make life miserable . . . has made building the states that make life worth living less of a priority. The time has finally arrived for a science that seeks to understand positive emotion, build strength and virtue, and provide guideposts for finding what Aristotle called the good life."—Martin E. P. Seligman

You'll see **Exercises** throughout this workbook. We encourage you to complete each of them because they'll help you think about your life and apply the principles you are learning. While reading and listening to ideas may help you understand the concept of change, true change can be yours only when you choose to be proactive. Completing the exercises and writing are two ways to do that.

JOURNALING

You remember Anne Frank whose diaries gave us a stunning perspective on the Jewish experience during World War II. She wrote, "I can shake off everything as I write; my sorrows disappear, my courage is reborn."

You can have a similar experience as you write about your experience in healing and as you engage in reflective writing exercises. Research shows that putting pen to paper helps you process difficult emotions and life events, gain clarity, and deepen your motivation to change.

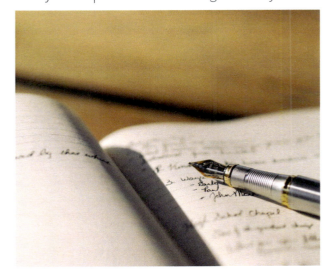

Recent studies have shown that writing thoughts and feelings is very therapeutic. In one study, researchers looked at the brain activity of people who were depressed and anxious. The MRIs showed an amazing amount of activity in the part of the brain that causes impulsivity. At the same time, other areas of the brain were blocked, causing confusion, memory loss, anxiety, and depression. Study participants were asked to write for five minutes a day about anything that they wanted—but they had to write by hand, not type. (You'll find out why in just a minute.) Most of them used this as a time to unload problems and negative feelings. Six weeks later the MRIs were repeated, and most of the participants' brains were completely normal.

Why such drastic results? Consider this: When you get physically ill from the flu or food poisoning, your body purges itself to get rid of the toxins. You vomit, sneeze, cough, and so on. If you eat again before the toxins are completely removed, you vomit again—the body can't handle the good until all the toxins are purged. The same thing happens to the brain. You have emotional toxins resulting from your experiences, messages (your own and those of others), and beliefs. Those toxic messages have built up through the years. Writing helps you purge those toxins, allowing your brain to accept and process new, positive messages

CAN'T YOU JUST TALK? WHY IS WRITING SO IMPORTANT?

When you share your thoughts and feelings by talking to others, you may not be honest because of the body language or facial expressions of the other person. You might also hold back because you're afraid of being judged or of causing damage to the relationship. You might think things like, "Oh, I shouldn't say that, "I'm too embarrassed or ashamed to admit that," or "That's stupid." But you can be honest on paper. The paper doesn't talk back or judge you. You can then fully clear out your feelings and thoughts. Writing also helps you clarify your decisions, figure out what you want to say to someone, and define your goals and your feelings.

> "Journal writing, when it becomes a ritual for transformation, is not only life changing but life-expanding."
> —Jen Williamson

Writing is one of the primary ways to reduce stress and get rid of psychological baggage. And here's why writing by hand is so important: compared to keyboarding, it has been shown by recent research to have other benefits. Writing by hand activates language areas of the brain that are not engaged with typing. It accesses both sides of the brain, which increases mental effectiveness, learning, and retention. Using both sides of the brain also encourages the expression of emotions. Emotional catharsis is often lacking in those with addiction issues, and writing will help with this. Research has shown that writing by hand makes what you're writing more personal and relatable to real life.

There are lots of ways to journal. As you progress through this workbook, your journal shouldn't be a travel log or a description of your day. Instead, it's meant to allow you to express your emotions and clarify how you're feeling. It can also help purge or eliminate negative thoughts. That's why we call the journaling used in this workbook **purging pages.**

HOW TO EFFECTIVELY USE PURGING PAGES (JOURNAL)

First, buy a notebook or journal with two separate sections (or clearly divide a single-subject journal into two sections). Write in each of these two journals every day. Here's how it works:

VENT-AND-PURGE THOUGHTS

In the first section, write for at least five to ten minutes a day about negative thoughts, feelings, and emotions. Let your feelings and thoughts flow as you write about the things that are on your mind. Give yourself permission to feel and think. This section is for purging, and **nothing is off limits.** No one is going to read your writing, because you're going to throw it away. That's right—you're going to toss it. You wouldn't keep your physical vomit, and you shouldn't keep your emotional vomit either. Keeping it **only** re-infects you and makes it very difficult to let it go. After you are done writing, empower yourself by throwing it away, shredding it, burning it, whatever—just get rid of it.

Kris shared her experience with purging pages: *"I usually don't write journal/diary entries. I have always written more 'legitimate' stuff like ideas, poems, quotes, stories, etc. I did my first purging exercise page and I just want to tell you how effective it really was. I wasn't sleeping well because I kept having nightmares. My nightmares are when those I love abandon me. I rarely have them nowadays but I had one last night and I woke up, having missed my Spanish class, feeling depressed and anxious. I sat down and wrote two and a half pages in my class notebook. I spent the first part purging and then I switched to the positives such as hopes, encouragement, affirmation, etc. I was shaking and crying when I first sat down and now I am level, calm, and have some hope. I am already a big fan of this process. I was a bit skeptical at the beginning but, I am pleasantly surprised."*

GRATITUDE THOUGHTS

At the end of the second section, write down at least three things a day that you are grateful for and why. Research shows that people who are grateful are less depressed, more creative, less anxious, and more focused. Feeling gratitude keeps you in the moment and prevents you from comparing yourself to others. You get rid of the "grass is always greener" mentality. Gratitude is a reflection of those things that are meaningful and positive in your life an awareness of those things that engender thankfulness in your heart.

HOW TO EFFECTIVELY USE THIS WORKBOOK

Each chapter of this workbook has been separated into learning modules that include five sections: specific principles of recovery, education and research pertinent to recovery, exercises, reflections and activities, and key takeaways. As you think about what you want to change and how you'll do it, we encourage you to take advantage of all the materials provided.

All the material has a purpose and can assist you on your path toward sobriety and greater life satisfaction.

1. PRINCIPLES
Modules begin with truth-based **Principles of Recovery** that will not only help your recovery but will enhance your well-being and coping skills. As you work through the content of each module, notice the underlying principles and consider how you may apply them to your life.

2. LEARNING MATERIALS
Each module contains the latest evidence-based research and concepts that will help you understand addiction and recovery. This includes information about factors that probably impacted your addiction and strategies that will help you make lasting change.

3. EXERCISES
Learning is not passive! Each of the exercises serves a purpose. Engaging in these activities with **effort and honesty** will help you change your addictive behaviors and adopt a healthier way of thinking, coping and being.

4. KEY TAKEAWAYS
The key takeaways at the end of each module briefly outline the concepts and principles emphasized in the module and those we hope you will apply to your life. This is a time to reflect on your next steps and how you will implement these ideas now and in the future.

5. RESOURCES
Lastly, lists of additional materials and resources we think will help expand your learning and recovery will be provided at the end of the workbook. Books, organizations, and online materials are provided that you can explore as a supplement to what this workbook provides.

KEY TAKEAWAYS

- Addiction is a brain disease that can be treated using a biopsychosocial approach.
- Positive psychology is the study of human thriving; applying it increases a sense of well-being and life satisfaction.
- "The good life" depends on positive emotions, engagement, relationships, meaning, and accomplishment.
- Emotional expression through hand-written journaling has significant therapeutic effects. You are asked to journal this way throughout this workbook.

MODULE 1
HAPPINESS, VALUES & THE BRAIN

PRINCIPLES

TAKE ACCOUNTABILITY FOR YOUR LIFE

Examine Yourself with Honesty and Responsibility

DISCOVER PURPOSE

Identify what Gives Your Life Meaning

THOUGHT QUESTIONS

What does happiness look like to you?
How would you describe it to someone who has never experienced it?
What does it feel like?
What invites it into your life?

Throughout this module, we talk about the influence of genetic factors on happiness and values. But your biology is not the only thing that affects your overall happiness; so does your mind. It is imperative in the process of recovery that you **examine yourself in an honest way and take responsibility for your life. Being accountable** for who you are allows you to take ownership for your life.

> As a reminder, all modules will begin with truth-based principles of recovery that promote self-efficacy and change through focusing on strengths and the good in your life. Not only will these help your recovery, but they will also enhance your well-being and coping skills.

I was working with teenagers from inner-city Chicago and Los Angeles: tough kids who had been involved in the "seedy" side of life. They had run in gangs and had participated in murder, robbery, and other forms of violence. One day in group, I asked the question, "How is it that you can take the life of another person without feeling remorse?"

A little guy no more than four-foot-eight stood up and said, "I'll tell you how. I come from a family of eleven kids. We all have different fathers. Our house, if you can call it that, is in a war zone. Bullets fly all the time. My mother is never home, and no one cares if I go to school, if I eat, or if I'm safe. No one except the local drug dealer, because I run drugs for him. But even to him, I am easily replaced. If no one cares about my life, why would I care about the life of another person? Life has no meaning."

"Without meaning or purpose, it can seem like life doesn't matter." It is easier to slip back into addiction when nothing matters. The good news is that you can experience happiness by **finding purpose and meaning.**

WHAT IS HAPPINESS

Though the definition of happiness may be different for each person, one thing applies to everyone: Happiness is a combination of how good you feel day-to-day and your overall satisfaction with life. Circumstances and moods can change from one day to another, but research shows that happiness levels tend to stay within a certain range. That's because a large portion of happiness is genetic—as much as 50 percent of your happiness is determined by your DNA. In other words, some people are born happier than others.

> "Probably the biggest insight . . . is that happiness is not just a place but also a process . . . Happiness is an ongoing process of fresh challenges, and . . . it takes the right attitudes and activities to continue to be happy." —Ed Diener

If half of your happiness is determined by DNA, what about the rest? About 10 percent is thought to be determined by life circumstances; the last 40 percent is caused by intentional activity—the things you decide to do.

It might seem a bit discouraging that half of your happiness hinges on your DNA, something you can't do anything about. But wait—that means that half of your happiness is in your hands! Here's what that suggests: You can change aspects of your circumstances and you can pursue activities that will boost your levels of joy. After all, bestselling author and meditation expert Sharon Salzberg wrote, "The difference between misery and happiness depends on what we do with our attention." And what you do with your attention is completely up to you.

An important aspect of happiness is accountability and being responsible for yourself and your own contentment. Stanford psychiatrist David D. Burns wrote, "There is only one person who could ever make you happy, and that person is you." You are the only one responsible for you and your decisions, actions, and thoughts. No one else is. It's easier to blame others when things go wrong, but when you do that, you give up your control to others. As Nathaniel Branden says, "You cannot respect or trust yourself if you continually pass on to others the burdens of your existence."

Happy people are more aware of positive experiences. They have negative experiences—we all do—but they don't pay much attention to those. Happy people are also proactive. If challenges occur, they ask themselves, "Is there an action I can take to improve or correct the situation?" If there is, they take it. If there isn't, they do their best not to dwell on what is beyond their control. They focus on the solution, not the problem. That's not always easy—but remember that **happy people have decided they want to be happy.**

> "If you believe your happiness is primarily in your own hands, you give yourself enormous power. You don't wait for events or other people to make you happy. If something is wrong, your response is not, 'Someone's got to do something,' but, 'What can I do?'"
> —Nathaniel Branden

Research shows the best predictors of a person's ability to be happy are (1) self-esteem and (2) the belief that we ourselves—rather than external forces—shape our destiny. If you believe that other things, like people or circumstances, determine your happiness, you give up control to that person or experience. Psychologist Sonja Lyubomirsky emphasized that when she said, **"Happiness is not out there for us to find. The reason that it's not out there is that it's inside us."**

THE LEVELS OF HAPPINESS

There are different levels of happiness, ranging from pleasure to happiness to joy, and they're not all the same. Let's look at those.

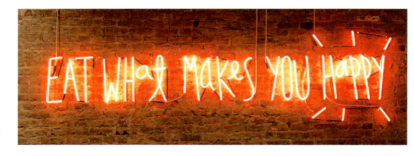

LEVEL 1 – PLEASURE

The first level of happiness is pleasure, feeling good in the moment. Where happiness is lasting, pleasure is fleeting, even though it can be intense. It involves the five senses and is manifested in something you see, hear, smell, taste, or feel. For example, pleasure might come from eating your favorite dessert or watching a beautiful sunset. While pleasure is not lasting, it is an important part of overall happiness when coupled with the other levels.

Because pleasure comes from external sources, you can adapt to it in ways you do not adapt to the other levels of happiness. In all areas of life, but especially with addiction, it takes more of the same activity or drug to produce the same amount of pleasure as you grow accustomed to it. This is called tolerance. Tolerance plays into the addictive cycle as the body and mind need more pleasure or more stimulation to feel normal. Those with addictions are usually stuck at this level because they are typically not used to putting in the effort it takes to feel happy.

LEVEL 2 – MEANINGFUL HAPPINESS

This level of happiness is based on a desire for connection and meaning, and it takes work. At this level, you're concerned about the well-being of yourself and others. It involves finding balance between work, family, hobbies, and other activities. This level can also include pleasure.

LEVEL 3 – JOY

This level involves a search for fullness and perfection. It means finding the right balance between the other levels. Renowned psychologist Abraham Maslow described this as **self-actualization**, which he defined as gaining meaning in life through fulfilling one's potential. This includes aspects of spirituality, a connection with the divine, and a connection to the larger universe. It also entails living authentically to your desires and talents. At this level, there is a greater appreciation and savoring of what life has to offer.

THE CHARACTERISTICS OF HAPPY PEOPLE

Research shows that happy people have four characteristics in common.

1. **Healthy Relationships.** Research indicates that healthy relationships are the number-one determinant of happiness. The people you surround yourself with and what you gain and give through daily interactions affect both well-being and mood. When recovering from addiction, it is particularly necessary to create connections and surround yourself with a healthy support system.

2. **Meaning or Purpose in Life.** Finding a meaning or purpose in life is extremely important to happiness. Without purpose or meaning, there is no direction or substance to life, which is a major factor in depression and anxiety. Meaning and purpose can occur in the form of an overall purpose, such as, "I want to be helpful and better the lives of those around me," "I want to be successful in my career," or "I want to leave the world a better place." You can also find meaning in day-to-day roles or activities, such as, "I find meaning in being a friend," "My purpose today is to help my child feel better about himself," or "Today I want to finish the project I've been working on." Meaning and purpose bolster resilience when challenges arise. It can be difficult to find meaning when you're overcoming addiction but doing so enhances your ability to remain addiction free.

   > "Happiness cannot be attained by wanting to be happy—it must come as the unintended consequence of working for a goal greater than oneself." —Victor Frankl

3. **Gratitude.** Research has shown that those who practice gratitude (beyond the simple attitude) have lower rates of depression, are healthier physically, and handle stress more effectively. Gratitude practice creates positive emotions and paints your world in a new light. You see life from a different perspective. By acknowledging and practicing gratitude for what you have, you will be more content and positive. When you're in recovery, it's especially important to look for what is right in life instead of what is wrong.

4. **Goals.** Goals keep you moving in the direction you want to go. When you reach a goal, no matter how small, your sense of self-esteem grows. Those with addictive thinking patterns tend to have a hard time setting goals, finding meaning and/or purpose in life, and remembering their dreams. Finding meaning and setting goals to reach those dreams is an important step to a healthy and fulfilling life.

MODULE 1

EXERCISE: Reflect on happiness in your life. Write about the following:
What is your definition of happiness?
If you aren't happy, what would be happening in your life if you were happy?
At what time in your life have you been the happiest?
Write specific things that you need to change to be happy right now.

VALUES AND HAPPINESS

Life sometimes seems like a boat without a rudder in the middle of a storm. At times, you feel like you're being tossed one way and then another, especially if you don't have values leading the way. Maybe you haven't given much thought to values, but they exist, regardless of whether you recognize them. And they make it a lot easier to navigate life.

> "Your core values are the deeply held beliefs that authentically describe your soul."
> —John C. Maxwell

When making decisions or creating change, you must clarify your values. To figure out what you value, ask yourself, "**What are my priorities in life? In what activities should I spend my limited time and resources?**"

"That's fine," you may be thinking, "but what do values have to do with happiness?"

In addition to contributing to happiness, values are important in the recovery process. Values impact how you will live your life and what you will become. They also determine what your legacy will be. **Will you be able to look back at your life and believe that you have lived with integrity**—true to yourself and your values—or will you feel like you have wasted your life or you weren't true to who you were? As Stephen R. Covey wrote, "We do make a difference—one way or the other. We are responsible for the impact of our lives. Whatever we do with whatever we have, we leave behind us a legacy for those who follow." Your recovery will be a lasting legacy of which you can be proud.

> "A joyful life is an individual creation that cannot be copied from a recipe."
> —Mihaly Csikszentmihalyi

WHAT ARE YOUR VALUES?

> **VALUES CLARIFICATION:** Review the list of values in the table. Underline every value that is important to you. You may want to add some that aren't on the list. Of those you've underlined, circle the ten most important to you. Then narrow those ten down to your top three to five values—those most important in your life.

You may want to share this list with a loved one or significant other and ask what he or she believes you value. Does his or her view of your values match your own, or is it different from how you see yourself? Are you really being honest?

Accountability	Balance	Optimism	Perseverance
Equality	Forgiveness	Time	Understanding
Job Security	Legacy	Community	Cooperation
Responsibility	Serenity	Gratitude	Humility
Achievement	Beauty	Order	Personal Fulfillment
Ethics	Freedom	Teamwork	Uniqueness
Joy	Leisure	Compassion	Courage
Risk-taking	Service	Growth	Humor
Adaptability	Being the Best	Nature	Power
Excellence	Friendship	Thrift	Usefulness
Justice	Love	Competence	Creativity
Safety	Simplicity	Harmony	Inclusion
Adventure	Belonging	Parenting	Pride
Fairness	Fun	Tradition	Vision
Kindness	Loyalty	Confidence	Dignity
Security	Spirituality	Health	Independence
Altruism	Career	Patriotism	Recognition
Faith	Future Generations	Travel	Wealth
Knowledge	Sportsmanship	Connection	Diversity
Self-discipline	Caring	Home	Integrity
Ambition	Generosity	Patience	Reliability
Family	Stewardship	Trust	Well-being
Leadership	Collaboration	Contentment	Environment
Self-expression	Giving back	Honesty	Initiative
Authenticity	Openness	Peace	Respect
Financial Stability	Success	Truth	
Learning	Commitment	Contribution	
Self-respect	Grace	Hope	

MODULE 1

EXERCISE: Write about the following: How have your values shifted since you began your recovery process? Consider how much time you spend on things of little importance to you. Do you need to adjust that so you are spending the most time on what you think is the most important?

JOURNAL - Write your obituary or legacy in your journal. Include what you would like to be remembered for when you are gone. Be thoughtful and honest. You may write that you want people to remember you as a kind, patient, and loving person or as a hard worker who spent time with your children and made them your priority. Next, think about how you are today. Again, be honest. Is who you are now consistent with how you want to be remembered? If not, what changes do you need to make?

THE BRAIN AND ADDICTION

The brain is a complex and remarkable machine. Within each brain region, we find dynamic systems of chemicals called **neurochemicals** and cells unique to the brain called **neurons**. Neurons are activated by information acquired through our senses. Each time we see, hear, smell, taste, or touch something, neurons release chemicals called **neurotransmitters** and neuropeptides that communicate with and strengthen connections with other neurons. Each release of a neurochemical strengthens the relationship between neurons. "Neurons that fire together, wire together."

"The human brain has 100 billion neurons, each neuron connected to 10 thousand other neurons. Sitting on your shoulders is the most complicated object in the known universe." —Michio Kaku

When you engage in enjoyable activities—eating, drinking, fun activities, and sex—a brain region known as the reward pathway is at work. Located in the center of the brain, it drives your motivation and sense of reward. The **reward pathway** is connected to other areas of the brain that then get information on what's happening outside your body. That strengthens brain circuits and reinforces positive behaviors. It also communicates with your memory. When you eat a delicious meal, the neurotransmitter dopamine is released in the reward pathway and alerts your memory—increasing the chance that you will eat that meal again.

This same thing happens with addiction. Drugs and addictive behaviors—such as gambling and pornography—alter the communication between neurons. As this happens repeatedly, dependence and addiction are established. **Repeated use of addictive stimulants (behavioral or substance) actually rewires the brain.**

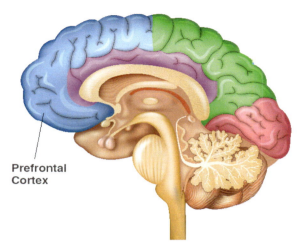

Prefrontal Cortex

Here's what happens: As addictive stimulants artificially raise the amount of dopamine or other neurotransmitters a need is created. That need can be met only through more of that stimulant. The brain's system of reward and enjoyment is overridden. In response to unnatural amounts of a neurotransmitter flooding the system, the brain decreases the number of receptors.

You probably know what that means: With fewer receptors, users no longer feel the stimulant's effects in the same way. Suddenly, the drug or behavior that once created excitement seems boring or not enough. The user needs to take or do more to get the same "high" that was once enjoyed. As that continues, the pathway created gets deeper and stronger. Using becomes easier and easier, and the habit becomes more difficult to break, even if the user no longer wants to engage in the behavior.

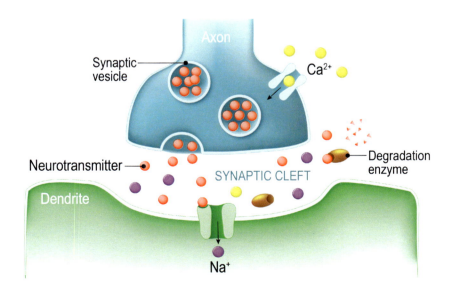

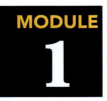

Each drug or behavior influences one or more neurotransmitters, which determines how the drug or action makes you feel. The following table matches commonly abused substances to the neurotransmitters and functions they affect.

Neurotransmitter	Functions Influenced	Addictive Behaviors/Drugs That Influence
Dopamine	• Pleasure/reward • Movement • Attention • Memory	• Cocaine • Methamphetamine • Amphetamine • Most drugs either directly or indirectly • Pornography/Sex • Gambling • Shopping • Gaming • Binge-eating • Internet
Serotonin	• Mood • Sleep • Sexual desire • Appetite	• Cocaine • Methamphetamine • Amphetamine • Most drugs either directly or indirectly • Pornography/Sex • Gambling • Shopping • Gaming • Binge-eating • Internet
Norepinephrine	• Sensory processing • Movement • Sleep • Mood • Memory • Anxiety	• Cocaine • Methamphetamine • Amphetamine
Endorphin/ Enkephalin	• Analgesia • Sedation • Rate of bodily functions (e.g., breathing) • Mood	• Heroin • Morphine • Prescription pain relievers (e.g., oxycodone) • Gambling • Binge-eating
Acetylcholine	• Memory • Arousal • Attention • Mood	• Nicotine/Smoking • Internet
Anandamide	• Movement • Cognition/memory	• Marijuana
Glutamate	• Neuron activity • Learning • Cognition/memory	• Ketamine • Phencyclidine • Alcohol

Copyright © 2021 by Trish Barrus and Jade Ozawa-Kirk

Gamma-aminobutyric acid (GABA)	• Neuron activity • Anxiety • Memory • Anesthesia	• Sedatives • Tranquilizers • Alcohol • Binge-eating • Internet
	• Memory • Bonding	• Pornography/Sex

> **EXERCISE:** Based on this chart and your experience, how have addictions affected your functioning? For example, Internet use has been shown to affect GABA and dopamine, both of which affect anxiety, memory, attention, and feelings of pleasure. An excessive Internet user may notice his attention span diminishing, becoming easily distracted and inclined to "multi-task" by playing a game on his phone while streaming a new episode of his favorite TV show. He may also think, "Just one more post" as he scrolls through social media—but one more post may turn into another hour without his noticing how much time has passed.

As addiction continues, new problems arise for the user. Fewer dopamine receptors result in difficulty experiencing happiness and pleasure from things that used to be interesting or pleasurable. Once favorite activities, such as sports or time with family, become boring, anxiety results until the high of using is experienced again.

MODULE 1

EXERCISE: Before you became addicted, what were your favorite activities? What did you feel when you engaged in these activities? What do you enjoy doing now? How would you like to find enjoyment in the future?

The process of addiction damages the brain. The prefrontal cortex (at the front of the brain) is one of the most quickly damaged and, in fact, shrinks with addictive behavior. The result is diminished impulse control and rational decision-making and increased impulsivity (the tendency to act on sudden urges, without pondering potential consequences or weighing pros/cons) and compulsivity (repeated behaviors to reduce anxiety). As impulsiveness and compulsiveness increase, it gets harder to say no to addictive behaviors—and using gets easier. Drugs and addictive behaviors can also affect people in different ways, depending on things like genetic make-up, environmental risk factors (divorce, death, neighborhood, job, abuse/trauma), and intrinsic resilience (the natural ability of someone to "bounce back" after experiencing trauma or challenges).

NEUROPLASTICITY

By now, you might think you've damaged your brain beyond repair from your addiction. But think again, because there's good news!

> "Picture your brain forming new connections as you meet the challenge and learn. Keep on going." —Carol Dweck

One of the brain's most extraordinary features is its ability to change and heal, something called neuroplasticity. Neuroplasticity is the brain's ability to form new neural connections across its lifespan. That plays a role in how addictions take hold, but it also explains how addiction can be overcome.

To more easily visualize that, think of hiking trails. Frequently used trails are worn down and smooth, free of vegetation. New trails, on the other hand, are usually overgrown with weeds; sometimes you can't even see the dirt path under all the foliage. But every time it's used, a new trail gets a little more worn in until it becomes as recognizable as the old trail.

That's very similar to how neural pathways and neuroplasticity work when you learn something new. Every time you have a new thought or engage in a new behavior, new paths are developed in your brain. That's why it's important to practice anything you want to master. The more often you do something, the more you remember, and the easier it is to do. Sadly, that works for better and worse. While practice can make you better at something, it can also reinforce the wrong things. Every time you rehearse a dialogue of negative thoughts—"I'm not good enough," "I'll never amount to anything," "I screw everything up"—you strengthen the pathway associated with those beliefs. And each time you engage in an addictive behavior, you strengthen the connections that may lead you to repeat it. As Aristotle said, "We are what we repeatedly do"—for good and bad.

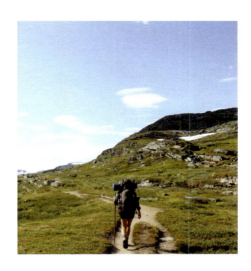

> "Every time we learn a new fact, a new skill, every time we give a new response; our brain changes. This is neuroplasticity! And this is true for adult brains too, so don't stop learning." —Aadil Chimthanawala

Here's why that's such good news: Through consistent effort, practice, and work, strong addictive pathways in your brain can be replaced. Deeply ingrained bad behaviors can be exchanged for fulfilling, good behaviors. In other words, you can overcome your addiction, alter your bad habits, and change your brain for good!

EXERCISE: What thoughts—positive and negative—do you tell yourself over and over? In other words, what are the well-worn paths in your brain? How can you reinforce the positive thoughts? How can you change the negative thoughts? Write some new thoughts you can use to replace those negative ones.

REPEATED THOUGHT	POSITIVE REPLACEMENT

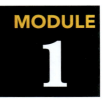

MODULE 1

LABELING AND STIGMA

Now you understand the power of words and neuroplasticity. Labeling is one way we all give power to words.

Labels can be divisive and negative or they can be uplifting and positive. Think about it. When you label someone, your perception of that person suddenly changes—for good or for bad. The same thing happens when you label yourself; you become defined by that label. Don't label yourself an **addict or abuser**—it's a trap that will emphasize your struggle and will leave little room for change. Instead, think of and label your addiction as a challenge; you are experiencing a drug or behavioral problem, but you are not that problem.

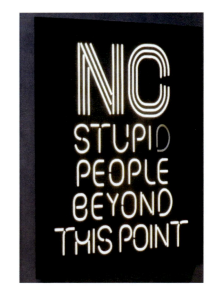

Put neuroplasticity to work by visualizing yourself in a new way. Label yourself positively— "I am a good person," "I am smart," "I am a wife, husband, or parent," "I am a good worker." You are what you see yourself as, and the more positive you see yourself, the better you will become.

> EXERCISE: Take a moment to think about labels. Though they often work against you negatively, you can also give yourself positive, helpful labels. Think back to the legacy you wrote earlier. Determine how you want to label yourself.

KEY TAKEAWAYS

- The experience of happiness is different from one person to another, and it is impacted by genetic and environmental factors.
- Happiness exists on a spectrum that includes pleasure, meaningful happiness, and joy.
- The four components of meaningful happiness are healthy relationships, meaning or purpose, gratitude, and goals.
- Values determine how you live your life and identifying your values can aid in recovery.
- Brain chemistry is impacted by addictive behaviors. Through neuroplasticity, old thought and behavior patterns can be replaced by new ones.
- The ways you label yourself can influence your life path.

MODULE 2
EMOTIONS

PRINCIPLES
TAKE ACCOUNTABILITY FOR YOUR LIFE
Examine Yourself with Honesty and Responsibility

DISCOVER YOUR PURPOSE
Identify What Gives Your Life Meaning

THOUGHT QUESTIONS
What emotions are you feeling at this time of transition and recovery?
How has emotional numbing played out in your life?
How has numbing clouded your vision for yourself, meaning in your life, and your purpose?

Several years ago, Sheryl Crow had a hit song entitled, "I Can't Cry Anymore." This song resonated with many because sometimes we all feel that way. Life gets us down, and we're tired of being down. But tears and emotions are useful because they help us relate to others. Emotions also provide you with good information and clarify how you think, desire, and feel. They validate what is **meaningful in life and help you understand your purpose** as you feel passionate about a certain direction or cause.

> "Human behavior flows from three main sources: desire, emotion, and knowledge."
> —Plato

Denying or numbing emotions is very unhealthy, both physically and mentally. When you deny emotions or blame others for the way you feel, you give up control of yourself because you aren't **taking responsibility or being honest with yourself.**

What is Emotion

Emotion is defined as:

- A mental state associated with the nervous system brought on by chemical changes in response to thoughts, feelings, behavior, and pleasure or displeasure.

- A person's internal state of being.

- Involuntary physiological response to an object or a situation, based on or tied to physical state and sensory data.

- A conscious mental reaction (such as anger or fear) experienced as a feeling, usually directed toward a specific object and typically accompanied by changes in the body.

Consider the feelings of this man:

> "Emotions make us human. Denying them makes us beasts." —Victoria Klein

"I killed my brother," he said. "It was an accident, I know, but all of these years [fifty-five] later, I still feel guilt at times. I think about him every day. My mom couldn't handle his death and became more and more depressed. She really never talked to me after the accident until I was in college. I was ten at the time of the accident. My dad escaped through work. I was basically alone. I cried until I couldn't cry anymore. And then I got angry. Angry at my brother for dying. Angry at my mom for not loving me and angry at my dad for escaping. Angry at being abandoned. Angry at everything.

"Anger and abandonment defined my marriage. Underneath, I just needed love and acceptance. But I was always afraid she'd leave; everyone else that I cared about had left. So, I pushed her away with my anger first, before she could leave me. And then I made excuses, like deciding that she wasn't good for me anyway.

"But she didn't leave. She loved and accepted. She finally broke through the hard veneer that I had formed. I cried, finally. I became vulnerable, finally. I admitted what was wrong, finally. And yes, I finally found a purpose besides being angry."

Thoughts cause emotions; emotions motivate behavior. At times, you repress emotions because they are uncomfortable or hurtful. When that happens, you numb yourself through dysfunctional behaviors or self-medication.

Most scientists agree that emotion is a brief conscious experience characterized by intense mental activity and physiological and behavioral changes. Emotions trigger major changes throughout the body that affect your behavior. You may feel a difference in your muscles or how fast your heart is beating. Your blood pressure may go up or down. Your energy level, tone of voice, and facial expressions may change. Anxiety and depression can interrupt feelings of pleasure and can cause feelings of pain.

In addition to their impact on the body, emotions have the power to enhance, distort, or totally disrupt mental processes. For example, happiness can increase your ability to focus and be productive, while anxiety makes it almost impossible to concentrate.

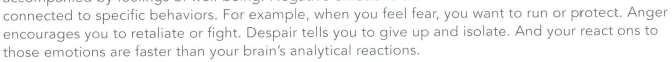

Obviously, there are positive and negative emotions. Positive emotions aren't linked to a resulting behavior; they are usually accompanied by feelings of well-being. Negative emotions are connected to specific behaviors. For example, when you feel fear, you want to run or protect. Anger encourages you to retaliate or fight. Despair tells you to give up and isolate. And your reactions to those emotions are faster than your brain's analytical reactions.

That's what helped our ancient ancestors survive. When they saw a bear coming, they reacted to the emotion telling them to run instead of analyzing, "Is that a nice bear or a bad bear?" "Will it hurt me or cuddle with me?" The problem is, your emotions still react ahead of your thinking brain, even though your "bears" are other kinds of stresses. Willpower can't change that. Fear, anger, disgust, and surprise will always be ahead of your analytic abilities. This can cause problems when you impulsively say or do something based on emotion, that is not well thought out.

MODULE 2

Is there an alternative to fear, anger, disgust, and surprise? Yes! And if you want to flourish today, you need to develop and expand positive emotions.

BROADEN-AND-BUILD THEORY

Positive emotions—including satisfaction, joy, amusement, and love—are good for you, and research shows just how much they can help. Psychologist Barbara Fredrickson proposed the Broaden-and-Build Theory, which suggests that positive emotional states have a vital role in our survival. When you experience positive emotions, you have greater awareness and can think more creatively. You see with greater insight and your perceptions are enlarged. Positive emotions also help you build your store of the physical, social, and intellectual resources that lead to well-being. In addition, positive emotions build on each other.

> "Feelings are much like waves, we can't stop them from coming but we can choose which one to surf."
> —Jonatan Martensson

Negative emotions, on the other hand, lead to narrow focus and a distortion of what may be neutral. It's what we call "tunnel vision" because it limits your perspectives about life. You may have learned to think negatively, and negative thoughts often give rise to negative emotions. This doesn't have to be the case, even if you think this is an entrenched habit.

It can be corrected. As you practice thinking positively, your emotions will be more positive, you will let go of automatic responses and emotions, increase your intelligence, creativity, health, and feelings of general well-being.

TYPES OF EMOTIONS

There are two types of emotions: primary and secondary.

PRIMARY EMOTIONS

Primary emotions are the body's first response to a situation. You are born with these and they are wired into your brain. Because of this wiring, you respond to specific emotions with certain physical reactions, such as sweating, increased heart rate, or a grimace.

Positive emotions broaden perspective and build on each other creating an upward spiral.

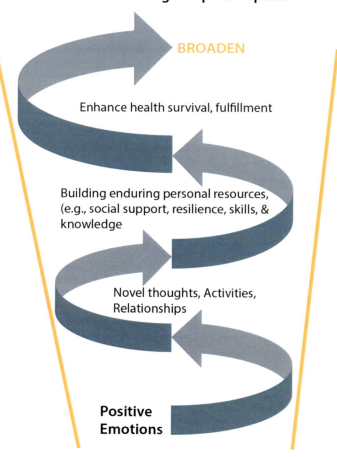

17 Copyright © 2021 by Trish Barrus and Jade Ozawa-Kirk

Researchers differ on what these primary emotions are, but most agree that the following emotions qualify:
- Anger: fury, outrage, wrath, irritability, hostility, resentment, and violence. (Some believe anger to be a secondary emotion–a reaction to other primary emotions.)
- Sadness: grief, sorrow, gloom, melancholy, despair, loneliness, and depression.
- Fear: anxiety, apprehension, nervousness, dread, fright, and panic.
- Joy: enjoyment, happiness, relief, bliss, delight, pride, thrill, and ecstasy.
- Surprise: shock, astonishment, amazement, astound, and wonder.
- Disgust: contempt, disdain, scorn, aversion, distaste, and revulsion.

SECONDARY EMOTIONS

Secondary emotions are the ones you learn from your upbringing and your environment. They are a reaction to your primary emotions, and they are not wired into your brain. As an example, you feel resentment because you fear your dad, who has abused you. Another example is a feeling of anger in response to shame or hurt feelings.

The key to dealing with a negative secondary emotion is to figure out the primary emotion behind your response. When you identify the primary reaction, you can take the necessary steps to resolve it.

Peter Salovey and John D. Mayer wrote that the ability to monitor feelings and emotions, your own and those of others, and to use that information to guide your thinking and actions is an indication of emotional intelligence. They further say that this type of intelligence controls who you are and helps build relationships.

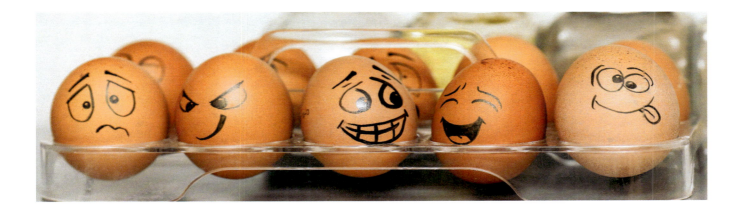

MODULE 2

EXERCISE: Write down an experience when you felt deep emotion. What was your primary emotion and what secondary emotion(s) were the result?

THE PURPOSE OF EMOTION

Emotions provide information on how we are feeling and they have four main purposes.

1. Protect. Emotions protect you when you are doing something that may be harmful. The feelings of fear you experience cause you to stop that behavior. In the same way, when you do something that goes against your values, uncomfortable emotions cause you to change direction.

> "Sometimes we put up walls. Not to keep people out, but to see who cares enough to knock them down."
> —Anonymous

2. Help with Decision Making. When you make a decision, emotions help you know whether your decision is right or wrong. Even in situations where you believe your decisions are rational and logical, emotions play a key role.

3. Provide Motivation. Emotions motivate you to act quickly and behave in ways that will maximize your chances of survival, well-being, and success. In recovery work, feeling disappointment in yourself, a fear of dying, or disgust that your life is not what you want it to be can motivate change.

4. Increase Communication and Connection. Emotions help you understand others, encouraging you to turn to connection. They give you clear information about how to respond in certain situations so you can have deeper and more meaningful relationships.

EXERCISE: Write down the emotions you are experiencing about your addiction or your recovery process. How have they motivated you, protected you, increased your communication or hindered your decision making?

EMOTION -

How it motivates. -

How it protects. -

How it increases communication. -

How it helps or hinders decision making. -

EMOTION -

How it motivates. -

How it protects. -

How it increases communication. -

How it helps or hinders decision making. -

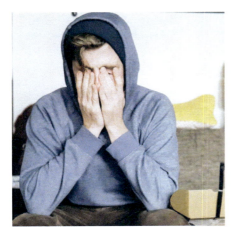
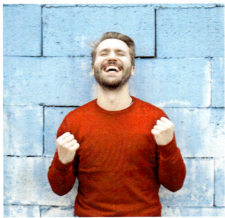
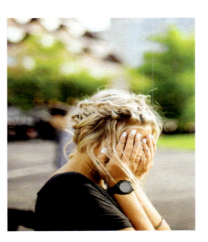

MODULE 2
EMOTIONAL NUMBING

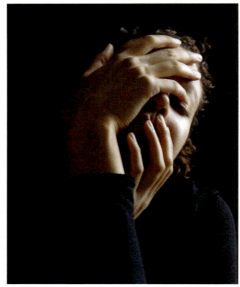

> "The single most prevalent form of denial in the human race is emotional denial. We do not want to accept the reality of our own emotions and we do not want to accept the reality of other people's emotions. As a result, we are constantly at war with ourselves and with each other." —Teal Swan

At some time in your life, you will likely experience tragedy or trauma, such as the death of a loved one, a horrible accident, serious illness, divorce, or abuse. If you don't deal with the emotions surrounding these experiences in a healthy way, emotional numbing may occur. Emotional numbing means you deny or repress your emotions, which may result in a loss of interest in things you used to enjoy, sadness, anxiety, sleep issues, depression, memory problems, feelings of being disconnected to yourself and others, and confusion. The trauma associated with Post Traumatic Stress Disorder (PTSD) can also cause emotional numbing because of wanting to escape and forget.

Emotional numbing can also occur if, as a child, you weren't allowed to feel emotion, or you were criticized or made fun of when you expressed emotion. Finally, emotional numbing is caused by limited self-care and ignoring important feelings. This is especially true for those with addictive thinking behaviors and patterns.

Researcher Brené Brown states that the problem with emotional numbing is **"We cannot selectively numb emotions; when we numb the painful emotions, we also numb the positive emotions."**

There is a significant link between emotional numbing and addiction. Most who engage in addictive behaviors do it because of the calming or euphoric feelings they get from use of the drug, alcohol, pornography, or other substance or behavior. This is especially true of those who are overly stressed, lonely, depressed, or isolated (feel like they just don't fit in) or don't have a good support system.

The recovery process and therapy can help you realize you've been denying your emotional needs and can help you begin to take care of those needs. That can be scary at first. You may have dulled or not acknowledged your emotions for years because of hurt, grief, loss, or other traumatic experiences. When you first start to feel emotions, it can be overwhelming. You may not initially know how to deal with them, and they can be associated with negative self-talk or triggers that can cause relapse.

It takes practice to understand how emotional triggers affect you and to learn how to cope with them without turning to drugs, alcohol, and addictive behaviors. Positive self-care, working on your dysfunctional beliefs, and figuring out what caused you to deny your emotions in the first place can create a safety net in which you can learn to experience your feelings in a more comfortable way and overcome the urge to return to the addictive behaviors.

HOW TO TREAT EMOTIONAL NUMBING

1. GIVE YOURSELF PERMISSION TO FEEL

You may be scared to feel emotions because they are too painful. They may remind you of trauma, abuse, loss, or other negative experiences in your life. Even positive emotions are hard to accept at times because you may believe you don't deserve to be happy. It's important that you allow yourself to feel—but even more important that you believe you can handle the feelings. You may not know how to handle them at first, but by believing in yourself, you will figure it out. The first step in treating emotional numbing is to give yourself permission to feel and show emotion.

> "Never apologize for being sensitive or emotional. It is a sign you have a big heart and aren't afraid to let others see it. Showing emotions is a sign of strength."
> —Bridgette Nicole

2. BE AWARE

Don't run from your feelings. Don't minimize or ignore them because "you shouldn't feel that way." Don't numb them because others are bugged by how you're feeling. Be tuned in to your feelings; give them credence and be comfortable in your truth. It's more empowering to admit your truth than to be dishonest with yourself.

> "What is necessary to change a person is to change his awareness of himself."
> —Abraham Maslow

Stay grounded in your surroundings and the here and now and pay attention to how you're feeling physically. A racing pulse, clammy hands, aching stomach, or muscle tension may all be signs of emotional distress. How are you feeling? What thought preceded your feeling? How is this affecting your body? When you acknowledge how you're feeling physically, you can change your thought process which will then change the physical. Here are some examples of this:

- I'm sad because I'm thinking about the past and my failed relationships. I feel tired and have no energy. I can't concentrate, and I feel like crying.
- My marriage didn't last, but I have 3 beautiful children and that makes me happy. When I think of my kids, I smile, and I don't feel as down.
- I'm angry. I feel attacked and it is so unfair. My heart is racing and I feel hot. My neck is a bundle of rock-hard muscles.
- I'm going to go for a walk and enjoy the sun. As I do, I'll think of five things I'm grateful for and concentrate on my breathing as I go. I will pay attention to what happens to me physically.
- I'm so happy. I just landed a great promotion. I feel calm and I can't quit smiling.

3. JOURNAL

Take a daily inventory of your emotions. By writing down what you feel and when, you may be able to identify patterns of emotional ups and downs. Remember it is also important to write down the thoughts that caused the feelings and how the feelings resulted in your physical reactions. If you have been emotionally numb for a long time, it may be hard to figure out how you are feeling. It is sometimes helpful just to start writing. Don't judge your words; let them come out on the paper without holding back. Remember to purge.

4. EXERCISE

Exercise has been shown to be the number-one factor in reducing depression and anxiety. When you get moving, the endorphins (positive chemicals) flood your body and brain.

5. PRACTICE GOOD NUTRITION

Research has shown that sugar and other foods affect mood. If you are anxious and depressed, poor nutrition can increase emotional numbing and make you want to isolate.

6. DEFINE THE PROBLEM AND SOLUTIONS

You might be upset and not even know why. Journaling can help define the problem, but make sure it is the primary problem. You might think you're annoyed at something trivial, but the problem might be much deeper. For example, you might get mad at your spouse for always being late for dinner, when in reality that is just a symptom. The real problem is that you don't feel you are a priority in your spouse's life. Once you have defined the real problem, give yourself time to let the emotions decrease and to think about possible solutions, then present them to your spouse. In addition, when difficult situations arise, it is important to assess how bad they really are before going into an emotional free-for-all. If you want to live a happy life, don't get all worked up over trivial matters.

7. BE VULNERABLE

Vulnerability is allowing yourself to be exposed to possible attack or harm, either physical or emotional. Brené Brown describes it as, "uncertainty, risk, and emotional exposure." It's that anxious feeling you get when you step out of your comfort zone or let go of your fears or uncertainties. It takes courage to embrace your strengths and your weaknesses, to be true to who you really are, and to share yourself with others. It takes trust in others. But more important, it requires trust in yourself that if you are rejected, you'll still be okay because you like who you are. This then results in the ability to trust others.

People with addictions tend to be fearful of opening up to others and being vulnerable. This may be you. You may have been hurt or rejected and so are overly concerned about what others think of you or you are overly protective of yourself. You may be a pleaser who just wants approval. You allow the wants and needs of others to become more important than what you want and need. You may live out of fear. Don't do this. Take care of your needs first and take courage in yourself. The remedy for this is really liking who you are.

Connect! Allow others into your world even if it's scary; they will have a different perspective that will teach you some important things. Emotional numbing can cause you to isolate and remain stuck in your own dysfunctional thinking patterns.
Others can lift you and help you to see a whole new and positive world.

EXERCISE: To start this process of learning to be vulnerable, open up to someone you trust. Tell that person your story. Record how becoming vulnerable felt to you.

8. MONITOR SELF-TALK

It doesn't matter what other things you do to heal emotional numbing if the things you say to yourself are negative. When you repeatedly tell yourself negative messages—like **"I'm not good enough," " I'm not very smart," or "I hate how I look"**—those messages become entrenched in your brain. Remember neuroplasticity. Practice new ways of thinking and talking to yourself. Research has shown that it is powerful to talk to yourself out loud in the third person because that is more real to you. It helps you be more aware of the negativity, stop it immediately, and replace the negative self-talk with something more positive.

> "Owning our story can be hard but not nearly as difficult as spending our lives running from it. Embracing our vulnerabilities is risky but not nearly as dangerous as giving up on love and belonging and joy—the experiences that make us the most vulnerable. Only when we are brave enough to explore the darkness will we discover the infinite power of our light."
> —Brené Brown

KEY TAKEAWAYS

- Emotions are one of your body's reactions to thoughts and experiences. They can affect recovery positively or negatively.
- Emotions serve to protect you and help you to connect with others.
- The Broaden-and-Build Theory explains how positive emotions expand creativity and help you develop even more positive emotions.
- Emotional numbing is the process of denying emotional experiences. This is detrimental to healthy functioning and can be a motivator for sustained addictive behavior.

MODULE 3
THE PROCESS OF CHANGE

PRINCIPLES

TAKE ACCOUNTABILITY FOR YOUR LIFE
Examine Yourself with Honesty and Responsibility

DISCOVER PURPOSE
Identify What Gives Your Life Meaning

CULTIVATE HOPE
Look for Possibilities and Be Optimistic

THOUGHT QUESTIONS

What is keeping you stuck in your desire to change?
What stage of change are you in?
How has blame affected your ability to change?
What can you do to increase hope and find meaning in change?

Neuroplasticity is the brain's main function; in other words, the brain is made to change. Desire and awareness of self are important first steps in change. These steps are made possible through being introspective and looking at ways you are not being **honest or responsible** for yourself. It is also important to look at what gives your life **meaning and purpose** and how this relates to the changes you want to make. Sometimes it is hard to be optimistic through challenges, but by **being optimistic and hopeful,** opportunities and possibilities become clearer.

"Laura came into my office five years after I had initially seen her for counseling. She was smiling and proud. "Remember me?" she asked. "I saw you five years ago. I was a senior in high school, and I was oppositional and didn't want to change."

"But," she continued, "I did it! I'm clean, and I got clean from heroin all by myself!"

I was impressed. Not many can do that. "How?" I asked.

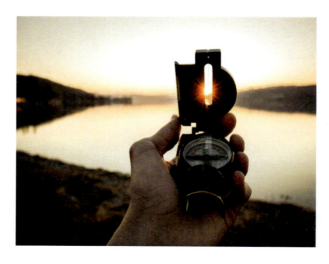

25 Copyright © 2021 by Trish Barrus and Jade Ozawa-Kirk

She responded, "The only thing I did during my senior year was sit around in the basements of people I hardly knew. I shot up all day long. I didn't know what the weather was like outside or what was going on in the world around me. I was completely oblivious. I never went to a prom or a ball game. All day long I sat there getting high. I had no purpose. I was a zombie without feeling. And worst of all, I blamed my parents and wouldn't accept their help. I thought they were trying to keep me from doing what I wanted to do, which was nothing. I finally woke up, I wasted all of those years, and I realized I can't do this for the rest of my life. I don't want to waste any more time. I had a baby, and that baby gave me great hope to change. I didn't want that baby to grow up seeing her mother as a druggie."

THE BRAIN AND CHANGE

Think back to what you have learned about neuroplasticity. Until recently, we thought the brain was static, meaning we believed that we are born with a certain number of brain cells and when a cell dies no new cell grows to replace it. We now know that the brain has the power to regenerate itself and create new cells. We also used to believe that after a certain point in development, the brain could not create new pathways of learning and connection (called neural pathways or neuropathways). Science has now proven that you can build new neural pathways when you learn something new or you try to change a thought pattern or behavior.

The more you focus and practice something, the better you become at the new skill you are learning or at overcoming an obstacle. As you do, new neural connections are created in your brain. But that doesn't seem to happen when learning experiences are passive—active engagement needs to take place. **When you want to change a habit, learn a new skill, or change a thought pattern, you can't just think about doing it. Action is required.**

And if you don't keep using what you develop, you'll lose it—your brain discards it to make room for more pertinent thoughts and behaviors.

CHANGE

C. Joy Bell said, "We can't be afraid of change. You may feel secure in the pond

> **Visualization**
>
> The same brain networks are at work when you imagine movement and when you actually move. Mentally practicing a movement can have the same effect on our minds as physical practice.
>
> Just as this concept works for high school basketball players practicing for a big game, it can work for you too! Mental visualization, sometimes called creative visualization, can decrease sensations of pain, reduce symptoms of anxiety and depression, and improve self-confidence.
>
> A few tips to get you started on strengthening your imagination:
>
> Use positive imagery. Rather than, "I don't want to stumble over my words," think, "I want to speak with eloquence and confidence."
>
> Use your own perspective, not that of an outsider. First-person point of view is paramount in the visualization process.
>
> Visualize every step of the process. Do this slowly in a step-by-step manner.
>
> Incorporate all five of your senses to make the mental experience as real and specific as possible. How will this scenario feel, look, smell, sound, and taste?
>
> Remember that visualization, like most things, takes practice.

MODULE 3

that you are in, but if you never venture out of it, you will never know that there is such a thing as an ocean, a sea. Holding onto something that is good for you now, may be the very reason why you don't have something better." Why do we hold on to the "sameness" of our lives even though we know it would be good to change? Here are some of the most common reasons. See which ones apply to you:

FEAR OF MAKING A MISTAKE. Though they may be scary or intimidating, mistakes are a part of life and they help you learn. Think about when you learned to ride a bike—you didn't do it perfectly the first time. You fell, wobbled down the street, crashed, and sometimes ended up in tears. But that's how you learned. Experience taught you, and each time you successfully rode that bike without falling, your confidence grew. Moving through the possibility of mistakes is necessary in order to accomplish anything!

NOT KNOWING HOW TO CHANGE. You might not know how you are going to make a change, but it is important that you believe in your ability to change. Instead of giving up out of fear, you can say, "I don't know how I'll do this, but I will figure it out." You can learn how to change in a variety of ways, including studying, reflecting about your situation and capabilities, asking for help from those close to you, and observing others.

CARING TOO MUCH ABOUT WHAT OTHERS THINK. You may tend to worry about how others see you because you want a connection and acceptance. But when you keep yourself from progressing because of fear of judgment, it is debilitating. Trust that accepting yourself is more important than seeking the approval of others. Trust that you know what is best for you, then do it. Any change that moves you closer to your ideal self and your ultimate goals is more important than criticism from others or even yourself.

LACK OF BELIEF IN YOUR ABILITY TO CHANGE. Change is possible for everyone. It takes boldness and effort, but it can happen! Remember the amazing things your mind has done already and remember it can do more (neuroplasticity). You can work towards a better way of life regardless of your past. It's never to late, things are never too bad, there is always an a way to change.

CHANGE CAN BE WONDERFUL, BUT FEAR KEEPS YOU FROM CHANGING. Take courage and learn from your mistakes, but don't fear them. Care what others think only so far as you really want a connection with them, and they are worthy of it. Work and learn to change. As David Schwartz said, "Believe it can be done. When you believe something can be done, really believe, your mind will find ways to do it. Believing a solution paves the way to the solution." Begin today.

EXERCISE: Take some time to think about what has kept you from change. Consider ways the four factors —fear of making a mistake, uncertainty on how to change, caring what others think, and lack of belief in your ability to change—may have contributed to keeping you from change Write your thoughts.

STAGES OF CHANGE

According to Prochaska and DiClemente's Stages of Change Model, the process of change takes place in these stages. Each stage represents a specific grouping of attitudes, beliefs, intentions, and behaviors that depend on how ready you are to move from one stage to the next. Change unfolds over time, and each stage reflects not only a period of time, but also a set of tasks required for moving to the next stage. Although the time you spend in each stage varies, the tasks you need to accomplish in that stage do not vary.

STAGE 1: PRECONTEMPLATION

In the precontemplation stage of change, you have no plans to make changes in your life in the foreseeable future. You might be unaware or under-aware of any problems or areas needing improvement, but your family, friends, neighbors, co-workers, or others close to you are often aware that you have challenges that need addressing. In this stage, you might initially go to the gym, to therapy, to the doctor's office, and so on because of pressure from others. But to successfully progress and move forward, you need to acknowledge that there is a problem and own that problem. In the addictive state, this is called denial. You don't believe you have a problem.

STAGE 2: CONTEMPLATION

In the contemplation stage of change, you're aware that a problem exists and are seriously thinking about overcoming it but have not yet made a commitment to act. The central focus of this stage is serious consideration of problem resolution. With addiction, the contemplation stage means you are evaluating and considering your options for treatment. To move forward in the cycle of change, you must avoid the trap of obsessive contemplation and make a firm decision to begin to take action. Small "baby steps" of preliminary action lead into the next stage.

> "Change is painful, but nothing is as painful as staying stuck somewhere you don't belong."
> —Mandy Hale

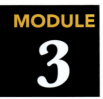

STAGE 3: PREPARATION

In the preparation stage of change, you begin to combine intention and behavioral changes. Those behavioral changes can be things such as seeking information for recovery treatment, smoking five fewer cigarettes per day or joining a gym. Although you make some movement toward reducing your unwanted behaviors in the preparation stage, you haven't yet fully engaged in activity to change—but are intending to take such action in the very near future.

STAGE 4: ACTION

In the action stage of change, you change your behavior, experiences, and/or environment in order to overcome your problem. Action involves the most behavioral changes and requires a considerable commitment of time and energy. If you are in treatment for addiction and are committed, you are in the action stage. You are classified as being in the action stage if you have successfully changed an unwanted behavior for a period of anywhere from one day to six months. At this stage, you likely have a high level of motivation and are doing the work for yourself, not because you feel pressure from others.

> "In any given moment we have two options: to step forward into growth or step back into safety."
> —Abraham Maslow

STAGE 5: MAINTENANCE

Being able to remain free of the chronic problem or addiction and/or to consistently engage in a new compatible behavior for more than six months suggests that you are in the maintenance stage. Stabilizing behavior and avoiding relapse are the primary signs of being in this stage.

EXERCISE: Based on what you've read about the stages of change, assess where you are in the process. Then go over your change assessment with your therapist for any feedback.

PROCESSES OF CHANGE

The primary benefit of recognizing where you are in the change process is understanding how to help yourself (or seek help from others) so you can move on to the next stage. Imagine you have a friend who received a wake-up call from his doctor at his last appointment. He was told that unless he lost weight, he would be high risk for a heart attack. The advice, encouragement, and help you give him would be different a few days after his doctor's appointment (in the precontemplation or contemplation stage) than it would be a few months into his gym membership and heart-healthy diet (action stage).

There are nine broad processes that can be used to facilitate movement from one stage of change to another. Each process can (and should) be tailored to your needs, preferences, and situation. Some are more useful in one stage than in another and can be used to help you progress toward recovery.

> "There are far better things ahead than any we leave behind."
> —C.S. Lewis

CONSCIOUSNESS-RAISING

Consciousness-raising is the most often used process of change and can be used at any stage of change. This process increases your awareness of what's going on inside (such as your emotions, thoughts, biases, and vulnerabilities) as well as what's happening externally (ranging from how family members are impacted by addictive behaviors to legal consequences of drug use). Consciousness-raising provides new knowledge about you or your problem and can provide information about consequences, causes, or solutions.

Consciousness-raising is usually the first strategy loved ones turn to when helping a precontemplator. They may confront or try to give direct feedback, or they may try to provide education. Media campaigns are an example of consciousness-raising.

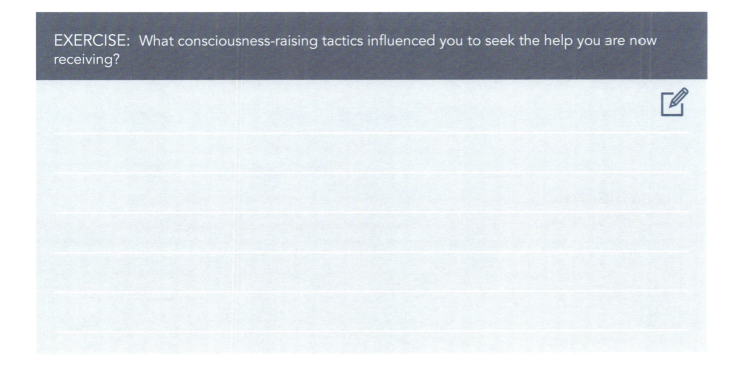

EXERCISE: What consciousness-raising tactics influenced you to seek the help you are now receiving?

MODULE 3

EMOTIONAL AROUSAL

Consciousness-raising and emotional arousal often go hand in hand, focusing on sharing information while heightening emotional response to the topic. Emotional arousal techniques can result in a sudden emotional release such as sadness, anger, or fear. Increased awareness and feeling around a topic can move you to action if you are in an early stage of change, such as precontemplation, contemplation, or preparation. Emotions generally motivate you to action.

Emotional arousal is sometimes most effective and most tragic when it results from real-life experience. For example, a family member or close friend may die of a drug overdose or suicide. Emotions can also be stirred through second-hand experiences, such as personal testimonies and movies.

> "Negative emotions like loneliness, envy, fear, and guilt have an important role to play in a happy life; they're big, flashing signs that something needs to change."
> —Gretchen Rubin

Most media campaigns use both consciousness-raising and emotional arousal.

EXERCISE: Think of a time when you were changed by an emotionally impactful experience related to your recovery. Describe that experience and what you learned from it.

SOCIAL LIBERATION

Social liberation relies on external environmental factors to help facilitate change. For example, low-fat or "heart-healthy" menu selections at restaurants can help make diet changes easier. Many social liberation techniques are brought about by advocacy groups. A changer's roles in social liberation include seeking out alternatives and options – such as, asking for a non-alcoholic drink menu or asking a doctor for alternatives to opioids for pain—and helping bring awareness of alternatives to the public.

Social liberation techniques may be perceived differently by those in different stages of change. They may seem annoying to someone in precontemplation, but incredibly helpful and comforting to those in the action stage. Increased awareness of them can also be helpful to someone in contemplation or preparation who is considering the necessary steps to take in the action stage.

> EXERCISE: Write about something that you feel extremely passionate about regarding recovery in general. It could be something like, "Doctors should be more responsible in their prescribing practices so that people don't become addicted to opioids." Talk about your feelings and how these could transform into an action plan.

SELF-REEVALUATION

Self-reevaluation requires a thoughtful examination of your life in light of your problem behavior. This requires a level of awareness and feeling that can be achieved through consciousness-raising and emotional arousal techniques. Self-reevaluation involves looking at your values and goals and contrasting them to the person you are because of your addictive behaviors or bad habits. This means honestly answering difficult questions about yourself.

Self-reevaluation can push someone on the cusp of change to commit. It is a process best employed in contemplation and preparation, but it's not limited to those; regular self-reevaluation will help remind you why you want to continue if you're struggling in the action stage and it will strengthen you in maintenance. Without proper self-reevaluation, failure is inevitable.

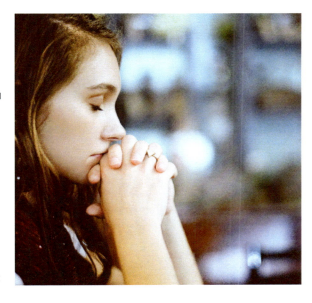

MODULE 3

EXERCISE: Honestly answer the following questions about yourself:
If I woke up tomorrow and I wasn't addicted, how would my life be different? What would I be doing, and how would I be thinking differently? How would my feelings be different? How would others be acting toward me?

COMMITMENT

Part of self-reevaluation is accepting responsibility for changing. This responsibility facilitates commitment to change. Commitment has both a private part and a public part. First, you must affirm to yourself that you have made the decision to change and that you will follow through with that decision. Then you let others close to you know about your commitment to a better life. Letting others in on your pledge will provide positive pressure to stick to the changes you have promised yourself. It is easier to renege on a commitment if you're the only one who knows about it.

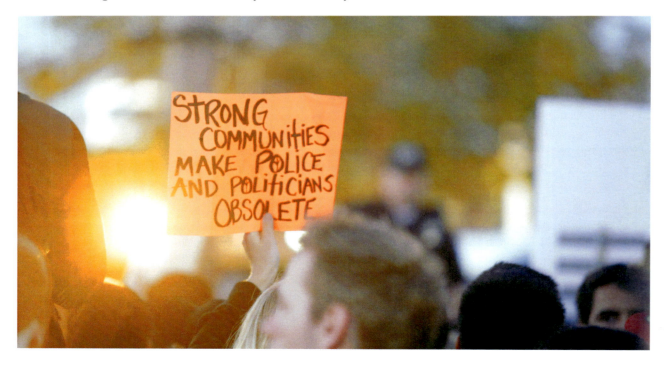

Commitment is a crucial part of moving into action. Through this process, many people who successfully create change are surprised by the type of resources and support others can provide to help them continue progressing. Accountability partners or mentors can be a reminder or reaffirmation of a commitment. It does not hurt to recommit throughout your change journey.

Commitment to Change Pledge

> EXERCISE: Write down your commitment about change and your recovery. Consider including one or more of the following:
> - A brief description of what you have determined to change.
> - Why you are making this change (such as wanting to improve relationships, improve health, or meet personal/career goals).
> - Steps you have already taken toward change.
> - Short-term and long-term steps you will take.

COUNTERING

Countering is the process of replacing unhealthy responses (or habits/reactions associated with an addictive behavior) with healthy ones. Just about any healthy activity can be used to counter a behavior you are trying to stop. For example, if you have a cigarette every day when you get home from work, you can establish a new routine of walking a lap around the block instead. If you're a drug user, when the urge to use hits, you can call a family member and ask about their day instead of using. Countering activities can be brainstormed ahead of time. It may be useful to keep a list of alternative healthy activities in a convenient place, such as in your wallet or on your fridge. You can tell family and friends about your countering activities so they can join or support you.

Countering is especially helpful in the action stage. Countering activities or healthy substitutes may also continue to be a part of recovery throughout maintenance.

MODULE 3

EXERCISE: Identify behaviors you would like to replace and brainstorm some healthy substitutes. Discuss these with your therapist. Write your healthy substitutes on a small card to keep in your wallet. (If possible, this card should be laminated.)

ENVIRONMENTAL CONTROL

Environmental control involves making changes to your environment to reduce triggers. It can be as simple as removing alcohol and tumblers from your home or as involved as creating new social situations and changing the friends who are pulling you down. Good environmental control can be paired with countering as you observe what times, places, and/or activities lead to your problematic habits and then make appropriate changes.

Environmental control techniques can begin in the preparation stage and should continue through the action stage. Though some environmental control practices—such as hanging a No Smoking sign in your cubicle—may be discarded after a period of time, others may be necessary to keep.

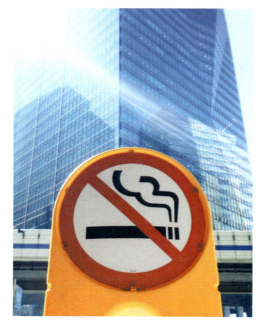

"You will become like the five people you associate with the most. This can be either a blessing or a curse." —Billy Cox

EXERCISE: Brainstorm environmental control techniques you can apply at home, at work, in your car and other places where you spend time. During your recovery both you and your environment will need to change. For example, if you always drank on the same recliner, replace it with a different piece of furniture. Even updating your living space with new paint or a new rug to represent the new can help keep your mindset moving forward in maintenance/recovery. You might also need to change your social network to people who are more supportive of your recovery.

REWARDS

Though punishment and reward are opposing sides of the same coin, reward is a much more effective tactic for lasting change. Punishment usually has only a temporary effect and may perpetuate feelings of shame. Rewards can come in many forms, from self-praise to a present that someone gives you when you reach a goal. Like countering activities, rewards can be planned. Planning a vacation with the money you have saved from not engaging in the addictive behavior is a great way to chart and maintain motivation throughout the action stage. You can also involve loved ones by asking them to help you with rewards throughout the process.

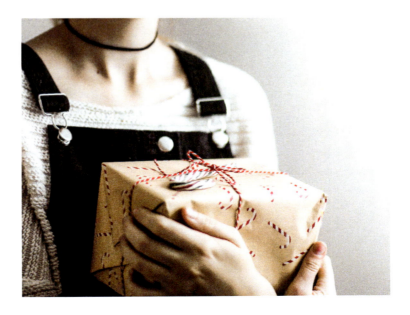

MODULE 3

EXERCISE: List some possible ways you could reward yourself for abstaining from your addictive behavior.

HELPING RELATIONSHIPS

A helping relationship is any supportive relationship that can assist you in small or big ways through your stages of change. Friends, family, acquaintances, sponsors, clergy, and professionals can all provide helping relationships. Helping relationships provide support, understanding, acceptance, resources and love. There is no need to grit your teeth and go it alone as you work to break free of problem behaviors. In fact, isolating yourself and keeping your struggle private may sabotage your efforts in the long run.

> "Teamwork is connected independence."
> —David Cottrell

> "To be fully seen by somebody, then, and be loved anyhow—this is a human offering that can border on miraculous."
> —Elizabeth Gilbert

The key is finding or choosing people who can adequately help you on your journey. Unfortunately, not everyone you would like to turn to for encouragement will be able to provide it appropriately. Test the waters to figure out who can really be there for you as you make positive change. Also, seek out those who are uplifting and emotionally healthy and not toxic or harmful to you. Unfortunately, sometimes people will support or even encourage you to continue with addictive behaviors because they find benefit from it in some way–a friend may not support you becoming clean and sober because they use with you, and perhaps you pay for the drugs.

EXERCISE: List all the helping relationships you have right now and the ways each supports you. Are there areas/ways you could use more support? Who can you turn to for that?

HOW WE CHANGE

> "Why waste time proving over and over how great you are, when you could be getting better? Why hide deficiencies instead of overcoming them? Why look for friends or partners who will just shore up your self-esteem instead of ones who will also challenge you to grow? And why seek out the tried and true, instead of experiences that will stretch you? The passion for stretching yourself and sticking to it, even (or especially) when it's not going well, is the hallmark of the growth mindset. This is the mindset that allows people to thrive during some of the most challenging times in their lives." —Carol Dweck

As mentioned, change doesn't happen all at once, nor does it occur in a straight line. There are ups and downs to change and ups and downs to recovery. Looking at the way we change helps us understand what's involved in change. According to researchers, there are three ways we change:

- Change comes from awareness and understanding of the past.
- Change comes from the present through rewards and punishments.
- Change comes from using understanding of the past and present to create a vibrant and motivational picture of the future.

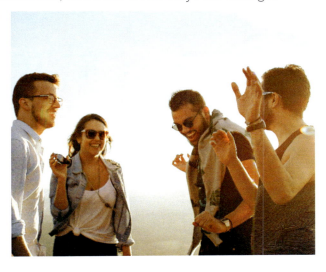

Of these theories, the weakest influence on current behavior is the past, because you can't change it. Dwelling on the past contributes to depression and feelings of hopelessness. Focusing on the present through rewards and punishment has been shown to be a much stronger facilitator of change.

MODULE 3

Understanding the past and using the wisdom you received as a result, however, is the most effective and empowers lasting change.

Progress happens when you begin to focus your attention on the "here and now" and how you can change your future life. You remove yourself from the rut of helplessness, hopelessness, and fear. You move, and as you move, your perspective changes. You become proactive. When you are proactive, you focus on the things you can change. Remember, you can change your thoughts, your emotions, your behaviors, and your intentions because they are internal things that are under your control. You can't change anything external to you, such as other people, the weather, and the stock market.

Fred Luskin talks about this in terms of unenforceable rules—things you want but can't control. They are things like, *Christmas should be happy. My spouse needs to lose some weight. Pain shouldn't be a part of life. Bosses should be respectful and listen. I want my recovery to be over now. I just want my life back.*

There are many things that irritate or annoy you every day, and these can consume a lot of your energy. Most of your frustrations arise from situations over which you have little or no control, such as another person's behavior. Dr. Luskin points out that it's fine to wish someone would behave differently or that the outcome would be different, but when your happiness depends on that wish coming true, that's when you get into trouble. The wish then becomes a demand in your mind–the "shoulds" and "oughts" in life turn into "I can't be happy unless. . ." "Unless my boss is respectful," "Unless my spouse loses some weight." When they become demands, these legitimate wishes increase your frustration levels, drain your energy, and can make the problem worse.

To be in control of yourself, stop worrying about things you can't do anything about. Look for ways you can control you which include the way you react to different situations and the demands you make on others and yourself. Stay focused on the future by changing the now. It's okay to have expectations but if those expectations are not met you can still be happy!

> EXERCISE: What are some of your unenforceable rules? Write down some of those that are keeping you stuck. Change them into thoughts that would help you. Here's an example: "Christmas is just stressful, but I will be happy even though others might not be."

> "Everything can be taken from a man but one thing: the last of the human freedoms—to choose one's attitude in any given set of circumstances, to choose one's own way."
> —Victor Frankl

LAPSES AND RELAPSE

Just as mistakes can be viewed as opportunities to learn and grow, lapses and relapse can provide a chance for self-examination, strengthened relationships, and movement toward a life of flourishing. They do not mean that you have failed or that you aren't changing. Let's look at the difference between the two.

LAPSES

A lapse occurs when someone with an addiction uses a small amount or engages in an addictive behavior and then stops. A lapse would include having a beer at the end of the day and stopping there, playing one video game for a few minutes and then stopping, or taking a hit from a joint when one is offered. **Lapses are short-lived and temporary.**

It is normal to experience slipups, and lapses are part of the process of change. The important thing is how you view them. **A lapse is not a relapse**, and it doesn't mean you have failed. When lapses are approached with guilt and self-blame, they are more likely to move into full relapse. Self-compassion is essential in the face of a return to negative behaviors. The path to recovery is rarely a straight line; for most, it's an upward spiral.

While lapses are a normal part of the change process, it's important to acknowledge them and take steps to prevent them from happening again or turning into a full-blown relapse. After a period of abstinence, even just a small amount of an illicit substance or looking at just a little porn can revitalize cravings for more use. Focus on positive thoughts and do not define yourself by the lapse. Be accountable to your support system and report to them quickly.

RELAPSE

Relapses occur when you purposely seek out drugs or addictive behaviors during the change process. This can be one session or a full binge. While you're in treatment, it's considered a relapse. Once you're no longer in treatment, it's considered a return to full-blown addiction.

Everyone has different reasons for relapsing, but for most people who are trying to recover and be healthy, relapses are prompted by uncomfortable emotions and stressful situations. These events or feelings are referred to as "triggers," and much of rehabilitation is centered around identifying personal triggers and devising strategies of how to avoid and/or manage them.

> "Becoming is better than being."
> —Carol Dweck

MODULE 3

For many, common triggers include:
- Encountering people they used with, gamed with, bought from, or going to places where they used to get drunk or get high.
- Isolating.
- Watching people on TV or in a movie abuse drugs, have sexual encounters, or drink.
- Hearing someone discuss their addiction in explicit or positive terms.
- Experiencing a difficult event (breakup, job loss, bereavement, argument, divorce).
- Experiencing extreme emotions (stress, anger, fear, frustration).

Since it's impossible to avoid most triggers completely, it's crucial that you learn how to cope with inevitable stressors while in treatment.

Relapse doesn't occur suddenly. There are many different physical, behavioral, and emotional relapse warning signs. Stay in tune with yourself and learn to recognize these common signs of relapse:
- Compulsive behavior
- Neglect of coping skills and healthy habits
- Return to previous habits, routines, or social groups
- Mood swings
- Cravings (a sign the brain is not healed)
- Sudden mood changes
- Depressed, anxious, or destructive thoughts
- Denial of events or behaviors that are leading down the addiction path again or thinking you are cured
- Secretive, bored, or isolating behaviors
- Increased irritability
- Making impulsive decisions
- Replacement of one addiction with another

A relapse or lapse does not undo previous progress made in an addiction recovery program. Learning to change addictive thinking patterns and focusing on positive thinking will continue to benefit you.

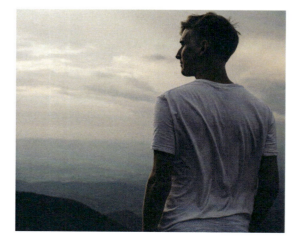

Relapse Triggers

| Friends, family, others that misuse substances |
| Stressful Environments |
| Relationship Issues |
| Feeling Bored |

EXERCISE: Think of a time that you relapsed after a period of being clean. What were you going through immediately before the relapse? What triggered your relapse? What is one step you will take to prevent relapse after this treatment is over?

KEY TAKEAWAYS

- The more you think or practice something, the stronger associated neuropathways become. This is the power of neuroplasticity.
- Change involves nonlinear movement through five stages: precontemplation, contemplation, preparation, action, and maintenance. Understanding your stage of change can help you identify what needs to happen to move you to the next stage.
- Nine processes of change promote change behaviors throughout all stages.
- Lapses and relapse are different, but you should approach both with self-compassion and see them as learning experiences.
- Awareness of relapse triggers can prevent a return to full addiction.

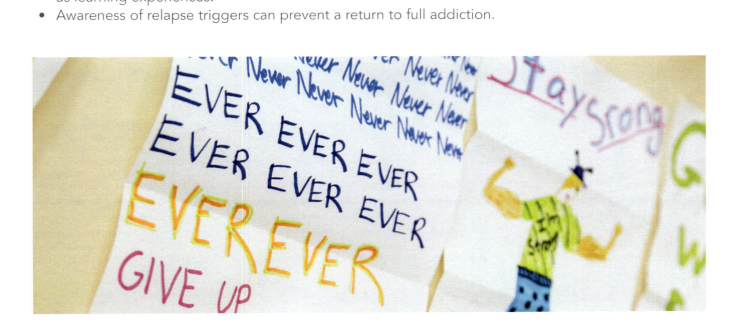

MODULE 4
POSITIVE PSYCHOLOGY & ADDICTION

PRINCIPLES

CULTIVATE HOPE
Look for Possibilities and Be Optimistic

PRACTICE GRATITUDE
Be Aware of Who and What Provides Goodness in Your Life and Show Your Thanks

CONQUER WITH COURAGE
Use Resilience to Overcome Weaknesses, Setbacks, and Obstacles

THOUGHT QUESTIONS

How optimistic and hopeful are you that this recovery will work for you this time?

What negative thoughts are continuing to keep you stuck?

How resilient are you and what does that mean to your recovery?

Hope, gratitude, and courage are all important concepts in positive psychology. When challenges and hardships in life occur, you can look at life in a positive way or you can be miserable. You can focus on the solutions to challenges and be resilient or you can stay stuck in the problem. I once heard a fourteen-year-old patient comment, "It is so much more fun to be happy than miserable." And it is! But at times, it takes a lot of courage to be happy when obstacles litter our path. That's why one of the principles to recovery is **"Conquer with Courage."**

Gratitude and hope have been found to increase positive feelings, happiness, and motivation. But you can't just give lip service to these two words. You have to **practice gratitude and cultivate hope** by being mindful of what you have and savoring the good moments in life.

Becca texted me, "I got it! I got the scholarship! Not only the regional one, but I placed first nationally. Thank you so much for the recommendation. This will change my life."

Becca had three kids with one on the way when she found out that her husband was cheating and had a serious drug problem. He hadn't been around much the past year and he had become increasingly annoyed with her and the kids, but she didn't suspect anything close to what he was doing. Their life hadn't been easy. He was a veteran who suffered from PTSD but the real blow came when he lost his leg in a terrible accident. Always resilient before, he seemed to take this challenge in stride, but he increasingly seemed distant and removed, what Becca described as "spacey" at times.

One day she found his computer open and realized she had been "duped." On his computer were the records of many drug deals, details and pictures of orgies with various women, and love letters to another woman. This all made her sick to her stomach. She was not only stunned but shocked. How could he do this? And now what?

Becca is an amazingly strong woman. She kicked him out and started her life alone, even in the face of pressure from in-laws and other family members to "give him another chance." She realized the depth of the problem and knew he didn't want to change. She began her life as a single mom with limited post-high school education, pregnant, and without money. Her ex-husband refused to help her and gave little child support each month.

A very spiritual person, Becca believed that God was watching out for her. She never wavered in her determination and positive attitude. She didn't just hope, she knew things would work out. Resentment and discouragement were not in her vocabulary even though life had not turned out the way she wanted.

> "Positive anything is better than negative nothing." —Elbert Hubbard

> "The aim of Positive Psychology is to catalyze a change in psychology from a preoccupation only with repairing the worst things in life to also building the best qualities in life."
> —Martin E.P. Seligman

With the help of family and friends, Becca made it through her first year of college with a newborn and three other children, but she didn't know how she would pay for the rest of her schooling or pay the bills. One of her professors suggested she apply for scholarships. Becca asked for recommendations. They came. Resilient, yes. Determined, yes. Happy and hopeful, yes. Courageous, yes. She gratefully acknowledged all of her blessings as she accepted two scholarships that would pay for the rest of her schooling.

In recent decades, the positive psychology movement has grown quickly. In contrast to models centered on mental illness and deficits, positive psychology has been described by researchers at the University of Pennsylvania as "the scientific study of the strengths and virtues that enable individuals and communities to thrive. The field is founded on the belief that people want to lead meaningful and fulfilling lives, to cultivate what is best within themselves, and to enhance their experiences of love, work, and play." You may have noticed mention of "the science of happiness" on social media and in articles, books, and videos. That's the science of positive psychology, and its powerful ideas can change lives.

As already discussed, addiction can be overcome, and even deeply ingrained behaviors and habits can be changed. Part of this "overcoming" will include examination of your own **strengths and virtues** and rediscovery of what you most value in life. It may also include working through pain left from past and present wounds. **Focusing on positivity does not mean denying negative aspects of this life. It means that you thoughtfully examine yourself, see your faults or weaknesses, and figure out**

MODULE 4

how to deal with them in a positive way. Finally, it involves creating a vision for your future.

Thinking positively is difficult because we are so used to thinking negatively. There are many reasons for that. Research has shown that we tend to be self-critical because we falsely believe being hard on ourselves will make us work harder and better. Many people grow up hearing messages that "they are not enough" or that "they will never be successful." Others try to protect themselves by assuming the worst so they won't be disappointed if things don't work out. And sometimes brain chemistry causes depression and negative thought states.

Does that mean you're doomed to thinking negatively? Absolutely not. With practice, practice, and more practice, you can learn optimism and positivity. You can literally rewire your brain through the power of neuroplasticity. Gratitude, optimism, and hope are three factors that can help. Mindfulness, flow, savoring, and resilience are other positive psychology principles that can aid your process.

GRATITUDE

You can replace a lot of the negative thinking that leads you to feel bad about yourself by being grateful for the good in your life. **But gratitude is not just a theory or an attitude; you need to apply it and practice it if you want it to have an effect on your life.** Practicing gratitude can help you meet your goals more often, feel better physically and emotionally, and increase your experiences of love, joy, and optimism. When what you already have becomes enough and you acknowledge the good others have brought into your life, you will feel better.

> "Gratitude goes far beyond saying 'thank you.' When we are grateful, we affirm that a source of goodness exists in our lives."
> —Robert A. Emmons

> "Gratitude unlocks the fullness of life. It turns what we have into enough, and more. It turns denial into acceptance, chaos to order, confusion to clarity. It can turn a meal into a feast, a house into a home, a stranger into a friend." —Melody Beattie

One proven way to apply gratitude is to record your thoughts in a gratitude journal every day. In one gratitude study, people wrote just once a week for ten weeks about five things they were grateful for that week. Those who participated reported that they:
- Felt better about their lives as a whole
- Were "more optimistic about the future"
- Reported fewer health complaints
- Spent significantly more time exercising

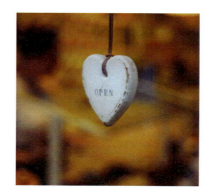

Studies conducted after the 9/11 terror attacks in the United States also showed that even in tragedy, focusing on gratitude made a difference. Those who lost loved ones who were grateful for the time spent with them, who were grateful for little things about their loved one, or who thought about their lives in a positive way recovered from grieving twice as fast as those who focused on the negative aspects of the tragedy.

Studies have also shown that you feel better about yourself if you both experience and express gratitude. This is an important quality in recovery, because addiction keeps you stuck in a place where you can't see the good.

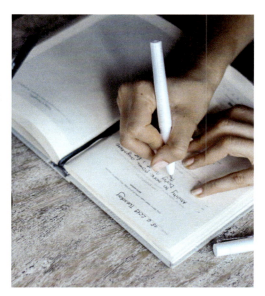

> "A basic law: the more you practice the art of thankfulness, the more you have to be thankful for." —Norman Vincent Peale

EXERCISE: Continue to **regularly write your gratitude thoughts in a journal each day.** List three to five things below that you feel grateful for today, especially in your recovery process. Make these things specific. It would be easy to repeat broad items daily *"I'm grateful for my dog, family, car, home, mind."* Your effort will be more effective when focused and unique. Expanding on the examples above, you could list:
1. I am grateful for my dog's friendship and smile. He is always happy to see me.
2. I am grateful that my family is supporting me through this recovery process. Knowing they are there makes me feel less lonely.
3. I am grateful that my boss appreciates how hard I am working.
4. I am grateful for my health.
5. I am grateful my mind brought to memory the good time I had hiking in the mountains last fall.

MODULE 4

OPTIMISM AND HOPE

Two important qualities stressed in positive psychology are optimism and hope. While they are quite similar in meaning, there are important differences between them. Though they are different, they are related; optimism and hope are usually experienced together. Let's look at both of them.

OPTIMISM

Optimism is the tendency to look toward the future with positive anticipation and confidence. Many people—maybe you're among them—think optimism is something you either have or you don't; either you are an optimist or a pessimist. **But research has shown that optimism can be learned through effort and practice.**

> "Optimism generates hope . . . hope releases dreams . . . dreams set goals . . . enthusiasm follows."
> —Martin E.P. Seligman

Learning to be optimistic requires you to actively question the negative beliefs and thoughts that are constantly chattering in your mind. Here's an example: Where did your mind go the last time you faced the difficulty of resisting the urge to use or you faced some other type of setback? A negative dialogue probably started in your head. Maybe you thought things like, "I'll never be able to do that" or "Things always turn out bad for me." Fighting against these thoughts one at a time, day-by-day, helps you establish a habit of optimistic thinking.

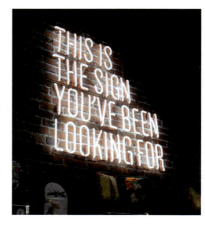

HOPE

Hope is a feeling that things will turn out for the best. When you have hope, you trust and believe that something you want will happen. You set goals, strengthen your tenacity and perseverance to pursue those goals, and believe in your own abilities to act. Along with hope comes a sense of self-reliance that instills in you the belief, "I can figure this out."

This might not seem to make sense, but **hope doesn't come from lack of hardship. In fact, it comes from facing and meeting difficulties.** If

> "Once you choose hope, anything's possible."
> —Christopher Reeve

things were too easy for you (especially when you were a child) and your caregivers solved all of your problems or kept you from challenges, you may not have learned how to be resilient. You may not have learned that you were competent enough to solve problems on your own. In that case, you may have had, and may still have, a harder time understanding how to hope. Hope is often taught by parents or caregivers who provide consistent support but let you experience things yourself. The dependability of parents and the success of a child in solving problems teaches the child that things will turn out okay. But if you didn't learn to be hopeful as you were growing up, it's not too late. You can put effort into developing both hope and optimism as an adult.

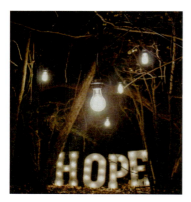

So, take hope if you're facing a real difficulty. You might not know how to change things right now, but you know you will figure it out. That is hope.

HOPE AND CHANGE

You might have found that when you try to change, it's easy to lose hope. Why does that happen? Finding your goals blocked can result in negative reactions and less hope. For example, being unable to progress toward a goal might cause real disappointment or discouragement.

When you've set goals but aren't getting good results, you may pass through several psychological stages. While they don't always follow the same pattern for all people, generally they progress from hope to rage, from rage to despair, and from despair to apathy.

> "Optimism is the faith that leads to achievement. Nothing can be done without hope and confidence."
> —Helen Keller

Less hope can also be caused by consistent negative messages and criticisms received while growing up. When you're constantly told that you don't measure up or that you are deficient, you might feel that what you do doesn't matter—or that you'll never be able to succeed because you don't have the ability. Hope can be destroyed before it even begins.

> EXERCISE: Did you receive messages in your past that have blocked you from feeling hope? What were those messages? How can you change them so you can feel hope?

HOPE AS A HABIT

Desmond Tutu wrote, "Hope is being able to see that there is light despite all of the darkness." Like so many other things in life, hope is a habit. To create this habit in your own life, start by practicing optimism to counteract your pessimistic thoughts. When difficulties come along, purposefully think about what you are gaining and learning from the experience. Remind yourself of times things have turned out well despite bumps in the road or unexpected turns in the path. Once you've established

MODULE 4

hope as a habit, it just happens without thinking. It's like every other routine that occurs daily without thought. For example, you brush your teeth, eat, and shower daily. Why not be hopeful every day?

Remember, it takes approximately twenty-one days to break a habit but sixty days to establish a new one. So, keep practicing and doing!

MINDFULNESS AND MEDITATION

Ancient Chinese philosopher Lao Tzu wrote, "If you are depressed, you are living in the past. If you are anxious you are living in the future. If you are at peace you are living in the present." And Abraham Maslow said, "I can feel guilty about the past, apprehensive about the future, but only in the present can I act. The ability to be in the present moment is a major component of mental wellness."

Not only are those statements extremely wise, but they sum up the general idea of **mindfulness–paying active attention to what's happening right now without judging it.**

Each day, your brain is inundated with significant amounts of information that comes at you from all directions. That makes it increasingly difficult to slow down, think, feel, and connect. The answer to that dilemma could be mindfulness. Overall, mindfulness creates space between us and our autopilot reactions: space to think, feel, and connect.

Research has shown that mindfulness improves immune function, increases gray matter density in the brain, increases positive emotions, and decreases negative emotions (anger, anxiety, and sadness). Research also suggests that mindfulness can do as much for depression as prescribed antidepressants!

To practice mindfulness, tune in to the present moment without assessing it as good or bad. Take time throughout your day to notice your body and its sensations, your thoughts, your emotions, and the world around you. As you do so, don't label or categorize what you notice. Instead, approach what

> "To keep the body in good health is a duty, otherwise we shall not be able to keep our mind strong and clear."
> —Buddha

you observe with curiosity and openness. For example, if you notice a nagging thought that keeps vying for your attention, you might think, "hmm. . . I seem to be going back to that idea. Maybe it is important to me," instead of thinking, "I can't stop thinking about that. I have other things to do and don't want this distraction. This is going to get in the way of my project."

Mindful curiosity promotes observing the world with openness and without expectations and biases. That's important because expectations of yourself and others set you up for disappointment and frustration. Similarly, your biases can cloud your perception and lead to judgment and labeling which, in turn, lead to stress and depression. Curiosity, on the other hand, keeps you from condemning yourself and others in ways that may stifle your progress or lead to unhappiness. It breaks up the clouds of automatic negative interpretation and allows for greater possibility.
Mindfulness even plays an important role in recovery. It not only minimizes negative emotions that may contribute to addictive behaviors, but also provides skills to help "surf" the wave of an urge to use or act out.

Various physical and emotional experiences will arise throughout your recovery process. As you approach these experiences and sensations with mindful awareness, you can move through them without being knocked over. Think of waves washing up on a beach. Tides ebb and flow, coming up on the sand and pulling back into the ocean. Emotions and cravings are similar. They come in, sometimes with great force, but if you pull back and wait mindfully (as opposed to choosing to rescue yourself from the discomfort by numbing or acting out), new opportunities and solutions will be yours.

Mindfulness can be practiced anywhere and at any time. It can take merely a moment of pausing to notice the sensation of your breath entering and leaving your body or it can be incorporated into your day by being especially aware of your thoughts and feelings. Each time you are in your car or as you perform a task, such as brushing your teeth or washing dishes, be mindful. Mindfulness can also be practiced more formally through mindful meditation, which involves setting aside specific time to notice thoughts or formally focus your attention on specific things.

EXERCISE: Start practicing mindfulness by incorporating one or more of the following exercises into your day.

1. **Slow down and notice your breath.** Observe and slow down your breathing for three to five minutes. As thoughts come to your mind and try to distract you, focus on a part of the physical sensation of breathing, such as the way air feels moving into your nostrils and out of your mouth or the rising and falling of your chest and stomach.
2. **Practice 5-4-3-2-1 Senses**. Here's how this works:
   - **What are 5 things you can see?** Look around you and notice five things you hadn't noticed before, such as a pattern on a wall, light reflecting from a surface, or a knick-knack in the corner of a room. You can also focus on one color; for example, you might notice five red things around you.
   - **What are 4 things you can feel?** Feel things like the pressure of your feet on the floor, your shirt resting on your shoulders, or the temperature of the air on your skin. Pick up an object and notice its texture.
   - **What are 3 things you can hear?** Notice all the background sounds you usually filter out, such as the hum of the air-conditioning, the chirping of birds, or the sound of cars on a distant street.
   - **What are 2 things you can smell?** Maybe you can smell flowers, coffee, or freshly cut grass. It doesn't have to be a nice smell. Maybe there's an overflowing trash can near you or the sewer, or maybe it's the subtle smell of yourself.
   - **What is 1 thing you can taste?** Pop a piece of gum in your mouth, sip a drink, eat a snack, or simply notice how your mouth tastes. "Taste" the air to see how it feels on your tongue.
3. **Choose an everyday task and observe it mindfully.** You can choose something as simple as putting on your shoes or opening a door. Use your senses to notice the details of the activity. Then pay attention to what you appreciate about the process from your hand's ability to move to the color of your shoes.

SAVORING

The Broaden-and-Build Theory, as mentioned in Module 2, maintains that positive emotions can be sought and created. Through savoring, those emotions can be prolonged and extended.

Savoring is the mindful process of paying attention to positive experiences. It requires slowing down to fully feel and engage in the good things happening to and around you. Doing so can bolster

MODULE 4

your resolve in recovery as you expand good feelings without the help of addictive behaviors.

Savoring is heavily connected to mindfulness, but there's an important difference between the two: **Savoring is not reserved for experiences that are going on right now.** The past and present can both be savored, too. Reminiscing on a happy memory can be an exercise in savoring, as can looking forward to an upcoming event.

Consider how savoring differs from the way you usually speed through life. If you're like most people, you often multitask. You rush from one "to-do" to another, checking off items as quickly as you can. You drive with your mind in a blur as you think about the last thing you did or the next thing you have to do. You allow certain tasks—such as preparing for the day or winding down for the night—to become routine and you allow conversations to become habitual. Sound familiar? If so, you're letting good—even great—moments pass you by.

> "I've always believed in savoring the moments. In the end, they are the only things we'll have."
> —Anna Godbersen

Savoring means slowing down, noticing and appreciating life around you. It combines positive sensations, emotions, perceptions, thoughts, and beliefs to create a fuller and even more enjoyable experience. Savoring means spending a moment to enjoy a job well done and to recognize a sense of accomplishment before moving on to the next task. It may look like observing a beautiful sunset with awe during your commute home, enjoying the warmth of the water as you shower, or the sensation of the weight of your comforter as you climb into bed. Savoring is engaging meaningfully in a conversation and feeling the joy that comes from connecting to another.

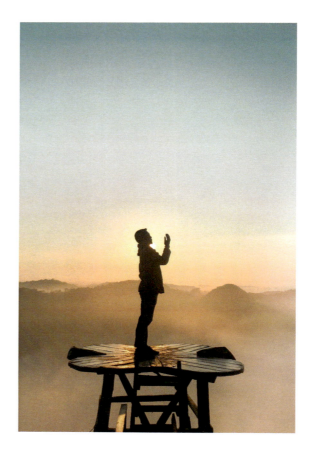

EXERCISE: Researcher Fred Bryant outlined four types of savoring. Reflect on your last week. Visualize moments during which you could have practiced savoring in one of the ways listed below. Write a few lines of reflection for each.
- Basking—enjoying the satisfaction of praise, accomplishment and blessings
- Thanksgiving—expressing gratitude and appreciation
- Luxuriating—taking pleasure (without restraint) in physical sensations and comforts
- Marveling—feeling wonder or astonishment

You're probably accustomed to society's fast pace and savoring will take effort. It may feel unnatural to slow yourself to a pace that allows for prolonged enjoyment. Just as with any skill worth developing, practice! Start with a moment set aside each day to immerse yourself in and savor the task or activity at hand. If nothing enjoyable is happening, turn to savoring the future or the past. Savor the successes you have experienced throughout your process of recovery. Savor the good times you anticipate as you maintain sobriety and reconnect with others and yourself. The act of savoring can remind you of and increase your motivation to continue progressing away from addictive behaviors.

There are six techniques that will help you practice savoring.
1. **Share with others.** Share your positive experience or thoughts with others by telling about them through words or your body language and facial expressions. This may be as simple as saying, "I feel great today!" This not only fosters connection but serves to deepen your experience of satisfaction.
2. **Build memories.** In the moment, take mental photographs of what you are enjoying. Use all your senses to create a memory. Reminisce on it later, on your own or with others, to further solidify the experience in your mind.
3. **Look forward with anticipation.** Think about something you are eagerly awaiting. This may be an activity or experience such as a vacation, or it may be the accomplishment of a goal. Think about what you will do, who will be with you, and, especially, how you will feel.
4. **Praise yourself.** Allow yourself to take pride in what you accomplish, great or small. Share with others! Try celebrating the character traits you are striving to develop, such as patience, perseverance, and gratitude. Congratulate yourself for a job well done and bask in the feeling.

MODULE 4

5. **Choose your focus.** Avoid the tendency to dwell on the negative by focusing on the positive. As you enjoy or think back on an experience, purposefully keep your attention on what went right and what felt best (rather than what went wrong).
6. **Become absorbed.** Allow yourself to become immersed in whatever you are experiencing. Gently move your attention back to what you are experiencing when your mind becomes distracted or It starts to chase thoughts that pop into your mind. Use all of your senses to fully focus on what you are doing and what is around you.

> EXERCISE: Choose one of these techniques and plan how you will use it in creating and capitalizing on positive emotions in your life this week. Write out the specifics of your plan.

FLOW

When you become completely absorbed in a task with full involvement, focus, and energy, you are in a state of flow. This is commonly called being "in the zone." A primary characteristic of flow is the way it causes you to lose perception of space and time. If you have ever been engaged in an activity for a while then looked at a clock to find hours had passed during a span of what felt like minutes, then you have experienced flow.

> "The happiest people spend much time in a state of flow—the state in which people are so involved in an activity that nothing else seems to matter; the experience itself is so enjoyable that people will do it even at great cost, for the sheer sake of doing it."
> —Mihaly Csikszentmihalyi

Activities that induce flow can vary person to person; for some it may occur when engaged in physical pursuits and sports; for others it may happen when using their hands or minds creatively in an art project; and still, others may experience it when they are immersed in and enjoying their occupation. Flow occurs when you do something you are skilled at and enjoy.

The primary researcher of flow, Mihaly Csikszentmihalyi, identified several features that are present during flow experiences.

Flow happens when you:
- Actively engage in a challenging yet doable task with clear goals (for example, win the basketball game) and you receive immediate feedback (points on the scoreboard).
- Are able to focus entirely on the activity with a sense of control and effortlessness.
- Move without worry or self-consciousness.
- Feel "one" with the task and/or environment.
- Lose your sense of time.

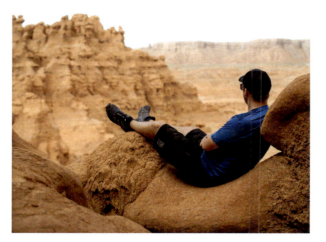

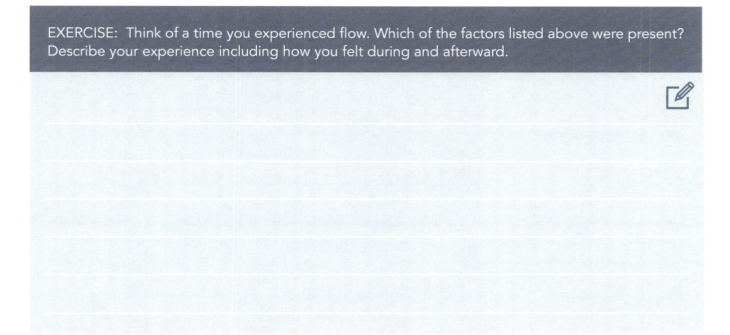

EXERCISE: Think of a time you experienced flow. Which of the factors listed above were present? Describe your experience including how you felt during and afterward.

Csikszentmihalyi's research found that **individuals who regularly engage in flow activities experienced greater instances of joy throughout their daily life.** Flow feeds a sense of meaning and fulfillment. It elicits positive emotions including peace, interest, pride, hope, and joy. Flow can also lead to greater learning and skill development as well as improved performance in flow activities. Each of these listed benefits can provide support throughout the process of breaking free of addiction. Flow activities can help you reconnect to what matters to you and leaves you feeling fulfilled and whole. They can also provide a positive distraction from using.

MODULE 4

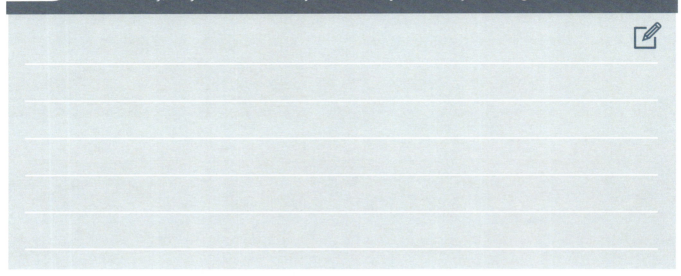

EXERCISE: Cultivate flow in your own life by examining activities you are passionate about or enjoy. Set a goal within this activity that includes a degree of challenge and stretching, but not too much. You might focus on a specific skill area or consider an outcome you would like to reach. Once you've chosen an activity and a goal, set aside uninterrupted time to do it. If you don't reach flow on your first attempt, try again another day, maybe with a few adjustments to your activity and/or goal.

MINDSET—FIXED VERSUS GROWTH

One of the most important concepts in recovery is what we believe about ourselves or, in other words, our perspective about how our own character determines our success. This has been called mindset. Carol Dweck found in her research that there are two types of mindsets: the fixed mindset and the growth mindset.

Those with a fixed mindset believe that their character, intelligence, and abilities are "carved in stone" and can't change. Those with this mindset must prove themselves over and over. They believe they have only a certain amount of intelligence, certain character traits, and certain abilities and they have to keep confirming those to themselves and others. They constantly wonder, "Am I good enough?" "Will I succeed or fail?" "Will I be rejected or accepted by the outside world?" These people see mistakes or losses as deficiencies instead of ways to grow.

Those with a **growth mindset,** on the other hand, believe that basic qualities can be cultivated through effort. People differ in their talents, abilities, interests, or temperaments, but everyone can change and grow. Those who believe in growth have a passion for learning rather than a need for approval. They don't acknowledge failure because they see all challenges and mistakes as opportunities for learning. Even if a goal isn't reached, at least progress has been made. Mistakes are to learn from, each leading to a bit more wisdom and

> "Love challenges, be intrigued by mistakes, enjoy effort and keep on learning."
> —Carol Dweck

experience. **Growth mindset is associated with greater happiness and achievement** because it is focused on the process rather than the end result.

This difference in perception becomes important, if not crucial, in the process of recovery. The path to sobriety is never a straight one, and it isn't easy. Most people can't just commit and desire to change one day and the next day be free of self-defeating and addictive behaviors. Growth mindset accepts that lapses are to be expected and that each day is a chance to do better and live cleaner. Those with a fixed mindset avoid risks and opportunities that may lead to failure. Playing it safe is preferred but that doesn't work in recovery because you must be willing to learn and take risks.

FIXED MINDSET		GROWTH MINDSET
- SOMETHING YOU'RE BORN WITH - FIXED	SKILLS	- COME FROM HARD WORK - CAN ALWAYS IMPROVE
- SOMETHING TO AVOID - COULD REVEAL LACK OF SKILL - FOSTERS THE TENDENCY TO GIVE UP EASILY	CHALLENGES	- SHOULD BE EMBRACED - AN OPPORTUNITY TO BE MORE PERSISTENT
- UNNECESSARY - SOMETHING YOU DO WHEN YOU ARE NOT GOOD ENOUGH	EFFORT	- ESSENTIAL - PROVIDES A PATH TO MASTERY
- CREATES DEFENSIVENESS - PERSON TAKES IT PERSONALLY	FEEDBACK	- USEFUL - SOMETHING TO LEARN FROM - USE TO IDENTIFY AREAS TO IMPROVE
- PROMOTES BLAME IN OTHERS - CAUSES DISCOURAGEMENT	SETBACKS	- USE AS A WAKE-UP CALL TO WORK HARDER NEXT TIME

MODULE 4

EXERCISE: One way to incorporate growth mindset into your recovery is to use the "power of yet." There may be instances where you feel discouraged because you aren't where you want to be. You may have lapsed or relapsed. Catch yourself and those intrusive negative thoughts. Add a gentle reminder that you are not there yet or you haven't yet completed your change. Use this idea outside of recovery as well. "Yet" embodies the growth mindset way of seeing possibility in the future as opposed to the fixed mindset of "this is just the way I am." It is hopeful and expects good things to happen in the future. List some negative thoughts and add "yet" to them.

"I'm not a patient parent."	"I'm not a patient parent yet."
"I haven't been promoted to manager."	"I haven't been promoted to manager yet."
"I haven't been sober for 90 days."	"I'm not 90 days sober yet."

RESILIENCE

Once there was a wise man who people visited from miles around. People complained about the same problems over and over again to the wise man. One day, he decided to tell a joke to the people who were gathered and they all roared with laughter. After a few minutes, he told the same joke. This time, only a few of them smiled. When he told the same joke for a third time, no one laughed or even smiled.

> "We all need resilience to live a fulfilling life. With resilience, you'll be more prepared to take on challenges, to develop your talents, skills, and abilities so that you can live with more purpose and more joy."
> —Eric Greitens

The wise man then smiled and said, "You don't laugh at the same joke over and over. So why do you always cry about the same problem?"

Brazilian novelist Paulo Coelho said that the secret of life "is to fall seven times and to get up eight times." **That "secret" describes resilience—simply put, the ability to bounce back. It involves coping with challenges life throws at you and then getting back up stronger than before.** Resilience means not being overcome by failures, setbacks, and disappointments. Rather, resilient people weather storms of difficulties, pick up lessons along the way, and press forward with a greater resolve. Following upsets and changes, they recognize that they may need to develop a new way of being.

Resilience combines the concepts of growth mindset: hope, effort and optimism. It is an important characteristic to hone during recovery because you're sure to experience setbacks and obstacles along your journey. Psychologist James Prochaska described the change process as an upward spiral. Resilience keeps you moving up even when you feel you've taken a step back.

Resilient people never give up. They just find a different way of doing things. From Walt Disney to Vincent Van Gogh to Thomas Edison, you can find people who had a dream, faced severe challenges but found a way to accomplish their dreams.

Walt Disney was fired from the *Kansas City Star* because his editor felt he "lacked imagination and had no good ideas." Steven Spielberg was rejected by the University of Southern California School of Cinematic Arts multiple times. Oprah Winfrey was born into poverty and overcame many challenges including molestation and abuse to become one of the most influential people in the world. Michael Jordan didn't make his high school basketball team and went on to arguably be the best basketball player of all time. He said, "I've missed more than nine thousand shots in my career. I've lost almost three hundred games. Twenty-six times I've been trusted to take the game winning shot and missed. I've failed over and over and over in my life. . . That is why I succeed."

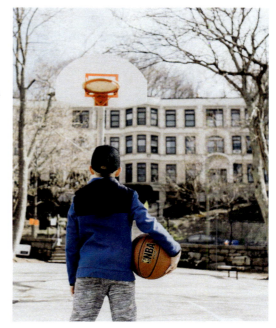

One of the most productive and imaginative inventors of all time, Thomas Edison was homeschooled until the age of sixteen when he entered the public school system. This ended when one day he overheard the teacher tell the inspector that he was "addled" or too stupid to learn, and it would not be worthwhile keeping him in school any longer. According to an interview given later in his life, he was so hurt by this that he burst out crying and went home and told his mother about it. He reported that she angrily confronted the teacher telling him that her son had more brains than he himself. Openly grateful for his mother's support and education throughout his life, Edison said many years later, "My mother was the making of me. She was so true, so sure of me, and I felt I had someone to live for, someone I must not disappoint." At times we need a cheering section to spur us on to greatness, but we have to have that inner will power and desire or all else will fail. Edison's many successes were tempered by the number of times he didn't succeed. When asked about the many thousands of failures he had when trying to create the lightbulb he famously said, **"I have not failed. I've just found ten thousand ways that won't work."**

MODULE 4

EXERCISE: Write down the strengths that you have which will help you face your recovery process.

To build resilience during your recovery process:
- Expect and accept change. Life is always changing. You are in the middle of big changes right now and you will definitely face more changes in the future. Recognizing the inevitability of change allows you to prepare yourself to stay afloat when waves of change surge.
- Learn from your past but don't stay stuck there. Resilience is strengthened by what you learn from the past. If you stay trapped in the past, you will feel hopeless and helpless. The only part of the past you can change is your relationship to it.
- View setbacks as positive experiences. When you realize that the past and your mistakes in the past are to be learned from, difficulties and misfortunes become growth opportunities and chances to turn toward others.
- Build hope and optimism, which is just one way to practice positivity. Expect good things to come into your life and be grateful for what you do have.
- Strengthen your support network. You are never alone on your path toward sobriety. Cultivate connections with your community, a faith organization, civic groups, family, friends, and others who are going through similar experiences. When your perspective or hope is waffling, borrow some of theirs.
- Have a goal in mind. Set realistic goals and move toward them in small, regular steps. Goals help keep your eyes facing forward and your feet moving in your intended direction.
- Care for yourself. Prioritize psychological, emotional, personal, physical, professional and spiritual self-care. This will prevent you from feeling depleted, rundown and more susceptible to being defeated by challenges.

KEY TAKEAWAYS

- Positive psychology practices build hope, motivation, and well-being while combating the detrimental effects of negative thinking.
- Positive emotional experiences expand creativity and problem solving.
- The regular practice of gratitude decreases depression and increases life and relationship satisfaction. The simple act of writing down things you are grateful for each day can have a profound effect.
- Savoring is mindfully enjoying positive emotions. This practice prolongs the experience of love, joy, wonder, gratitude, pride, and other beneficial emotions.
- Flow, or focused engagement, enhances joy and satisfaction.
- Mindfulness is nonjudgmental awareness of the present moment. It pulls your thoughts to now, away from the past and future places where you tend to dwell. Mindfulness can be practiced in many ways each day.
- Growth mindset sees challenges and mistakes as opportunities for learning and progression.
- Resilience is a necessary characteristic for successful recovery. It includes growth mindset and hardiness against challenges.

MODULE 5

SELF-ESTEEM

PRINCIPLES

TAKE ACCOUNTABILITY FOR YOUR LIFE
Examine Yourself with Honesty and Responsibility

DISCOVER PURPOSE
Identify what Gives Your Life Meaning

FIND YOUR IDENTITY AND NURTURE SELF-WORTH
Live from the Inside Out and Not the Outside In

THOUGHT QUESTIONS

Do you really know who you are and your purpose in life?

Do you base your feelings about yourself on accomplishments or on intrinsic characteristics?

Do you accept who you are and try to live with integrity–true to yourself?

One of the underlying principles of each of these modules is **responsibility and accountability**. This module is no different. As you take responsibility for your life, your feelings of empowerment and confidence grow. This increases feelings of respect and esteem for yourself. **Finding purpose** is also a principle that is outlined in several of the modules. When you have **purpose and meaning** in your life, you tend to live consciously and engage in self-acceptance. You understand with more clarity who you are. Your **identity and self-worth** (or who you are) is evident not only to those around you but to yourself. **Never give up on your dreams.**

An older man who was financially broke lived in a tiny house; one of his sole possessions was a beat-up car. He was surviving on ninety-nine dollars a month from social

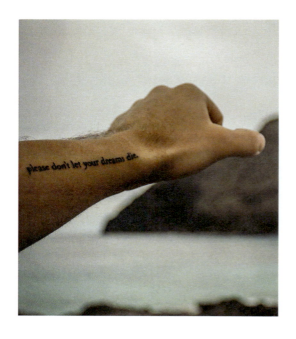

security checks. At the age of sixty-five, he decided things had to change and so he thought about what he had to offer the world. His friends raved about the chicken he made and he decided that selling that recipe was his best shot at making a change.

He left his home and traveled to different states telling restaurant owners about his mouthwatering chicken recipe. He even offered to give them the recipe for free, asking only for a small percentage of the items sold.

Unfortunately, none of the restaurants took him up on his offer. He heard "no" more than a thousand times. Even after all those rejections, he didn't give up. He believed his chicken recipe was something special. He was rejected 1,009 times before he heard his first yes.

With that one success, Colonel Harlan Sanders changed the way Americans eat chicken, and Kentucky Fried Chicken, popularly known as KFC was born.
Remember, never give up and always believe in yourself despite rejection.

> "Of all the judgments we pass in life, none is as important as the one we pass on ourselves. Self-esteem is the disposition to experience oneself as competent to cope with the basic challenges of life and worthy of happiness." —Nathanial Branden

love that

WHAT IS SELF-ESTEEM

Despite the many books, articles, and seminars devoted to the subject of self-esteem, there has been little consensus or agreement about what it means. Is it simply a feeling that you are of worth? Is it a compassionate feeling toward yourself? Is it having self-respect? Is it something you are just born with?

In his book *Honoring the Self*, psychotherapist Nathanial Branden, an expert in the psychology of self-esteem, defines it this way:

> "Self-esteem is the disposition to experience oneself as being competent to cope with the basic challenges of life and of being worthy of happiness. It is confidence in the efficacy of our mind, in our ability to think. By extension, it is confidence in our ability to learn, make appropriate choices and decisions, and respond effectively to change. It is also the experience that success, achievement, fulfillment—happiness—are right and natural for us. The survival-value of such confidence is obvious; so is the danger, when it is missing."

Sometimes it's easier to define a concept by looking at what it isn't. Those who lack a healthy respect or love for themselves or who lack a belief in their abilities usually engage in self-defeating behaviors or things that don't promote success in life. They may engage in destructive behaviors, such as chemical dependency or other addictive activities. They often feel like they aren't "good enough." People with low self-esteem tend to sabotage their lives. They may have a good job but believe that others are going to eventually "see them as they really are" and they will get fired. They then engage in negative behaviors, such as being late, arguing with their boss, or other sabotaging behaviors that lead to job loss. People with low self-esteem generally do not look at life in a positive way; they are often depressed or anxious and may have little motivation to change.

MODULE 5

Self-esteem does not involve demeaning others to make yourself feel better. That is a false sense of feeling good. Remember that someone else's success does not hamper your success. You can feel good about yourself and be successful on your own terms.

Without self-esteem or self-love, life is not as satisfying. **The way you feel about yourself determines how you treat yourself and others.** Self-esteem is reinforcing. When you feel good about yourself, you act like it, which then reinforces your good feelings. And here's what happens as a result: you succeed more often. Your expectations for yourself increase. You are more motivated to be actively engaged in life. You have more confidence. On the other hand, if you lack self-esteem, you give up easily, make more mistakes, and aspire to less. And that means you get less of what you want.

To achieve a healthy level of self-esteem, you must be able to **accept who you are and be confident about your decisions and behavior.** Self-esteem has to do with what you think of you and not what anyone else thinks of you. Even though accomplishments are very important and in some sense are indicative of your character and personality, you are not your accomplishments.

Here's an example that illustrates that principle: Upon meeting one of her clients for the first time, a psychologist asked him to describe himself. He said, "Oh, I'm on the board of regents of a local university; I'm vice-president of a local company; I've won this award and that award." In response, she stopped him and asked, "Those are nice accomplishments, but if you take them away, does that mean you're nothing?"

The psychologist was trying to help him understand that he was not his accomplishments. He was able to accomplish because he had certain strengths. He was probably organized, he was likely a good people person, and he seemed to have vision. His strengths determined what he was able to accomplish. It's the same way with you: when you review your life, it is very important to define yourself in terms of your abilities, and strengths which will then determine your accomplishments.

HOW YOU ACQUIRE SELF-ESTEEM

Self-esteem doesn't come from affirmations or from looking in the mirror to greet yourself each day with, "Good morning, Beautiful!" It cannot be gained by being showered with praise, because if you don't have self-esteem, you won't believe the praise you get anyway. Self-esteem doesn't come from wealth or money or from the college your children attend and the awards they receive.

> "Dare to love yourself as if you were a rainbow with gold at both ends." —Aberjhani

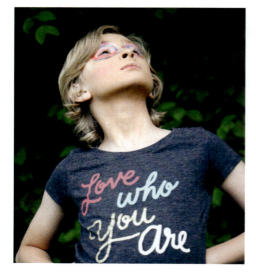

Self-esteem does not come from peers, belief in a higher power, or participating in service, even though all of these contribute to self-esteem. Self-esteem is not about your accomplishments; it stems from those internally generated practices that make it possible for you to achieve. It comes from work, understanding yourself, and being true to who you are. It is about your character and having enough integrity to live true to your values and beliefs. When you stick up for yourself and your beliefs or engage in activities that others are fighting against, your self-esteem grows stronger—even though what you think or believe may not be adopted by others.

Self-esteem involves all aspects of your person: the emotional, the cognitive, and the behavioral. It also necessitates you looking hard and deeply at yourself. Like many, you may have just put yourself on automatic pilot and refused to look at who you are in a detailed or honest way. You may be in denial about who you are. If so, how do you expect to change?

Life is about listening to other's ideas, opinions, and thoughts and then coming to an understanding about what **you** think or feel. But it goes beyond that: too many people remain stuck in this "intellectualizing" and don't "do" what they think or talk about. That can lead to feelings of inadequacy, incompetence, or just plain hopelessness.

To increase good feelings about yourself, you must be proactive. You must practice life.

In *The Six Pillars of Self-Esteem*, Nathaniel Branden writes that practicing "implies a discipline of acting in a certain way over and over again—consistently living our core truths." He describes self-esteem as the ability to:

- Practice living consciously. Pay attention to information and feedback about your needs and goals. Face facts that might be uncomfortable or threatening. Refuse to wander through life in a self-induced mental fog.
- Practice self-acceptance. Be willing to experience whatever you truly think, feel, or do, even if you don't always like it. Face your mistakes and learn from them.
- Practice self-responsibility. Establish a sense of control over your life by realizing you are responsible for your values, your choices and actions at every level, the achievement of your goals, and your happiness.
- Practice self-assertiveness. Be willing to appropriately express your thoughts, values, and feelings; to stand up for yourself; and to speak and act from your deepest convictions.
- Practice living purposefully. Set goals and work to achieve them instead of living at the mercy of chance and outside forces. Find meaning in life. Choose
- Practice integrity. Integrate your behavior with your ideals, convictions, standards, and beliefs. Act in congruence with what you believe is right.

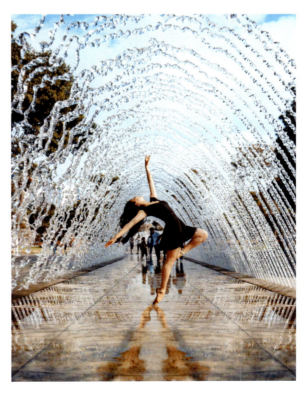

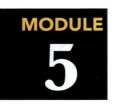

MODULE 5: THE PRACTICE OF LIVING CONSCIOUSLY

Most of us sleepwalk through life; we put ourselves on automatic pilot and we go. We wake up, go to work, eat lunch, come home, eat dinner, play with the kids, and go to bed. We have obligations, and we fulfill them. But the sameness of the routine promotes not living consciously or mindfully. That means we aren't aware of our surroundings, our thoughts, our feelings, our behaviors, and our relationships. At times, we can't even answer the questions, "Why am I doing this?" "Is this good for me?"

> "You have brains in your head. You have feet in your shoes. You can steer yourself in any direction you choose. You're on your own. And you know what you know. You're the guy who'll decide where to go."
> —Dr. Seuss

How you perceive the world is all about your level of awareness and your thoughts about it. Truth is an individual thing. You're hot while someone else is cold. Whose truth is right? Law enforcement officials will tell you that when there is an accident, each witness will often report different things. If there are seven witnesses, there will be seven different perspectives depending on factors like proximity to the accident, the angle from which the accident was viewed, the witness's own experience, biases, and common sense. If someone is a few feet away, his perspective is going to be much different than that of the person who views the accident from a block away. Bias colors perception as well. A witness who thinks women are terrible drivers will assign blame to the woman, while it may have been the man's fault. Expectations can also color perception; you often see what you expect or want to see.

Living consciously means being aware not only of your surroundings but of all the things that can affect what you "see"—and it is a choice. You can pay attention and be fully present when you are making critical decisions like whether to have another drink when you're trying to stay sober, feeling emotions instead of repressing them, or exploring how much you desire to change. Or you can be physically present but mentally absent during these activities. Either way, you are responsible for the level of consciousness you bring to any experience or feeling—and you are responsible for the results.

Living consciously entails seeking and being open to any information, knowledge, or feedback that affects who you are, what you think and believe, and what you feel. It is about being aware of how your environment affects you, and how that in turn affects your behaviors and emotions. It is being honest with yourself and letting go of how others influence your beliefs about the world and about yourself. It is defining who you are and not being defined by others. It is deciding who you want to be and then, no matter how you are treated, acting congruent with what you have decided about yourself. Then you will be in control of yourself, and no one else will be in control of you.

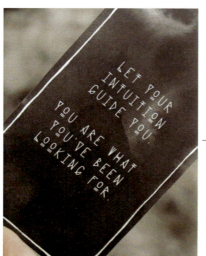

For example, imagine that someone flips you off on the freeway and you feel the anger rising. You can either participate in road rage or you can calm yourself. Road rage not only leads to destructive tendencies but it puts the other person in control. If you are in control of you, don't let it bother you. You shrug it off.

10 Principles of Recovery

In recovery, it is important to be very real with yourself and to practice control. Knowing and accepting your truth will lead to better decision-making abilities. That means you need to realize the extent of the problem you are dealing with and to avoid denial. Look at all the factors that have contributed to the addiction and your thinking patterns. It is imperative that you choose to confront with authenticity what is keeping you stuck instead of being driven by fear or other negative emotions. When you are authentic with your feelings, you experience greater self-efficacy and self-respect and less stress.

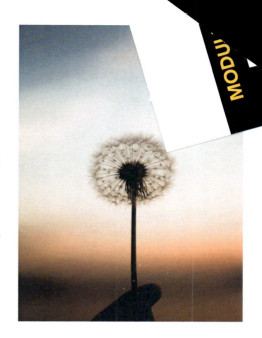

Living consciously also means that you know yourself well enough to recognize when you aren't living your values. At times you can get distracted by "life" and overlook what really matters to you. When that happens, you need to refocus on what is really important and that may mean disconnecting from the world and taking time for yourself.

Distractions are a barrier to living life more consciously, which is why it is important that you start to identify what distracts you, wastes your time, causes procrastination, and keeps you from doing what needs to be done.

EXERCISE: What are the major distractions in your life that keep you from what you value? How will you deal with these? Write each down and write a plan for dealing with it them.

Handwritten response:
- Social media and comparing myself
- Body Image - my body
- Brying shift
- Feeling like I need to be social
- Pleasing others
- Food - Obsessing over it.
- Feeling inadequate

5

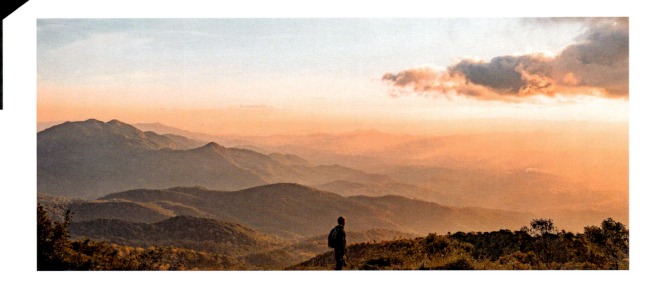

THE PRACTICE OF SELF-ACCEPTANCE

Practicing self-acceptance means that you own and take responsibility for your thoughts, feelings, and behaviors. You are real with yourself and accept who you are, regardless of past mistakes or choices. Unfortunately, the human mind focuses on negativity which means you naturally focus more on what you aren't than what you are, on your weaknesses instead of your strengths.

> "When you acquire enough inner peace and feel really positive about yourself, it's almost impossible for you to be controlled and manipulated by anybody else." —Wayne Dyer

How do you practice self-acceptance? Accept that you are doing the best you can. Think about this: you are doing the best you can with your current knowledge, energy levels, and desire, or you would do something else. Remember a day when you just had no energy. You didn't accomplish much, and you started to feel guilty because you had so much to do. Could you have done better? Sure, but with the energy level you had and the place you were mentally, you did the best you could. At times like that, give yourself permission to just be lazy and realize you have little desire or motivation. It is what it is.

FORGIVE YOURSELF

"Have a crusty day"

Self-acceptance can be crippled by regrets about the past. Whether it's something you've done or if your personality rubbed someone the wrong way, it's important to learn from your mistakes and accept that you can't change the past. Forgive yourself and move on. Your mistakes and imperfections are not failures or indications that you are defective, they are growing opportunities for learning, healing, and growth. Focus on the positives in your life.

> "You don't have to prove yourself because you are proof of yourself when you are true to who you are." —Trish Barrus

BE TRUE

Feelings of unworthiness or feelings of being "not good enough" are far too common when you try to prove yourself to others. You shouldn't change who you are just to please someone else; that's not being "you," and it never feels good. Don't be hard on yourself because you don't think you're measuring up to your own expectations. Silence your inner critic and focus on what you are doing well.

This is hard for me

> EXERCISE: List some of the proud moments in your life. What motivated you to do them? As you think about what you're proud of, list some of the characteristics you used in those moments that you really liked.

My first black diamond!
Having each baby

PERFECTIONISM

> "You wouldn't worry so much about what others think of you if you realized how seldom they do." —Eleanor Roosevelt *yep*

Thinking you need to be perfect to be of worth can lead to unhappiness and is often accompanied by depression, anxiety, or other mood disorders. Perfectionism usually starts in childhood as children get the message that they need to perform or meet the expectations of others to be accepted. That message can last a lifetime and often results in the belief, "I will never be good enough."

MODULE 5

> "Understanding the difference between healthy striving and perfectionism is critical to laying down the shield and picking up your life. Research shows that perfectionism hampers success. In fact, it's often the path to depression, anxiety, addiction, and life paralysis." —Brené Brown

Perfectionistic Thoughts	Whole & Healthy Thought Patterns
The following is a list of perfectionistic thought patterns. How many do you experience?	Now look at the list of whole, and recognizing healthy thought patterns. Do any of these describe you?

Perfectionistic Thoughts:
1. Unreasonable goals or goals that vastly exceed performance. ✓
2. Can't find pleasure in working toward the goal; focus is only on the outcome.
3. Worth is based on achievements. ✓
4. Worth is based on comparisons with others. ✓
5. Doesn't feel satisfied. ✓
6. Doesn't feel loved or validated unless performing well. ✓
7. Can't share mistakes without excessive shame.
8. Experiences excessive, chronic, and pervasive fear of failure.
9. Believes in external standards for success. ✓

Whole & Healthy Thought Patterns:
1. Sets obtainable, realistic goals.
2. Believes inherent self-worth.
3. Adheres to goals which can self-reward.
4. Places "emphasis" on "recognizing" individual uniqueness.
5. Accepts self as valuable while acknowledging human weaknesses.
6. Can accept failure as part of learning process. Able to keep trying.
7. Derives goals from inner awareness.
8. Goals reflect growth to the next stage of progressive development.
9. Enjoys the "journey."
10. Emphasis on keeping life in balance.

The goal is to define yourself the way you would like. **Remember, you don't have to prove yourself, because you are proof of yourself when living true to your values.**

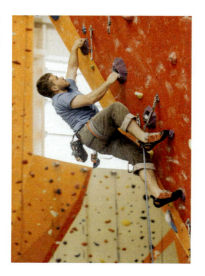

EXERCISE: After reviewing the list of perfectionistic thought patterns and healthy thought patterns, which best describes you? How do you need to change the way you think so you feel fully accepted by yourself?

accept! Love baseline lizzy more, even before I make all the changes and meet my goals. I'm still ok and loveable right now

THE PRACTICE OF SELF-RESPONSIBILITY

> "It is easy to dodge our responsibilities, but we cannot dodge the consequences of dodging our responsibilities." —Josiah Stamp

Self-responsibility is the idea that you are the author of your choices and actions and that your happiness, or lack thereof, is in your control. Being responsible means that you are okay admitting your errors and faults instead of blaming others for your problems or mistakes. You want to be in control of your life, and you understand that you give up control when you blame others.

Those with addictions may use drugs or other addictive behaviors as an excuse to be irresponsible or may blame others for their addiction. They may believe that their upbringing or life circumstances are responsible for their addiction. Another key perception of addictive thinking is the belief of never being wrong. This is reinforced by other addictive thinking patterns, such as projection, rationalization, denial, manipulating others, and self-victimization. The reality is that everyone makes mistakes. Facing missteps with honesty and integrity is an important part of recovery. This can be facilitated by noticing how others overcome their mistakes and by adopting the mantra, "A mistake is not the end of the world."

While you shouldn't blame others or let them control you, you should guard against the tendency to be "a pleaser," which is common among those with addictive thinking. Pleaser's believe that they are in charge of others' happiness. Making others happy becomes their life mission. They believe that the more they do for someone, the more approval and love they will receive. Of course, this is not true.

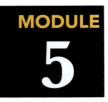

MODULE 5

No one can make you happy, just as no one can make you sad. And people approve and love you because of what they do for you.

Practicing self-responsibility means that you set boundaries and don't take on the job of fixing other's problems. When you try to be a caretaker in that way, you send the message, "Let me help you get out of this mess because you aren't competent to do it yourself."

Living responsibly means you think for yourself and explore what you believe and value. You don't blindly accept whatever your culture, parents, or society tell you your values should be. Self-responsibility helps you realize that no one is going to come along and rescue you or fix your life. If you want to get something done or solve a problem, you need to be proactive. Don't sit on the sidelines and hope that someone else figures it out for you. You'll be waiting a long time.

Recovery necessitates facing behaviors, ways of thinking, and uncomfortable emotions. If you don't change addictive thinking patterns, you will likely go from one addiction to the next. In fact, recovery might feel impossible if you're still trapped in the same thinking patterns, habits, and behaviors. Remember that trust in yourself grows, if you do not pass on to others the responsibility for your life.

> EXERCISE: Watch for times when you blame someone else for your behavior. Ask yourself, "If I was behaving responsibly right now, how would I change my behavior?"

- getting to church on time.
- friendships

THE PRACTICE OF SELF-ASSERTIVENESS

Being assertive means being authentic and true to who you are, treating others with respect (which includes listening to their ideas), and realizing that you deserve just as much respect as you give to others. It is being confident without being aggressive. It is realizing that your ideas are just as

yes →

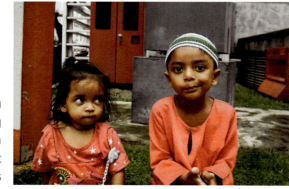

71 Copyright © 2021 by Trish Barrus and Jade Ozawa-Kirk

important as someone else's and that you need to stand up for yourself in appropriate ways without fear of rejection or judgment.

Being assertive means not being passive. Passive people tend to let others call the shots, they have little respect for themselves, and they don't have boundaries. They are sometimes referred to as doormats. Being assertive does not mean being aggressive. Aggressive people are bullies. They have no respect for the feelings or ideas of others. They tend to be toxic and hard to be around.

If it's difficult for you to be assertive, you probably have a fear of being judged or rejected even if you know you are right. You may have a problem saying "no," even though you realize it's in your best interest. You may feel like you're being rude if you stick up for yourself.

Those with addictions often have trouble being assertive <u>because they believe they have let people down and don't deserve to be valued</u>, even though they may desperately want the approval of others. They then tend to hide and isolate themselves from social interaction.

You'll need to practice being assertive if you're not that way naturally. Here are some tips to help you be more assertive:

- Be aware of what you're feeling and thinking. Give yourself permission to feel, think, and express feelings and thoughts to others.
- Practice listening to understand. Provide others with the same courtesy that you would like by listening attentively. Don't jump in and cut them off. Try to understand their viewpoint and perception. You may learn something.
- Have the courage to speak up even when others may not agree. They may learn something.
- Say "no" when someone asks something of you that you don't want to give. It's okay to advocate for yourself in this way. If they dislike you because you said "no," it is about their lack of boundaries, not your failings.

> EXERCISE: Write about a situation where you did not feel assertive. Then visualize yourself being assertive in that situation. How do you look? What do you sound like? What is your body language saying about you? How do you feel when you are assertive? Write about this new experience. Once you've completed that analysis, practice being assertive with one person in a situation where you would normally find it hard.

MODULE 5
THE PRACTICE OF LIVING PURPOSEFULLY

Living purposefully means <u>setting goals that matter to you</u> and then working to achieve them. It is finding meaning and purpose in life. If you don't have meaning and purpose in life, you have a hard time being or staying motivated. Abraham Maslow said, "The only happy <u>people I know are the ones who are working well at something they consider important</u>."

Living purposefully incorporates living consciously and responsibly. It means that you are aware of what gives your life meaning and that you take responsibility for setting goals that contribute to this meaning. It then requires that you follow through and achieve those goals. Nathaniel Branden wrote, "Living purposefully is a fundamental orientation that applies to every aspect of our existence. It means that we **live and act by intention**. It is a distinguishing characteristic of those who enjoy a high level of control over their life."

> "When you connect to the silence within you, that is when you can make sense of the disturbance going on around you." —Stephen Richards

Those with addiction frequently have a hard time finding meaning. The addiction often takes over their thoughts, desires, and brain chemistry, making it impossible to think or act rationally. The addiction becomes so powerful that the only thing that gives meaning is getting the drug or engaging in the addictive behavior.

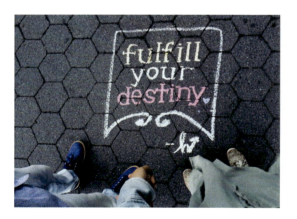

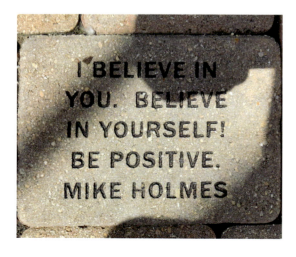

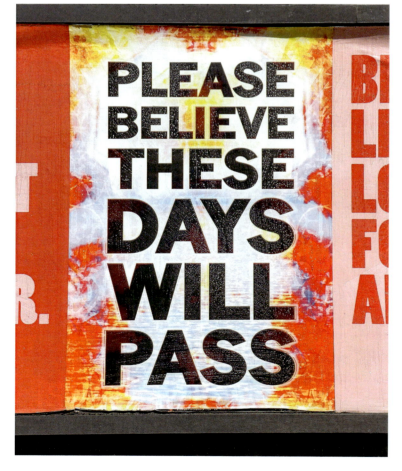

73

Copyright © 2021 by Trish Barrus and Jade Ozawa-Kirk

EXERCISE: Write answers to the following questions. Think back on the legacy you wrote previously.
1. What am I trying to achieve in life?
2. How am I trying to achieve it?
3. Who am I trying to be?
4. How am I trying to be that?
5. What is something I am passionate about?
6. How do I spend my spare time?
7. What do I think about when no one else is around?
8. What gives my life meaning or purpose?
9. What five hobbies do I enjoy?
10. What did I dream of becoming when I grew up? Did I give up on that dream? Is it still something I want? Is it something I could resurrect?

I am only trying to be ME. And learn boundaries with those whose energy sucks mine. I will not allow myself to be brought lower.

THE PRACTICE OF LIVING WITH INTEGRITY

Living with integrity means that you are true to who you are. It is aligning your behaviors, values, beliefs, and thoughts and acting in congruence with what you know to be right. **It is listening to your own truth and not allowing others to define that for you.**

You may have been taught from an early age to pay far more attention to signals coming from other people than from within. You then looked for the approval of your parents, teachers, and other significant people. As a child, you may have been encouraged to ignore what you wanted and needed because authority figures knew far more about what was best for you. That caused you to focus on living up to the expectations of others. It is important to be aware of and respect your own insights, intuition, and perspectives. If you don't, it's very difficult to be happy and content.

"How hurtful it can be to deny one's true self and live a life of lies just to appease others." —June Ahern

MODULE 5

Erik Erickson, a famous psychologist and peer of Sigmund Freud, proposed that people's personalities develop in stages from infancy to old age. The last stage of life is integrity versus despair. Erickson maintained that if we live a life true to ourselves—in other words, if we are motivated from within instead of being what others want us to be—we will live with integrity. If not, we will likely suffer despair.

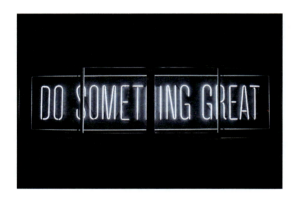

EXERCISE: In past modules, you have learned about values and how they have affected your life—especially how they have affected addictive behaviors. Now that you have learned about self-esteem, would you change anything you have previously written? What do you need to change in your life or keep doing to have integrity?

KEY TAKEAWAYS

- Healthy self-esteem is an essential part of a satisfying life. Without it, people tend to engage in self-defeating behaviors, including addiction.
- Self-esteem can be acquired through deliberate practice.
- Elements of self-esteem include self-acceptance, responsibility for one's own actions, and appropriate assertiveness.
- Self-esteem is bolstered by living consciously and mindfully. It is also increased by finding purpose, meaning, and integrity based on one's values.
- In recovery, self-esteem can act as a buffer and motivator against relapse.

MODULE 6

SELF-COMPASSION, CONFIDENCE, & SPIRITUALITY

PRINCIPLES

TAKE ACCOUNTABILITY FOR YOUR LIFE
Examine Yourself with Honesty and Responsibility

DEFINE AND STRENGTHEN YOUR SPIRITUAL SELF
Connect with Your Higher Power

FIND YOUR IDENTITY AND NURTURE SELF-WORTH
Live from the Inside Out and Not the Outside In

THOUGHT QUESTIONS

How do you, or do you, practice compassion for yourself?

Do you truly have confidence in yourself and who you are, or do you doubt?

What are the main needs in your life? What does spirituality mean to you?

French philosopher and priest Pierre Teilhard de Chardin said, "We are not human beings having a spiritual experience. We are spiritual beings having a human experience." Whatever that **spiritual experience** means to you, it is critical that you define it. And in that process, you must **discover who you are and connect fully with yourself and your higher power.** This process also entails nurturing or having compassion for yourself. It is replacing criticism with kindness and realizing that mistakes will be made but that mistakes aren't failure. The only time you fail is when you fall down and stay down.

Ramon was thirty-four years old when he died and twenty-one when he became seriously ill with polio. He was one of the last people in the state of Utah to contract the disease before the vaccine was released.

Growing up, Ramon worked hard at whatever he did. He toiled alongside his father on the family farm. He was a leader in high school and served as student body president his senior year. He earned all-state honors in almost every sport. He also worked hard to develop his character; he was humble and well-loved by his fellow students.

Polio changed his life. He could no longer walk or play the sports he so passionately loved. He could no longer run with his two-year-old daughter or hold his newborn son without help. He was hospitalized for three years struggling with the disease and eventually regained enough strength to live. Paralyzed from the neck down, he made a decision. If this was his life going forward, he would make the best of it. Ramon was a very spiritual man and he could have turned on his God and thrown a spiritual temper tantrum, demanding "Why me?" But his faith in God had strong roots, so when the hard times came like the sun scorching the earth, his testimony of God's love survived and thrived.

This is the legacy that my father left me, for I was that two-year-old. Never once did I hear my father ask "why me?" or hear him utter a foul or unkind word. Never did I hear a word of self-pity come out of his mouth. Never did I hear him question what he knew in his soul and his heart to be the truth of our existence. Never once did he question his circumstances to me or others, even though I'm sure in the loneliest part of the night he despaired. He smiled a lot and told corny jokes. He loved and empathized with those around him, especially those who were worse off than he was. He had the confidence to get an engineering degree—but because of discrimination against the handicapped in those days, no one would hire him. This did not deter him. He knew who he was. Polio hadn't changed that.

Finally, after many months, a firm in Las Vegas hired him. He became their star employee as he invented and secured dozens of patents. He couldn't participate in sports, but he coached young men's church basketball teams. He zoomed up and down the court in his electric wheelchair, urging the boys on just as he taught and encouraged me in everything I attempted. His strength helped to build mine.

> "Be nice to yourself. . . It's hard to be happy when someone is mean to you all the time." —Christine Arylo

A big part of self-esteem and honoring yourself is self-compassion. The ability to nurture yourself is critical in helping you feel cared for, accepted, and secure. Negative emotions promote feelings of worthlessness and incompetency. **Self-compassion,** on the other hand, enables you to **shift your focus from what you aren't to what you are, from your weaknesses to your strengths, from helplessness to hopefulness.**

One important element of compassion is kindness. Just as you are kind and understanding toward others, it is important to be kind to yourself when you make mistakes or feel inadequate. Rather than ignoring your emotions and needs or being self-demeaning, you need to take a balanced, mindful approach to your negative emotions so that your feelings are neither suppressed nor exaggerated. What if you can't avoid negative emotions? The healthy way to manage unavoidable negative emotions is to fully experience them in a nonjudgmental way while practicing self-soothing techniques, such as introduced in the mindfulness section. Facing negative emotions head-on helps you see them from a different perspective and they eventually lose their powerful and often debilitating grip.

Being kind to yourself may be a foreign concept to you, especially if you have experienced trauma or abuse or grew up with critical caregivers. You may have coped by using substances or addictive behaviors. Self-medication inevitably ends in self-deprecation; you think, "Why did I do that? It's not good for me," or, "I'm such a loser because I can't control myself." These thoughts and other similar ones add to the negativity surrounding addictions. If you want to progress and recover, you must value and be kind to yourself. You may have been taught as a child that valuing yourself and being confident is arrogant or conceited. But there is a huge difference between arrogance and confidence. Arrogance is caused by insecurity and the need to prove yourself to others. It is believing that you are better than

MODULE 6

others. Confidence means you know who you are, and you approve of yourself. You don't have to play the "I'm better than you game." You treat yourself and others with respect.

CONFIDENCE VERSUS SELF-DOUBT

According to the latest world happiness report, we are in the middle of an addiction epidemic, not just opioid addiction. An estimated one-half of the population suffers from one addiction or another.

Chalk part of that up to doubt. Doubt affects your confidence and, therefore, your self-esteem. What's true and what isn't? Who do you believe? Addiction often results from an effort to medicate doubts, fears, and insecurities.

Self-confidence, on the other hand, comes from learning to believe in yourself and your ability to overcome challenges. The more you try something and have success at it, the more you feel competent. The more competent you feel, the more your confidence grows. The more confident you are, the more success you experience. It's called the **Confidence/Competency Loop.**

> "Inaction breeds doubt and fear. Action breeds confidence and courage. If you want to conquer fear do not sit home and think about it. Go out and get busy." —Dale Carnegie

Without confidence, you experience fear. When you are fearful, you become tentative. You delay. You procrastinate. Eventually, you don't act at all.

MYTHS ABOUT CONFIDENCE

> "If for a while the harder you try, the harder it gets, take heart. So, it has been with the best people who have ever lived." —Jeffrey R. Holland

You might have heard—or might even believe—some of these myths about confidence:

- Confidence is a personality trait. Sometimes you look at a person and think, "He has so much confidence; he must have been born with it." Even though some people have an inherent ability to be confident, it is not a personality trait; it can be developed.
- Confidence is all about thinking positively. Even though thinking positive thoughts will feel good in the moment, it will not create confidence. Positive thoughts can motivate you, but action is key. You need to think positively and then act.
- If I have confidence, I'm confident in all situations. In fact, confidence is situational. Some people might have the ability to be confident in all situations, but that is rare. The more you work on a challenge and solve it, the more your confidence builds and the more you believe in your ability to solve other problems and challenges.
- Confidence is determined by others, situations, or your environment. This is completely untrue. Being confident is a choice. Be the architect of your own fate and take an honest inventory of your life. How have you created happiness in your life? How have you created misery? Self-reflection will

help you focus on the power that you have instead of feeling helpless and victimized. As you focus on your capabilities and strengths, your confidence will grow.

DOUBT

Self-doubt is the opposite of self-confidence. It is the decision not to try because of fear of failure, of making a mistake, or not feeling good enough.

> "Each time we face our fear, we gain strength, courage and confidence in the doing." —Theodore Roosevelt

THE FOUR D'S OF DOUBT:

- Delaying. Delaying or procrastinating action is triggered by uncertainty or overthinking. The more you delay, the more you overthink and overanalyze, and you eventually talk yourself out of moving ahead. The more optimistic you are and the more you motivate yourself to move, the more positive thoughts will build on each other and you'll see things from a different perspective.

- Disappearing. When triggered by fear, you tend to hide from others and from life because you don't have confidence that you can deal with it. This leads to further feelings of not being capable. Disappearing results from focusing on the negatives instead of the positives, what's wrong with you instead of what's right, and your weaknesses instead of strengths. Disappearing instead of being proactive leads to feelings of powerlessness as well as a sense of isolation and loneliness.

- Disapproving of self. Being hypercritical of yourself is a learned behavior and usually comes from feeling defective, an idea that began when you were young. You might have felt that you weren't good enough because you thought you could never measure up to your parents' expectations. Interestingly, that's not always a result of criticism; it can also result from being overly praised. When a child gets constant praise but doesn't feel deserving, he begins to worry that he has to hide his true self so that others won't be disappointed in him. Some parents also live through their children; children then feel they must be successful so their parents will be fulfilled. Such a child takes on the responsibility of making her parent happy and becoming who the parent wants her to be. The eventual result is an adult who is a pleaser and who is overly critical of themselves.

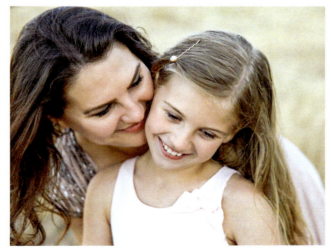

- Feeling discouraged. It's normal to occasionally feel discouraged. The problem comes when you blame others or your environment for what is going wrong. Sometimes you know the solution but you don't act on it because you are stuck. At times like this, it helps to ask yourself, "Where am I now?" and "What do I need to do to get to the next step?"

MODULE 6

EXERCISE: Write down areas in your life where you lack confidence. What habits of self-doubt are stopping you from feeling confident?
How will you change these habits?
How has doubt affected your good feelings about yourself?

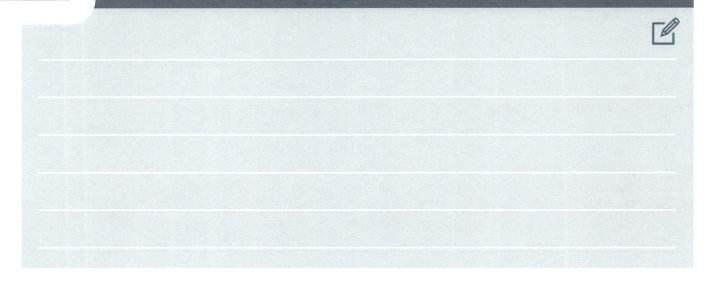

THE MODEL OF SELF-LOVE

THE THREE STEPS OF LOVE

Self-esteem has to do with what you think of yourself, not what anyone else thinks of you. It's not based on comparison or being better than someone else. As a Positive Psychologist, Trish Barrus has identified steps that can help you think well of and value yourself. They are known as the Three Steps of Love.

STEP ONE: GET TO KNOW YOURSELF

We don't love what or who we don't know. To love someone, you need to know their strengths, weaknesses, values, beliefs, and so on. The same thing is true regarding self-love: If you want to love yourself, learn to know yourself, including what you need, and what you believe. As part of the "getting to know you" process there are several exercises outlined below. Take time to really think about these exercises and be honest with yourself. Notice we don't ask you to list your weaknesses or qualities about yourself that you don't like. That's because most of us are aware of our weaknesses and focus too much on them.

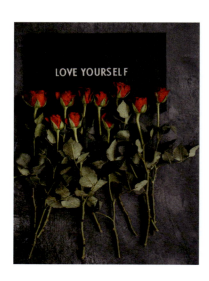

EXERCISE: Write down your strengths in the following six areas. These should be your "being" strengths—the ones that define your character, not those connected to what you do or accomplish.
- Social: strengths in social situations or relationships, such as being honest, loving, kind, and loyal.
- Physical: physical attributes you like about yourself (smile, hair, physique), the way you take care of yourself (hygiene, exercise, diet, health), and strengths in fashion.
- Career/education: work or school-related strengths, such as being creative, a team player, or a hard worker.
- Spiritual: not specific religious practices, but strengths, such as, wisdom, compassion, faith, forgiveness, and the ability to commune with nature.
- Cognitive: strengths in thinking abilities, such as being smart, analytical, or a good problem solver.
- Emotional: your emotional strengths, including your ability to feel deeply, to be passionate about life, and to be emotionally stable.

MODULE 6

EXERCISE: Now that you have identified and written a list of your strengths, write your challenges with recovery. Determine how your strengths will help you meet and overcome these challenges. For example, you may have the strength of persistence; focus on the fact that even though you don't see immediate results in the recovery process, you can keep going and persist.

Another aspect of "getting to know you" is knowing what your values are so that you can use them in everyday life.

EXERCISE: Write down your values and beliefs about life and relate them to your recovery process. For example, you may value hard work or time with family and friends. Define what this means to you and determine how these values will help you recover and become who you would like to be. You were asked to do this in Module 1. Do you see your values differently?

In the early 2000s, Ed Deiner and Martin Seligman, the fathers of positive psychology, conducted groundbreaking research regarding personality and found that everyone possesses twenty-four character strengths to different degrees. Gender, socio-economic class, culture, or other attributes do not matter. We all have a truly unique character profile of twenty-four strengths. Your top five strengths are those most routinely used and are called the "core signature strengths".

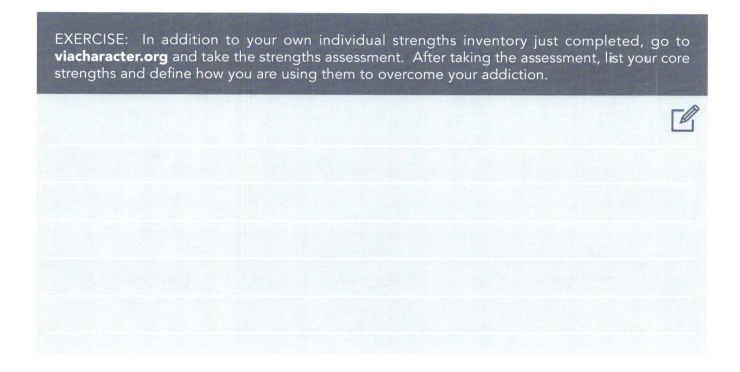

EXERCISE: In addition to your own individual strengths inventory just completed, go to **viacharacter.org** and take the strengths assessment. After taking the assessment, list your core strengths and define how you are using them to overcome your addiction.

STEP TWO: UNCONDITIONALLY ACCEPT YOURSELF

The second step in loving is to unconditionally accept yourself. As mentioned in Module 5, this is a very important part of self-esteem, loving others, and loving yourself. If you really want to love someone, you unconditionally accept who that person is—strengths, weaknesses, needs, and all. You might not like some of the things the person does but without acceptance, there is no love. If you love only that person's potential, you love only what the person might become, not the person.

The same thing applies to self-love. You need to unconditionally accept yourself. You may not like everything you do, but you need to be willing to look at yourself **honestly**, take responsibility for and accept who you are and where you are in life. If you don't accept who you are, how can you change? Denial keeps you stuck.

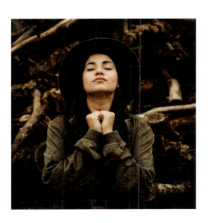

MODULE 6

EXERCISE: What are some things about yourself that you just can't accept? What will it take for you to act with intent and accept and then change these things? Write your reflections.

> "If you really put a small value upon yourself, rest assured that the world will not raise your price."
> —Unknown

STEP THREE: HONOR YOURSELF BY MEETING YOUR NEEDS

You don't love a person for what that person does for you; you love that person because you sacrifice for and serve him or her. You get to know what the person needs and you help meet those needs. A parent's love for their children provides a good example of this principle.

To truly love yourself, you must discover what you need in life and in your relationships and then you must work to meet your own needs by doing for yourself. Focusing on yourself doesn't mean you are narcissistic or selfish. Honoring yourself means you take responsibility for yourself and for meeting your own needs and you don't expect others to take responsibility for you. You respect yourself enough to not let others control who you are.

MASLOW'S HIERARCHY OF NEEDS

Instead of studying what goes wrong with people, psychologist Abraham Maslow focused his research on a more positive perspective of human behavior. He was interested in human potential and how we fulfill that potential by focusing on needs and motivations. He proposed that human motivation is based on people seeking fulfillment and change through personal growth. This process is ongoing and non-linear, meaning people revisit their needs many times throughout their lives.

According to Maslow, needs are organized in a hierarchy. In other words, more basic needs must be addressed before one can focus on higher needs. He also said that most behavior is simultaneously determined by more than one need. Here's how it works: the first-level needs are basic and sustain life; they include things like food, clothing, sleep, and shelter. If you are hungry, it is difficult to work on fulfilling your potential or finding meaning in life. Those with addiction often struggle at this level since basic needs are often overridden by the need for the substance or behavior. As another example, the next level deals with safety and security needs. Those with addiction often get stuck at this level as well. Paranoia about life in general and a dysfunctional perspective keep people with addictions trapped because they seldom feel safe or secure. The hierachy of needs is outlined below:

1. **Biological and physiological needs:** air, food, drink, shelter, warmth, sex, sleep, and so on.
2. **Safety needs:** security, stability, order, law, protection from elements, and so on.
3. **Love and belonging needs:** friendship, intimacy, trust, acceptance, and receiving and giving affection and love. This includes affiliating and being part of a group of family members, friends, or co-workers.
4. **Esteem needs:** Maslow classified these into two categories: first, esteem for yourself, including dignity, achievement, mastery, and independence; and second, the desire for reputation or respect from others, such as status and prestige.
5. **Self-actualization needs:** realizing personal potential, achieving self-fulfillment, and seeking personal growth, peak experiences, and spiritual development.

Self-Actualiization
Desire to become the most that one can be

Esteem
Respect, Self-esteem, Status, Recognition, Strength, Freedom

Love and Belonging
Friendship, Intimacy, Family, Sense of Connection

Safety Needs
Personal Security, Employment, Resources, Health, Property

Physiological Needs
Air, Water, Food, Shelter, Sleep, Clothing, Reproduction

MODULE 6

EXERCISE: List your needs. After you review your needs, set goals on how you are going to meet them, especially those dealing with your recovery. Make sure your goals are motivated from within. What do you need to work on to feel true self-fulfillment and purpose in life

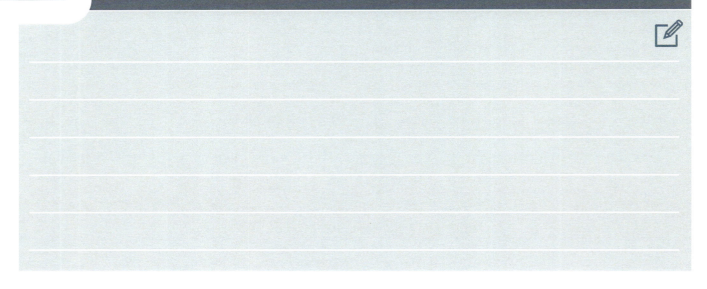

ADDICTION AND SPIRITUALITY

Maslow's last level of needs is self-actualization, which includes spirituality and religion. He believed that all of us have a need to expand beyond our own selves and experience spirituality. Some feel uncomfortable with the word spirituality because they align it with religion. But these two terms are very different: Religion is organized around a set of beliefs, customs, and rituals and includes the practice of worshiping a God or Gods. Religion often includes a component of spirituality, but you do not have to be religious to be spiritual. Spirituality is a feeling that there is something bigger than yourself; it includes the idea of being connected to other living things, humanity, or a higher power. It entails what gives your life meaning and purpose, and it requires you to get in touch with your values, your truth, and your beliefs.

> "Spirituality is about seeking a meaningful connection with something bigger than yourself, which can result in positive emotions, such as peace, awe, contentment, gratitude, and acceptance."
> —Unknown

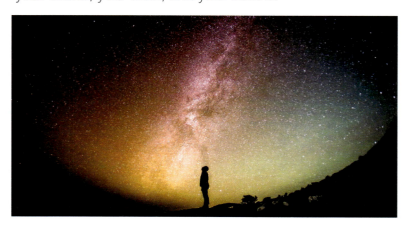

Spirituality involves receiving sustenance from nature, a higher power, or humanity and then giving back for the good of all. It is about faith, love, and hope.

Connection with something greater than yourself, whether it is communion with God or a higher power, nature, humanity, a cause, or some other purpose, activates a certain part of the brain that creates a greater sense of love. Spiritual experiences have also been shown to involve a perception of life that lessens the effect of stress and increases self-esteem.

> "Science is not only compatible with spirituality; it is a profound source of spirituality. When we recognize our place in an immensity of light-years and in the passage of ages, when we grasp the intricacy, beauty, and subtlety of life, then that soaring feeling, that sense of elation and humility combined, is surely spiritual. The notion that science and spirituality are somehow mutually exclusive does a disservice to both."
> —Carl Sagan

Addiction takes away your ability to be spiritual because it disconnects you from meaning and purpose. It also disconnects you from others because your entire focus is on the addiction and using. Your reward center is short-circuited, and everything is about the next high or experience. An important element of the human condition, the ability to choose, is also taken away by addiction. You become a prisoner of your desires and your brain becomes diseased.

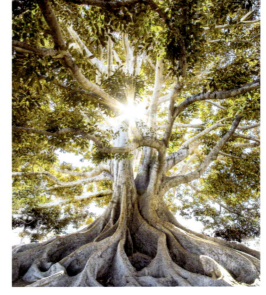

Spiritual people are connected to and love others. But how do you love others when you don't love yourself? Spirituality is about progressing, changing, and becoming a better person. Addiction takes that away. Spirituality is about hope, but addiction keeps you stuck in feelings of helplessness and despair. Spirituality is about being grateful for the little things in life, but because of damage done to neurotransmitters by addictive behaviors, nothing satisfies you but your addiction.

Healing the brain allows you to see things from a different perspective and introduces spirituality into your life. Being spiritual restores all the things addiction takes away. But spirituality doesn't just magically emerge; it's the result of hard work, difficult decision making, endurance through challenges, and prayer or meditation. It comes from giving up the carnal and being focused on the good and uplifting in life. It comes from being in tune with your value system again and moving away from self-indulgence.

> "Spiritual light rarely comes to those who merely sit in darkness waiting for someone to flip a switch." —Dieter F. Uchtdorf

MODULE 6

EXERCISE: Prayer, meditation, or mindfulness are coping skills that can help replace negative behaviors. They also help you accept things as they are, in the moment. Take time to be still and quiet. Reflect on your feelings regarding a higher being or power. List the things you may need to do to feel more spiritual in your life.

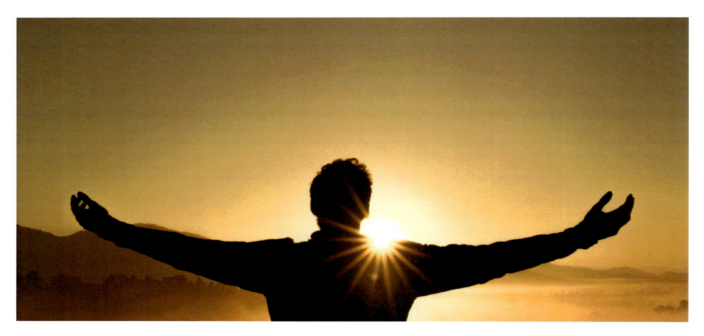

KEY TAKEAWAYS

- Self-compassion helps build regard and esteem for the self. It replaces self-criticism with kindness.
- Confidence is a learned skill that contributes to motivation and efficacy. There is a difference between confidence and arrogance.
- Self-love can be developed through awareness, acceptance, and deliberate effort to meet your needs.
- Spirituality enhances love for yourself and others and can provide motivation and support throughout recovery.

MODULE 7
BARRIERS TO CHANGE

PRINCIPLES
CONQUER WITH COURAGE
Use Resilience to Overcome Weaknesses, Setbacks, and Obstacles

FORGIVE YOURSELF AND OTHERS
Release Yourself from the Past

THOUGHT QUESTIONS
How has shame impacted your life? Have you truly forgiven yourself and others?

What thoughts or behaviors do you still hang on to that are damaging to you?

There are always barriers and obstacles in life that keep us from changing as soon or as much as we would like. Some of those are toxic relationships, mental health issues, abuse, forgiveness, shame, and guilt. It takes **courage to face these issues** and even desire to go on after trauma has occurred. But our courage and resilience to bounce back and keep going is what defines us. Shame is a big factor for those who suffer with addiction. You may feel that you have destroyed your life and the lives of others. It may be hard for you to **forgive yourself.** You may have been horribly hurt from being abused, and it can be hard to **forgive others**. But peace comes when you face your demons and **draw on the power of forgiveness and courage.**

Some years ago, a group of scientists went to the jungle to capture monkeys for research purposes. They tried several different ways to catch the monkeys, including using nets. But finding that the nets could injure such small creatures, they finally came upon an ingenious solution. They built many small boxes and in the top of each, they bored a hole just large enough for a monkey to get his hand into. In each box, they put a nut that the monkeys especially liked.

They then set these boxes out under the trees. When the men left, the monkeys came down from the trees to examine the boxes. Realizing that there were nuts to be had, they reached

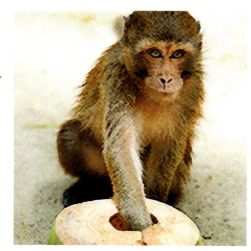

into the boxes. But when a monkey grabbed the nut and tried to pull his hand back out, he couldn't. His little fist with nut in hand was now too large.

At about this time, the men came out of the underbrush and converged on the monkeys. And here is the curious thing: When the monkeys saw the men coming, they shrieked and scrambled about in an attempt to escape, but as easy as it would have been to get away, they would not let go of the nut so that they could withdraw their hand from the box and escape. The men captured them easily.

Moral of the story: Holding on for dear life to those things that are keeping you trapped will not bring happiness.

Unfortunately, most of the traps in life are those we create for ourselves. Just like the monkeys, we hold on for dear life to things that aren't in our best interest. Addictive behaviors are a good example of these. We also hold on to past mistakes; we cling to fears; we won't let go of anger and resentment; we become attached to people that drag us down; and we feel shame. If you're going to find happiness in life, you need to examine what you hold on to. Take a close look at the attachments in your life. Are they building you up or tearing you down? Are they contributing to your happiness or fueling your misery?

TRAUMA AND ABUSE

According to data from the National Center for Post-Traumatic Stress Disorder and the Department of Veterans Affairs, as many as 75 percent of abuse and violent trauma survivors develop substance abuse issues. Addictive behaviors, including eating disorders, also influence many victims of trauma and abuse.

> "Radical acceptance rests on letting go of the illusion of control and a willingness to notice and accept things as they are right now, without judging."
> —Marsha Linehan

Traumatic events affect the brain's processing center (the hippocampus), causing intrusive memories to play and replay through daily life, perhaps as nightmares or flashbacks. Trauma also interrupts the brain's executive control command center (the prefrontal cortex), diminishing the ability to inhibit behavior and making addictive behaviors more difficult to resist.

Initially, a victim of trauma or abuse may turn to a substance or negative behavior to cope with resulting emotions or thoughts and the euphoric rush may give temporary relief. Because of the brain's reduced ability to stop the use after trauma, addiction can quickly develop. The difficult emotions remain and without better coping skills and tools, relief from the use of addictive substances/behaviors seem to be the only way to get through feelings like sadness, anger, fear, or guilt.

If your history includes trauma and/or abuse, you'll need to address that as part of your recovery process. Working through a history of trauma may include individual therapy with trauma-centered approaches, including Eye Movement Desensitization and Reprocessing (EMDR), cognitive and/or behavioral therapy, and ketamine treatments. It is important to be honest with yourself and aware of how your mind and body may be holding on to remnants of the past. These events can be overcome and you can feel whole again.

MODULE 7

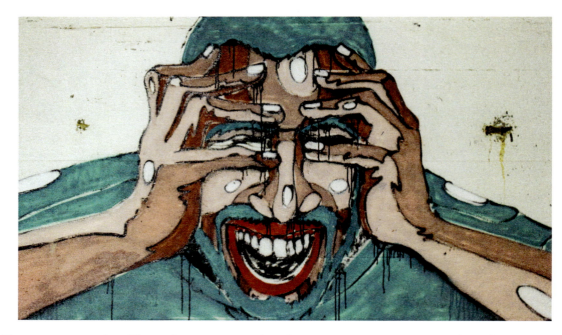

Not all traumatic effects are negative. Though some may develop post-traumatic stress disorder (PTSD), most also develop Post Traumatic Growth (PTG). PTG entails growth and change from insights about the world, relationships, meaning, values, and the self.

PTG relieves many of the detrimental effects of trauma, including the sense of helplessness that often occurs. Using various forms of coping to build something new from what was tragic, **PTG is facilitated by concepts like courage, spirituality, hope, and gratitude.**

If you have traumatic events in your past, it is likely that the principles and skills you have covered in this workbook thus far have contributed or are contributing to your development of PTG. It may be helpful to review gratitude, resilience, and other topics that stood out to you, and consider them again with your traumas in mind. Other ways to facilitate post-traumatic growth include these:
- Don't push away emotions (negative or positive), especially those related to your adversity. Processing emotions is part of working through the past. This can't happen if you repeatedly stuff down or numb away hard feelings. Allow yourself to feel even if it hurts. In the most difficult moments, it can be helpful to have a supportive person with you or on the phone.
- Share about what happened to you with trusted people. Research calls this "constructive self-disclosure." Constructive self-disclosure helps you fully process traumatic events. On the other hand, keeping things bottled up or ignored can lead to prolonged or worsening symptoms. This is where individual therapy can be especially helpful if not crucial.
- Remember your strengths and notice how they helped you through the trauma. What skills, talents, qualities and characteristics got you through the adversity? You can revisit your VIA Character Strengths and look for those specifically. Remind yourself that you are strong. You are fighting and recovering!

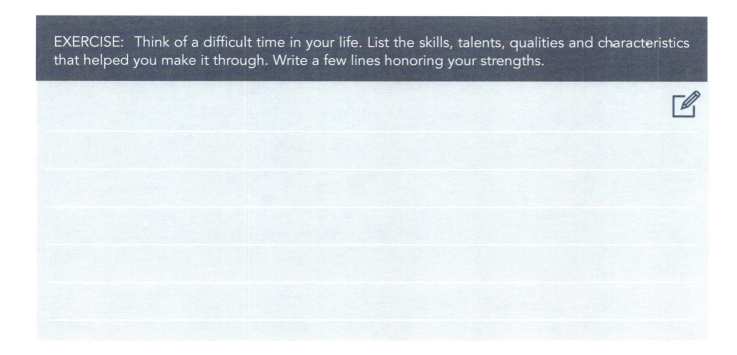

EXERCISE: Think of a difficult time in your life. List the skills, talents, qualities and characteristics that helped you make it through. Write a few lines honoring your strengths.

One way to make sense of past traumas is to write. Consider exploring specific impactful events in your Purging Pages. Write in a place that is secure and private so you can be open and honest. Writing about your past should be for you (and possibly your therapist), not for loved ones or others. Research has found that writing about a traumatic event for twenty minutes over as few as four consecutive days can provide clarity, healing, and a new perspective. It can also reduce depression and distress around the event/memory. Do this writing at your own pace when you feel ready. It's a good idea to share your plans with a licensed professional and check in if you begin to feel loss of control as you look closely at aspects of your history.

MODULE 7

EXERCISE: View your past in a new light. Choose an impactful or traumatic event from your life. First, practice a moment of mindfulness to relax your mind and body. Bring the incident to mind as you breathe deeply. Let the event play out in your mind as a film. If you notice your body reacting more than you feel you can handle, stop and do this exercise at another time or with a therapist's coaching and help. After playing out the event from beginning to end, shift your attention to where you are now. Identify:

- Three strengths you used during or in reaction to the event.
- Three insights gained or things learned from what happened to you.
- One thing you have done differently (for the better) than you may have if you had not experienced the event.
- One thing you will do differently going forward.

TOXIC RELATIONSHIPS

Someone once said, "Stop setting yourself on fire to keep someone else warm." That's an apt description of a toxic relationship. A toxic relationship is one that involves negative patterns, including jealousy, control, manipulation, and more; it can be a romantic relationship, a friendship, or a family relationship.

Toxic relationships can hurt in many ways. They can feed addiction and impede recovery. Toxic relationships pave the way for addictive thinking and other roadblocks to progression. They can magnify existing effects of trauma and abuse.

Toxicity in a relationship is more difficult to see when you are in it. It's a lot easier to see the toxic nature of a friend's relationship than your own. The following are signs that you are in a toxic relationship:
- You feel bad more often than you feel good being around the person. After interactions with this person, you are more likely to feel upset or drained rather than comforted.
- You or this individual attempt to manipulate or control the other.
- You try to hide your relationship problems from other people. When around family or friends,

you "put on a happy face" to mask the distress you are experiencing. You may feel inclined to defend this person or your relationship to others.
- You do not feel like you can trust or depend on this person.
- You feel pressured to change to fit this person's desires. You cannot be the authentic, best version of yourself around the person.
- You feel obsessed or preoccupied with making this person happy or with fixing your relationship.
- You feel more fondness for previous times in your relationship than hope for the future. You feel a longing for how things used to be, without belief that you can feel as fulfilled in your relationship again.
- You are afraid of this person and avoid triggering the person's anger or jealousy. The person lashes out violently toward you or others.

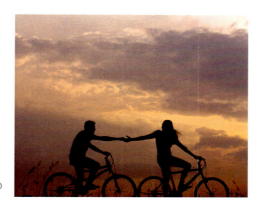

Healthy Relationships	Toxic Relationships
You create time for yourself to do what you like. You have friendships outside this relationship.	You are together all the time. You feel hurt when alone time is requested. One partner can't live without the other.
You both share your fears, dreams, concerns, and other personal thoughts openly. You are both honest about your actions.	One or both of you keep information from or lie to the other. You are not honest or forthright with one another.
You are considered equals. Both of you contribute to decisions and share responsibilities.	One of you dominates the relationship, telling the other what to do.
Conflicts are managed through communications and become a way to better understand one another.	Communication shuts down when conflict arises. The silent treatment is common.
Both of you trust one another.	You are unable to trust. You insist on checking up on each other (through phones, social media, by asking others, and so on) to ensure honesty.
Both of you are accepted as yourselves.	One of you is pressured to change to fit the other's ideals.
You celebrate each other's accomplishments.	You feel jealous or insecure when the other succeeds.
You are both physically safe. Each body is respected. Sexual activity is according to each partner's comfort.	Force is used, including hitting, shoving, or grabbing. One of you is pressured or forced into unwanted physical/sexual acts.
You enjoy the relationship. You have fun or find fulfillment through interacting with each other.	You take precautions to avoid upsetting the other. Contempt and criticism take joy away from the relationship.

MODULE 7

If you suspect you are in a toxic relationship, it is important to realize that individual healing must come before a relationship can heal. You might need to take time away from your relationship to focus on your own goals and recovery. Recovery can be difficult to maintain when the same patterns and dynamics that were present during times of heavy addiction continue after the addictive behavior has stopped. Many times, it is hard to end a toxic relationship because it has become so familiar.

In a dysfunctional relationship, the other person may work to get you back to the "way you were" because that's what works for them. For instance, many times families are co-dependent with the addicted person. The addiction may be serving a purpose. For example, the family member doesn't have to worry about their own problems because they are so enmeshed in the addicted person's issues; or they may have a compelling need to feel needed and this is satisfied by the addicted person. When healing occurs, the dynamic changes and everyone involved is affected. Some may not like the change and they may work, even unknowingly, to sabotage the recovery. It is important to look for these patterns and realize that it is not selfish to prioritize your own mental health when harmful patterns exist in your friend and family relationships. Use appropriate boundaries (discussed in Module 9) to protect your sobriety.

If you suspect your relationship is beyond toxic and is, in fact, abusive, talk to your therapist about this immediately.

> **EXERCISE:** Identify a toxic relationship you have had or currently have. What makes it toxic? How do you plan to improve or remove yourself from the relationship?

SHAME AND GUILT

Though they are often used interchangeably, shame and guilt are not the same. **Guilt** is a judgment about a behavior or action ("That action was not right"); **shame** is a judgment of the self ("I am worthless"). Guilt can work well

> "Shame corrodes the very part of us that believes we are capable of change." —Brené Brown

for you; in the right dose, guilt can act as a motivator for changing and making amends. Shame, on the other hand, rarely works in your favor resulting in feelings of inferiority, inadequacy, and self-hatred. It is linked to hopelessness and depression.

Shame propels you toward withdrawal and secrecy. Why would you show to others a version of yourself that you despise. They may have a similar judgment of you. Unfortunately, secrecy and isolation are places where shame thrives and grows.

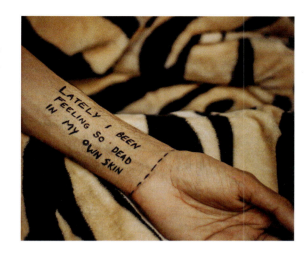

The harshness and criticism turned inward because of shame causes so much pain that those who experience it will do anything to get away from it. This leads to shame's cyclical relationship with addiction; a substance or behavior provides a temporary escape from the pain of shame but only increases shame in the long run. With each use, shame sinks in a little deeper and grows a little darker. This pushes the addicted to use again for more relief from the discomfort, and the downward spiral continues.

Shame can have a major impact on recovery: It may cause you to feel unworthy of treatment and a life without addiction. **Recognizing shame and breaking its cycle is imperative in the process of recovery and healing.**

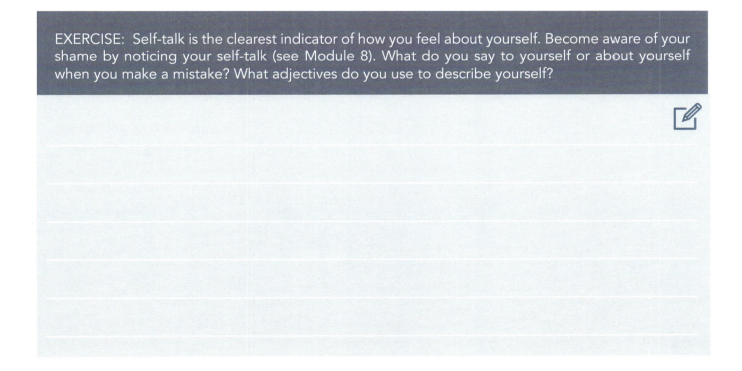

EXERCISE: Self-talk is the clearest indicator of how you feel about yourself. Become aware of your shame by noticing your self-talk (see Module 8). What do you say to yourself or about yourself when you make a mistake? What adjectives do you use to describe yourself?

As you become aware of the shame messaging within your mind, take steps to stop it in its tracks:
- Notice your shame triggers. Are there people, places, or things that prompt unkind feelings toward yourself? As you realize what triggers your shame, make appropriate changes. This may

MODULE 7

mean enforcing boundaries with toxic individuals, processing past events with your therapist, or checking the reality of what is upsetting you.

- Reframe how you view mistakes. Remind yourself that mistakes do not speak to your value or character. They are part of the process of life. Remember the growth mindset principles discussed in Module 4.
- Speak your shame. Shame loves to be kept hidden; it withers in the light. Share your feelings with someone you trust or someone who has gone through similar experiences. This is where recovery support groups can be helpful.
- Talk to yourself like you'd talk to someone you care about. Rarely would you talk to another person the way you talk to yourself. Catch your shaming self-talk and ask, "What would I say to my best friend if s/he was in a similar situation? How would I support him/her?"
- Develop self-esteem and self-love. Care for yourself with kindness. Highlight your strengths and celebrate your successes. Reread Modules 5 and 6 and revisit them often.

The greatest remedy for shame is empathy gained through connecting with others. When you feel like turning away, turn toward the helping relationships you have found. Mentors, therapists, family members, and friends can remind you of your worth and act as listening ears. Let them bolster you. And when you feel shame, be there for someone else. Expressing empathy can help you see your own experiences in a new light with greater gentleness.

EXERCISE: What are your shame triggers? Think through the times you felt the most shame. Write down the shameful thoughts you had. How can you reframe those thoughts and approach yourself in a gentler way?

FORGIVENESS

On October 2, 2006, a tragedy occurred in Lancaster County, Pennsylvania. Charles Roberts walked into an Amish schoolhouse armed with three guns and shot ten young girls, killing five of them and himself. In a suicide note to his wife, Charles claimed that he had taken the lives of innocent children to make up for the loss of his first child. The couple's first child had died in 1997, just twenty minutes after she was born three months prematurely. "In some way he felt like he was getting back at the Lord

for the loss that we had sustained," said Charles's wife in an interview with the Daily Mail.
Although Charles had committed this heinous crime, the Amish community and the loved ones of the deceased demonstrated forgiveness. They attended Charles's funeral and comforted his widow. One family lost not one but two of their daughters to this crime. Charles's mother recalls that the parents of these girls were the first ones to greet her after the funeral. She couldn't believe their love and acceptance. She asked them if they could ever forgive her son. They replied, "Is there anything in this life that we should not forgive?"

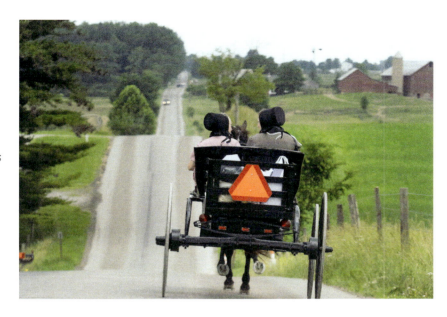

If you don't forgive, bitterness and hate can consume you. **Forgiveness is the deliberate and voluntary act of changing feelings toward an offense or offender.** Forgiveness expert, Fred Luskin, explains that it's like making peace with the word "No." It involves releasing resentment, bitterness, anger, and vengeance regardless of whether an individual or group "deserves" forgiveness. When you forgive others, you dignify yourself. You free yourself of the negative feelings another's actions have stirred up in you. You take back control and have the ability to move forward.

When you forgive, you don't deny the offense or downplay its seriousness. You don't forget what happened or condone someone's bad behavior. Forgiveness does not require reconciliation, nor does it mean you welcome a toxic person back into your life. It is possible to forgive while maintaining legal or other consequences of a perpetrator's actions.

Forgiveness can be healing for both the victim and the offender. Through forgiveness, you can break away from emotional pain including anger. It facilitates psychological healing by providing a degree of closure. It has been shown by research to bring about improved physical and mental well-being, including lower blood pressure, stronger immunity, and fewer anxious and depressive symptoms. Forgiveness allows you to move forward with peace and possibility. Forgiveness is letting go of the idea that you could have had a different past.

MODULE 7

EXERCISE: Consider who may have hurt you over the years. Who might you forgive? Did you include yourself on the list?

Fred Luskin teaches a nine-step process of forgiveness. This process takes time and effort, and it may be best facilitated with a loved one or therapist. You may find yourself revisiting steps throughout your process. Like the Stages of Change, these steps do not need to be linear. Move at your own pace and practice self-compassion as you work to let go of the grievances you have carried.

1. **Be aware of your feelings toward what happened.** Be able to describe what was not okay about the situation and tell those you trust about it.
2. **Commit to feel better.** Make this commitment to yourself for yourself.
3. **Remember that forgiveness does not mean reconciling.** It means finding peace and understanding, blaming less, taking less offense, and living a good life despite the ways you have been wronged.
4. **Stay in the moment.** Recognize that it is not the event that is causing you to be upset now; it's dealing with the feelings, thoughts and physical sensations associated with the event.
5. When emotions and feelings arise, **practice stress management** and appropriate self-soothing. Do what helps you calm down and re-center.
6. **Let go of expectations** that others may not be able to or may not choose to meet. Remember that you can hope for good things in life but cannot demand them from others. As taught in Module 3, unenforceable rules only cause you to suffer.
7. **Seek another way** to have your needs and goals met rather than through the experiences that hurt you.
8. **Live well.** This is the best revenge. Dwelling on painful feelings gives power to the person who hurt you. Instead, put energy into appreciating what you have and creating the life you want.
9. When looking at your past, **remind yourself of the strength you've shown** in overcoming. See yourself as a heroic conqueror who chose forgiveness.

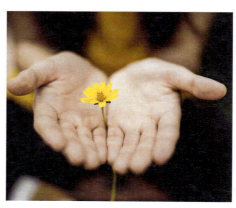

101

Copyright © 2021 by Trish Barrus and Jade Ozawa-Kirk

EXERCISE: Choose a person or situation where you would find greater peace through forgiving. Spend some time pondering on your feelings about what happened. Identify what bothered you or was not right about the situation. Write some of your thoughts and feelings. Then, write a commitment to find greater calm through forgiveness. If it is too disturbing to do this exercise alone, do it with someone you trust.

FORGIVENESS IN RECOVERY

Addiction can be triggered by trauma, abuse, or other hurtful actions that are hard to forgive—not only because of the damage done but because of the lack of control you feel when you are preyed upon. However, research shows that failing to forgive causes a constant state of anxiety or depression that inhibits the healing process and can cause relapse.

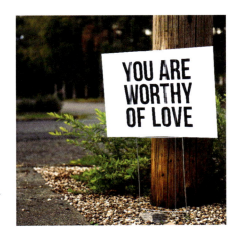

It can be difficult to forgive, especially during recovery. You may not want to deal with the negative emotions that the forgiveness process involves. As your resentment and anger build up, the events themselves may be exaggerated in your mind. But that almost doesn't matter. After a while, you're not so much impacted by what happened to you as you are by your feelings about what happened. **Remember that you cannot control the actions of others, but you can control how you feel and perceive them.**

Forgiveness is something you do for yourself so you can be in a more positive state. It promotes self-control. Failing to forgive or letting go of a grudge can result in feelings that ignite relapse. If you don't let go of emotions from the past that may trigger relapse, that person or experience still has control over you. When you forgive, you rid yourself of the hurt and resentment that so easily weighs you down and keeps you from living a full and joyful life of recovery.

MODULE 7

FORGIVENESS OF SELF

It's hard to forgive yourself when your actions have hurt others, destroyed relationships, or created hardships for you. You may feel guilt, shame, fear, or hopelessness that those relationships can never be repaired or that your situation cannot be improved. Even when you have made mistakes (and still make them), you must intentionally choose to be happy and focus on the positives instead of the negatives. Forgiving yourself is crucial if you want to move on with your life. Here are some specific tips on how to do that:

- Be aware of and admit your wrongs. You can never hide from yourself. If you don't admit your mistakes or you try to bury the feelings associated with your past actions, you stay in a negative cycle.
- Correct your wrongs. You can't go back and fix the mistakes you've made, but you can stop doing what is wrong and be proactive in doing good. You can also make restitution for any mistakes where possible.
- Forgive others. Forgiving others is a necessary step in forgiving yourself. When you harbor resentments and ill feelings toward others, it's hard to act differently with yourself. Sometimes people will not forgive you for mistakes you've made. That's okay, because you've done your part.
- Let it go. Don't keep punishing yourself for past mistakes. This doesn't help anyone. Understand what is really bothering you and then focus on letting it go. Focus on who you are and what your strengths are instead of on what you're not.
- Purge your feelings. Write about your past and the circumstances around your mistakes and then destroy these writings. This is a good purging exercise and can be very therapeutic.

EXERCISE: Write a letter of forgiveness to yourself. Use compassion and kindness about your mistakes, what you have learned and what you will do going forward.

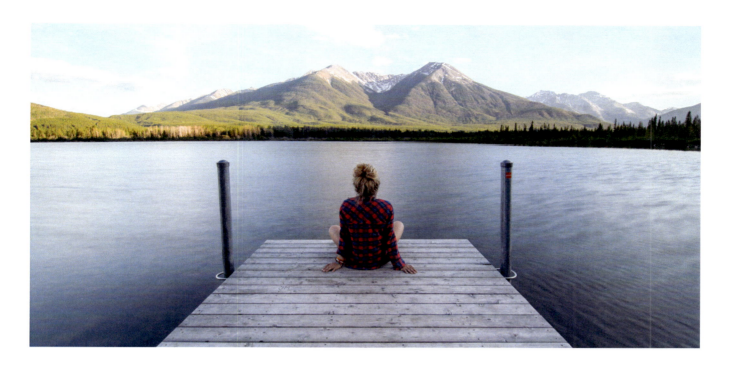

SELF-DEFEATING BEHAVIOR

Self-defeating behaviors are any maladaptive or unhelpful behaviors you engage in repeatedly that prevent your success and growth and are barriers to change. They are a form of sabotage. Any behavior that moves you away from what you want or that gets in the way of reaching your goals is self-defeating.

> "Excuses are the explanations we use for hanging on to behaviors we don't like about ourselves; they are self-defeating behaviors we don't know how to change." —Wayne Dyer

Each person has a number of self-defeating behaviors. The ones that plague you may be different from those haunting the person next to you. In the short term, self-defeating behaviors may seem to serve a purpose: They may distract from or cover up unpleasant consequences. They might temporarily relieve anxiety or depression, but in the long run, self-defeating behaviors prevent progress and contribute to a lack of self-esteem and self-efficacy. Their "helpfulness" is usually short-lived and followed by more serious consequences.

Common self-defeating behaviors include:

- Avoidance
- Aggression
- Attention seeking
- Pride
- Passiveness
- Perfectionism
- Impatience
- Procrastination
- Arrogance
- Emotional numbing
- Stubbornness
- Fear
- Extreme guilt
- Negative self-talk
- Hopelessness

MODULE 7

Your addiction may have begun as a self-defeating behavior—maybe as a way of avoidance or emotional numbing. These behaviors often start small but intensify over time. They may seem like a good idea or an acceptable way to meet a need in the moment but their ultimate outcome is not worth it, especially when compared to more adaptive behaviors.

To overcome self-defeating behaviors, like negative self-talk, begin by noticing them. Awareness is always the first step to change. One way to increase your awareness of self-sabotaging is to think about a recent goal (including past attempts at recovery). What stopped you from reaching the goal or made your path toward it more difficult? Ask yourself, **"How did I get in my own way?"**

After identifying these forms of self-sabotage, recognize your triggers. Certain circumstances, especially difficult emotions, may tend to lead you to self-defeating behaviors. Some interactions or people may set off a domino effect of negative self-talk and unhealthy forms of self-soothing. Awareness of triggers can help you stop self-defeating tendencies before they start. You can plan for them and choose alternatives. Next, think about behaviors you would like to see replace the self-defeating ones in your life.

What behaviors would really help you on your path to recovery or toward other goals?

What behaviors are typical of the person you want to be?

Consider why these behaviors are more desirable, and plan for specific ways you could use them. Visualize how you intend to use new behaviors the next time a trigger for self-defeat presents itself.

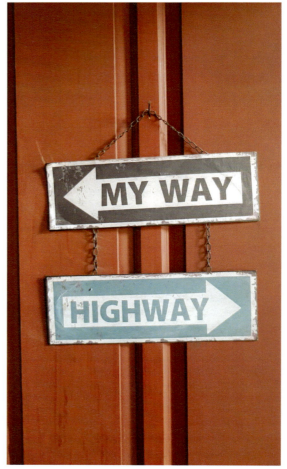

> EXERCISE: Complete the following chart. List self-defeating behaviors you tend to engage in and alternative behaviors with which you would like to replace them. Reflect on how you think this alternative may provide better results and formulate plans of action. After a few weeks of conscious effort in replacing your self-defeating behaviors, reflect on your actual outcomes. An example using procrastination as a self-defeating behavior has been provided.

Self-Defeating Behavior	Alternative Behavior	Desired Outcomes and Benefits	Plan of Action	Actual Outcome
Procrastination	Manage time and remove distractions	Less stress, real change in habits I've put off working on, sense of accomplishment	Make timeline for next deadline, download distraction blocking app	

MENTAL HEALTH DISORDERS

It is common for addiction to occur with other mental health concerns or disorders, including anxiety, depression, post-traumatic stress disorder (PTSD), bipolar disorder, and attention-deficit hyperactive disorder (ADHD). When an addiction and another disorder occur together, it is called dual diagnosis or co-morbidities. Addictive behavior is difficult to stop in any case and becomes even more challenging when paired with mental health disorders.

Dual diagnoses are important to understand because they greatly impact each other. Addiction often

MODULE 7

develops as a means of self-medicating severe anxiety, depression, schizophrenia, or other mental health issues. Sometimes the addiction occurs first, increasing the risk for a mental health disorder. Drug use often causes depression and anxiety, especially when associated with withdrawal.

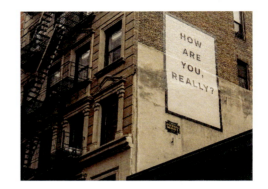

Understanding the symptoms of mental disorders can help you determine if you should speak to your therapist about the possibility of a dual diagnoses.

Disorder	Symptoms
Depressive Disorder	Low mood, feelings of hopelessness and helplessness, sleep and appetite disruption, lack of interest in activities, sense of isolation, fatigue, trouble concentrating, crying spells, irritability
Anxiety Disorder	Excessive or persistent worry, feeling on edge or keyed up, hyper-vigilance, racing thoughts, irritability, fear, heart palpitations, upset stomach
Bipolar Disorder	Mood swings that include depressed mood and mania (racing thoughts, risky behavior) and delusional thinking (including invincibility and grandeur, rapid speech, impulsivity)
PTSD	Flashbacks, nightmares, heightened reactions, agitation, irritability, isolation, anxiety, fear
ADHD	Difficulty concentrating and focusing, hyperactivity, fidgeting, impulsivity, short attention span, depression, anxiety, mood swings
OCD	Persistent thoughts and obsessions, compulsive (sometimes ritualistic) behaviors, agitation, fear

> **EXERCISE:** Do any of the symptoms in the chart above affect you at times when you are not using or engaging in addictive behaviors? Do they worsen when you are involved in addictive behaviors?

Recognizing addictive behaviors as a means of managing an underlying diagnosis can be empowering. It can help you treat yourself more compassionately as you see your addiction as a mistaken means of coping with difficult moods or memories. Gaining awareness of this way of self-medicating will empower you to choose different means of dealing with negative emotions. Well-researched interventions and treatments are available for all the diagnoses listed above. If they affect you, addressing them will aid in your recovery process.

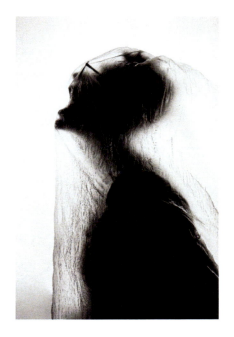

KEY TAKEAWAYS

- Experiences of trauma and abuse often contribute to addictive behaviors. These should be processed through individual psychotherapy.
- Toxic relationships get in the way of recovery and perpetuate addictive thinking patterns. It sometimes takes an outside perspective to identify them.
- Empathy is the strongest antidote for the paralyzing emotion of shame.
- Forgiveness is for the forgiver. It can free you from anger, resentment, and despair. Forgiving yourself is an important step in maintaining recovery.
- Dual diagnoses are crucial to understand for effective addiction treatment.

MODULE 8
ADDICTIVE THINKING

PRINCIPLES

TAKE ACCOUNTABILITY FOR YOUR LIFE
Examine Yourself with Honesty and Responsibility

CONQUER WITH COURAGE
Use Resilience to Overcome Weaknesses, Setbacks, and Obstacles

LIVE WITH INTEGRITY
Move Forward with Authenticity and Determination

THOUGHT QUESTIONS

Are you in denial or deceiving yourself about your addiction?

Do you make excuses or rationalize your negative behaviors?

Look at the messages that you send to yourself every day. Are they positive or negative?

What patterns of addictive thinking do you still hold onto?

THE FIGHT OF TWO WOLVES

One evening, a grandfather told his grandson about a battle that goes on inside all people.

He said, "My son, a battle goes on in all of us. The battle is between two wolves. One wolf is bad; he is anger, envy, sorrow, regret, greed, arrogance, self-pity, guilt, resentment, inferiority, lies, false pride, superiority, and ego. The other is good; he is joy, peace, love, hope, serenity, humility, kindness, benevolence, empathy, generosity, truth, compassion, and faith." The grandson thought about the words that his grandfather had spoken. After a moment he asked, "Which wolf will win?"

The grandfather simply replied, "The one you feed."

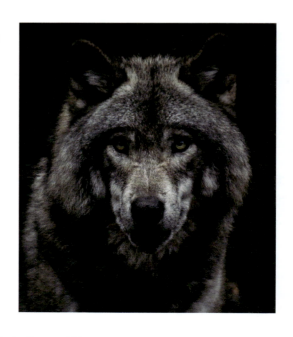

109

Addictive thinking is a faulty way of preceving life and how to get your needs met. It can be learned by observing others, imitating their behavior, and modifying according to feedback/reactions received or thinking errors can be formed by simply finding a behavior rewarding because it addresses an urgent need, and then addiction is formed.

> "The roots of addiction can be seen in our search for happiness in something outside of our self, be it drugs, relationships, material possessions."
> —Lee L. Jampolsky

Addictive thinking takes many forms but it is basically the notion of living from the outside in instead of the inside out. It is the idea that experiences, relationships, chemicals, or other external things can bring you relief or happiness. But that's not true! When you believe this, you are constantly needing something external to make you happy. You then need more and more of it because your tolerance levels have gone up. Even if the behavior is damaging to the rest of your life, you continue to engage in it.

Addictive thinking patterns begin with obsessions and compulsions. **Obsessions** are continuous thoughts about the positive effects of engaging in a behavior, such as drug use, gambling, or overeating. Obsessions may appear as an attachment to an object, person, chemical, or activity, even when it is harmful or may lead to your downfall. Even in the face of losing your job, relationships,

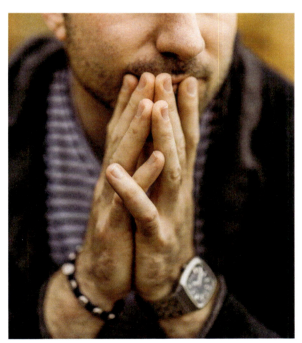

health, or other important things in your life, you can't stop thinking about the object of your obsession. **Compulsion** is an irrational urge or craving to use the drug, visit the refrigerator, or get on the internet even though the pleasure you get will not last long even if the behavior may result in a negative outcome Still, you go in search of a reward—such as pleasure or escape from pain—and the use of denial and rationalization allow you to continue to engage in the behaviors.

These patterns are unconscious and protective. They become truth to those in addiction. Because of this, they cannot be reasoned away simply or with facts.

In the long run, addictive thinking damages your capacity to cope and learn the skills you need to live a healthy lifestyle. Everyone has some form or degree of addictive thinking. For those struggling with substance or behavioral addictions failing to address these dysfunctional thinking patterns will lead to moving from one addiction to another rather than fully recovering from addiction all together.

Essential steps in undoing and overcoming addictive thinking include gaining awareness of your thinking patterns and taking responsibility for them. Use mindfulness skills as you observe yourself with curiosity (rather than judgment) and realize the messages you repeatedly tell yourself and the patterns you use to interact with the world. **Awareness is the first step to change!**

> "What many fail to realize is that being attached to what we think we want and don't have while resisting what is happening in the moment is the cause, not the cure, of much personal suffering and interpersonal conflict."
> —Lee L. Jampolsky

MODULE 8

After noticing your addictive thinking, take accountability for your part. No one else can control or choose your thoughts. Though external circumstances may have impacted the unhealthy ways you cope through addictive thinking, you are in the captain's seat when it comes to taking action and making changes.

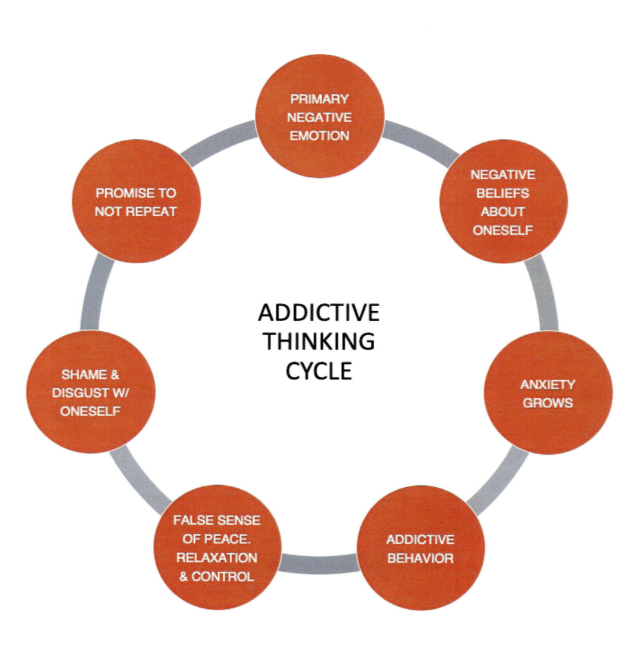

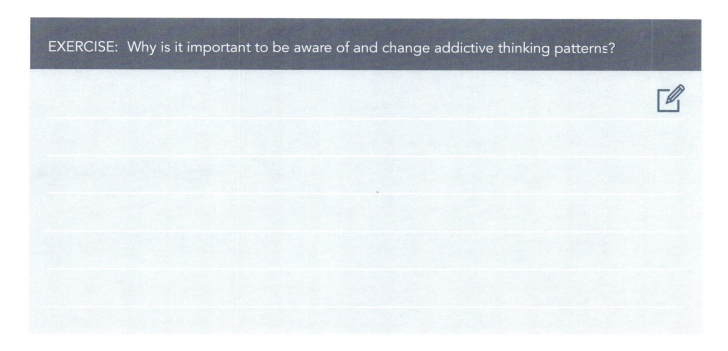

EXERCISE: Why is it important to be aware of and change addictive thinking patterns?

As mentioned, addictive thinking can take many forms. Consider each of the following patterns and how they may affect your life path. A crucial part of the recovery process is honest examination of the ways of thinking and being that got you where you are.

SELF-DECEPTION

Self-deception is the process of allowing yourself to believe invalidated or untrue thoughts, feelings, or situations as truth. For example, a man who feels like his parents are the cause of his addiction convinces himself that there is nothing he can do to change. Accepting that untrue belief as truth, he chooses to continue on his path of irresponsibility and refusing help. Meanwhile, his addiction worsens.

> "Above all, don't lie to yourself. The man who lies to himself and listens to his own lie comes to a point that he cannot distinguish the truth within him, or around him, and so loses all respect for himself and for others. And having no respect he ceases to love."
> —Fyodor Dostoevsky

Self-deception may come in the form of excusing away evidence opposed to your falsely held belief. This form of addictive thinking prevents you from being able to see your situation as it really is. It gets in the way of being able to recognize your responsibility, the consequences of your actions, and the behaviors contributing to your circumstances. The opposite of self-deception is **self-awareness** or **self-knowledge,** which acknowledges the truth of a situation and allows you to take responsibility and make better decisions.

Self-deception is the backbone of many addictive thinking patterns. It presents in many ways throughout the course of addiction or any negative behavior. For example, a student with a big deadline looming may tell himself, "I can go out with my friends for just an hour and still have plenty of time to finish the paper." In reality, he knows he will be out for three or four hours and will be too tired to work when he returns home. Another example is a girl who says to herself, "If I really had a problem with drugs, my boyfriend would be insisting that I get into treatment. Things must not be as bad as he says they are."

MODULE 8

DENIAL

Denial is refusing to admit or accept the truth or reality of a situation. For example, a woman denies that alcohol is affecting her ability to care for her kids—even though her drinking has gone from just evenings after putting her children to bed, to afternoons as they nap, to mornings while they play.

Denial is often used to protect yourself from pain, fear, and difficult realities. Facing the truth, especially if doing so requires **taking responsibility** for hurtful actions, can be incredibly difficult. It is easier to deny or ignore the truth.

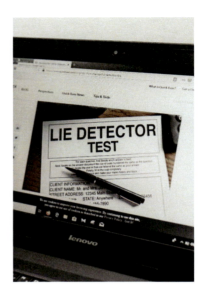

> "Denial is the worst kind of lie because it is the lie you tell yourself."
> —Michelle A. Holme

Denial starts small. It may begin with a lie you tell yourself about how much you use before feeling the effects of the drug. It grows gradually to protect your addictive behavior so you can convince yourself and others that you can continue the behavior. Eventually, you will reach a point of crisis in which reality becomes undeniable. At this point, you must choose to continue addictive use or turn toward reality and recovery.

EXERCISE: What things do you tell yourself when you are in denial? What have you told family or friends when they have tried to help you seek recovery in the past?

Something that may keep you in denial or away from self-awareness is your fear of failure. As mentioned throughout this workbook, **mistakes are not failures. Mistakes are how you grow.** Failure occurs when you quit. A good way to help yourself in a situation where you made a mistake is to say, "I made a mistake. I have this weakness. I'm not going to be in denial about it."

EXERCISE: How has fear resulted in your denying the truth? Write down some actions you will implement to stop denial.

RATIONALIZATION

Rationalization is trying to explain or justify behaviors with seemingly plausible or logical reasons that are untrue. Sometimes, the reasons may seem good, or they may be outright ridiculous. Either way, they mask or distract from the real reasons behind a behavior.

"Rationalization is a process of not perceiving reality, but of attempting to make reality fit one's emotions."
—Ayn Rand

You can think of rationalizations as excuses. The process of rationalization often starts after a decision or action has already been made. For example, you may purchase a new pair of shoes on a whim and then later come up with a list of reasons (rationalizations) why buying more sneakers was a good idea.

One way to notice rationalizations is that they come in clusters. Usually, a good or true reason for doing or not doing something is singular. For example, "I'm not going to the party because I don't feel like being around people tonight." Rationalizations, on the other hand, are often poured out as many reasons behind a decision: "I'm not going to the party because the shirt I planned to wear is dirty, I really should spend some time with my dog, and I've put off cleaning the kitchen long enough."

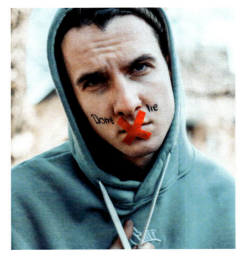

Rationalization reinforces denial by explaining away reality. It provides reasons to persist in self-deception. Because it provides reasons behind a behavior, it is used to continue an addiction or bad habit. As with self-deception, **overcoming rationalization requires awareness and willingness to see the truth as it is.**

MODULE 8

EXERCISE: Write an honesty contract with yourself; in it, commit to being honest about your thoughts and actions. Addiction is easier to overcome when brought into the light while keeping secrets allows addiction to fester.

PROJECTION

Projection involves blaming others for things that are your responsibility. A prime example of projection is the claim, "He makes me do it. If you had such a horrible husband, you would drink, too." As another example, a man who has been hiding his pornography use becomes distant and cold toward his spouse, claiming she is the one withholding affection and engaging in less conversation.

As you project fault onto someone else, you can more easily deny the need to change. Projection creates a false sense of helplessness which maintains the status quo. The need for change is placed on a different individual. You can't change others' behavior (and in the case of projection, the other does not truly need to change at all), so you are left to continue your addictive behavior as a means of coping.

> "Everything we say about other people is really about ourselves."
> —Merrit Malloy

> "Our minds influence the key activity of the brain, which then influences everything; perception, cognition, thoughts and feelings, personal relationships; they're all a projection of you."
> —Deepak Chopra

SELF-VICTIMIZATION

Self-victimization is thinking you are the victim of someone else's actions. For example, a woman botches a big presentation at work partly because of nerves and partly due to lack of preparation. Rather than determining to spend more time getting ready for her next assignment, she becomes angry at her boss, convincing herself and a coworker that he sabotaged her delivery.

> "Whenever you think something or some person is ruining your life, it's you. A victimization mentality is so debilitating." —Charlie Munger

Self-victimization is a way to justify bad behaviors, gain sympathy from others, and move attention away from negative acts. By taking the stance of a victim, you excuse yourself from your own actions and may receive enabling attention. Self-victimization is demonstrated in comments such as "It's not my fault" and "Why do these things always happen to me?" Feeling like a victim leads to entitlement, blaming, feelings of powerlessness, and refusal to take responsibility. However, at times you may find yourself in a situation in which you are being mistreated or abused. In these situations, change is easier said than done; yet, labeling yourself as a victim gives other people control.

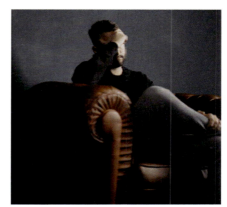

> "Never be bullied into silence. Never allow yourself to be made a victim. Accept no one's definition of your life; define yourself." —Harvey Fierstein

EXERCISE: In what ways do you see yourself as a victim? Being aware is the first step to change.

MODULE 8

> "We live in a world where unfortunately the distinction between true and false appears to become increasingly blurred by manipulation of facts, by exploitation of uncritical minds, and by the pollution of the language."
> —Arne Tiselius

MANIPULATING OTHERS

Manipulating others means using deceptive or corrupt methods to influence them to change their perceptions or behaviors for your personal gain. For example, Terry knows that if she cries, her husband will stop any difficult conversation. When he brings up topics she does not want to discuss, she quickly becomes tearful so he will postpone the exchange.

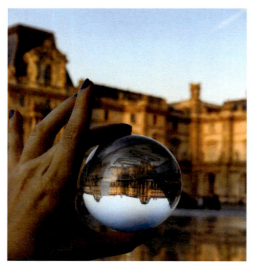

Manipulators use emotional threats at times to get what they want. For example, a substance abuser tries to convince his parents that if they don't provide money for his treatment, he may overdose; in reality, he is planning to use the money to pay for more drugs.

Manipulation is highly related to other forms of addictive thinking. Unlike addictive thinking patterns commonly seen in average people, manipulating others is likely to develop only once an addiction has set in. At first, it may be used to hide an addictive behavior or rationalize destructive actions. Eventually, manipulating others becomes second nature and may happen even when someone with addictive behaviors knows better. This can be the form of addictive thinking that is most difficult to manage.

People in addiction can also become the victims of their own manipulations. That is, they may come to a point of manipulating themselves, often through self-deception, rationalization, and denial.

COGNITIVE DISTORTIONS (TWISTED THINKING)

> "I think the greatest tragedy of mankind is that people have ideas and opinions in their heads but don't have a process for properly examining these ideas to find out what's true. That creates a world of distortions." —Ray Dalio

Cognitive distortions are misperceptions or inaccurate thoughts that affect your way of processing what you feel and experience. Also known as "twisted thinking," cognitive distortions are a way your mind reinforces negative beliefs about yourself and the world. These thought patterns convince you of things that are not true and keep you stuck in pessimism and hopelessness. Cognitive distortions are referred to as "automatic negative thoughts" because they happen so quickly, they feel involuntary.

Identifying twisted thinking patterns is the first step in overcoming them. As you become aware of and notice your cognitive missteps, consciously put effort into replacing distortions with more realistic, uplifting alternatives. Listed below are examples of twisted thinking patterns

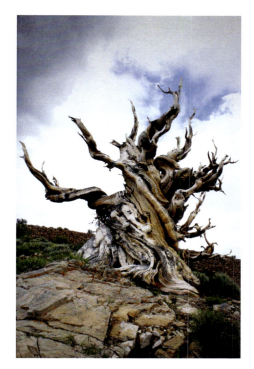

BLACK-AND-WHITE THINKING

Seeing things as all good or all bad, with no room for middle ground or gray area.
> Example: "If this performance isn't perfect then I'm a total failure."
> Example: "Jesse was unkind. He's a terrible person!"
> Example: "I had one drink. Know I'm total failure."

STRATEGIES TO CHALLENGE:

- Rather than labeling with absolutes ("total," "always," "never"), grade situations on a scale of 0–100 (with 0 being the absolute worst and 100 being the very best). In your assessment, realistically consider the bad and the good. You'll often find through the "scale score" that few things are entirely bad or the worst-case scenario.
- Define the labels you are using. In the examples above, what makes a "total failure" or a "terrible person"?
- Judge yourself the same way you would judge others and be kind

FILTERING

Ignoring positive aspects of a situation to focus on and magnify the negative.
> Example: "My sister's harsh comment ruined the entire dinner."
> Example: When tackling a big task, all you can think about is the hardest part.
> Example: "Everything about this recovery process is difficult and horrible."

STRATEGIES TO CHALLENGE:

- When you catch yourself focused on the negative, redirect toward the positive by thinking of three to five good aspects of the situation.
- When arriving at work, get the unpleasant tasks out of the way first.
- Be realistic about the negative side of things but follow up by thinking through what you learned or gained as a result.

OVER-GENERALIZATION

Using one incident or limited evidence to draw a broad, general conclusion. "Isms" such as racism, sexism, and ageism are based on over-generalization.
> Example: "My father treated me poorly, so all men are evil."
> Example: Someone has let you down once, so you never trust or turn to that person again.

MODULE 8

STRATEGIES TO CHALLENGE:
- Remember that everyone makes mistakes, and often those mistakes are accidental and not because of an intent to hurt you.
- Remind yourself of positives you have experienced with a person, group, or situation you are tempted to avoid.
- Think of the exception. When you catch yourself saying "always" or "never," consciously remember the time that "always" or "never" wasn't the case. For example, you might think, "Jenny is always so inconsiderate! . . . Except the many times she's brought me a cup of coffee without my asking for it.

HEAVEN'S REWARD FALLACY

Believing that any good act you commit must be repaid or rewarded.
    Example: "If I eat what she wants for dinner, she'd better be nice to me tonight."
    Example: "I'm not putting in any extra work until my boss expresses his appreciation."
    Example: "If I make changes for the better, everyone should forgive me immediately."

STRATEGIES TO CHALLENGE:
- Savor the feelings that come from within when you work hard or do good.
- Become aware of your intention. If you are doing something for outside praise or reward, consider changing course to do something for yourself and your own regard

PERSONALIZATION

Believing others' words or actions are a reaction to you or directed toward you. Internalizing is another word for this.
    Example: "John seems really out of sorts tonight. I must have done something wrong."
    Example: When you receive negative feedback about your performance (a meal you made, a memo you wrote), you interpret it as a comment about your value or character.

STRATEGIES TO CHALLENGE:
- Be clear with yourself about what is in your control and what is not. How others react, behave, and feel is NOT in your control.
- Adopt the following two mantras: "It isn't about me" and "I am not my performance."
- List all the alternative/external reasons something may be so; for example, why John seems out of sorts or why you got negative feedback about something you did.

EMOTIONAL REASONING

Assuming negative feelings demonstrate reality.
    Example: "I feel worthless, so I must be worthless."
    Example: "It feels like I'll never be able to stay clean. I might as well go back to using."

STRATEGIES TO CHALLENGE:
- Become familiar with your feelings and emotions and recognize them for what they are. Let yourself feel them but remind yourself that they will pass.
- Repeat these two mantras: "Feelings come, and feelings go" and "Feelings are not facts."
- Access your logical brain and strip out the emotion by giving yourself time to cool down or

gain control. This can be done by writing and purging your emotions. Ask yourself "What are the facts?"

JUMPING TO CONCLUSIONS

Becoming convinced of something without adequate (or any) evidence to support it.
    Example: "John did not call me during his lunch break. He must be angry with me."
    Example: You get a sense that your neighbor doesn't like you. Each time your dog barks, you think, "Sam must hate our puppy. He's probably sitting over there feeling angry at us."

STRATEGIES TO CHALLENGE:
- Give yourself and others the benefit of the doubt.
- Consider the opposite of your initial conclusion. Remember that both may be true, but that something in the middle is probably most realistic.
- Get more information. Practice assertive communication. Get comfortable asking what others are thinking and/or feeling.
- Consider, "If I did that, what would the reason be?"

FALLACY OF FAIRNESS

Expecting absolute fairness in all situations.
    Example: "If one of us gets a pay raise, we must all get a pay raise, or I will throw a fit."
    Example: "I felt miserable for years because he is a terrible communicator. He should now experience the same amount of pain that I have."

STRATEGIES TO CHALLENGE:
- Ask yourself how helpful is this thinking? Will it make things better?
- Put the shoe on the other foot. If you were in the more advantageous position (getting the raise or having made your partner miserable by your behavior), would you want the same outcome you are wishing on others?

SHOULDS

Holding to personal rules of how you and others should behave, including always needing to be right and expecting others to change for you without compromise.
    Example: "To be happy in life, I should have the nicest clothes and vehicles."
    Example: Beating yourself up repeatedly for mistakes you have made, constantly thinking, "I shouldn't have done that."

STRATEGIES TO CHALLENGE:
- Think about what has informed your "shoulds." What has influenced you to believe these rules?
- What factors in your upbringing, your culture, your experience have contributed?
- Ask yourself," Is this based in fact or in judgment/opinion?" Exercise self-compassion.
- Change your words. Replace "should" and "must" with "wish" or "want." If appropriate, take steps toward what you want.
- What are other ways to look at this?

MODULE 8

EXERCISE: Make a chart and write the negative thoughts you have throughout the day. Choose which cognitive distortion is associated with your negative thought and spend a few minutes thinking through a different perspective

Thought	Cognitive Distortion	Different Persepective

NEGATIVE SELF-TALK

Self-talk is the way you yourself in your mind. Your brain provides a near-constant monologue or narration of the day's happenings without you even realizing it. This chatter is called self-talk. It's made up of your conscious thoughts and underlying, unconscious beliefs and assumptions. A lot of self-talk is neutral or even positive, but much of it can be negative and self-defeating. It often contains the cognitive distortions listed above. Sometimes self-talk is completely false.

Think about what emotion you feel right now. Are you happy? Sad? Discouraged? Engaged? Curious? Why do you feel this way? You probably think of your feelings as being caused by circumstances, including environment, people or events. But research shows that feelings are actually the result of self-talk. You can use this knowledge to work backwards in challenging negative self-talk. Try to notice the next time you feel a negative emotion—sadness, anger, shame.

Once you catch it, pay attention to the thoughts going through your mind. They are likely the source or the culprit of your negative mood.

The mind is flexible and can be changed which applies to self-talk. When you challenge self-talk, negative thinking can be overcome and replaced with more helpful, reasonable and kind thoughts. This skill can be learned and practiced until you start to easily notice negative self-talk and choose a more realistic or encouraging mindset.

After you've identified negative thoughts going through your mind, push against them in one of these five ways:
- Do Reality Testing- Ask yourself if there is evidence for or against your thinking. Are your thoughts based on fact or perception? Is there a way to test for truth?
- Consider Alternatives- Could this situation be viewed differently? If your mood was different, would you interpret the situation in a more positive way?
- Put Things into Perspective- Consider whether your stance could be extreme. Can you find anything good within a situation that seems all bad? How much does this situation matter in the long run?
- Turn Toward Goals- How do your thoughts relate to your goals? Are they helping you progress? Is there anything to be learned from them or the situation?
- Think of a Friend- Would a friend or loved one speak to you the way your mind is? If not, what would they say right now?

> **HOW TO CHALLENGE SELF-TALK**
>
> Use the following list of guiding questions to help you challenge your negative self-talk. You may want to post these questions somewhere so you will see them often and remember to use them.
>
> - How accurate is this thought?
> - What evidence do I have?
> - Is thinking this way helpful?
> - What would someone else say about the situation?
> - Am I making assumptions?
> - Am I holding myself to an unfair or double standard?
> - What are the exceptions?
> - What are other ways to look at this?

After you challenge your self-talk, replace it with something more positive. One researcher suggests using the 5 to 1 ratio (Five positives to every negative) with your partner. Try that with yourself. When you say or think something negative about yourself, think or say five positive things. It may be helpful to have a list of a few positive affirmations on hand to repeat to yourself and drive negative thoughts away. These could be tailored to recurrent negative self-talk. For example, if you often catch yourself thinking, "I can't do anything right" after you make a mistake, replace that thought with," I am capable and worthy. I get back up after mistakes and setbacks." Thoughts of gratitude, reflecting on past successes and strengths, and journaling can also help in this process.

> "Don't be a VICTIM of negative self-talk—remember YOU are listening."
> —Bob Proctor

Other strategies to combat negative self-talk:
1. **Write your purging pages every day.** Get the negative talk out onto paper so it does not follow you around. Make sure that you throw it away. You'll find there is something therapeutic about this ritual.
2. **Soften the wording.** Fully replacing negative thoughts with positive may feel impossible. "I

MODULE 8

hate this" may never realistically be "I love this." But replacing extreme wording with a more neutral phrase can help. When you find yourself thinking, "I hate this," replace it with "I don't like this." Replace "This is impossible" with "This is difficult."

3. **Time yourself.** Give yourself a specific amount of time to engage with the negativity. Set a timer. When the time is up, tell yourself it is time to move toward brighter and better things.

4. **Say it out aloud.** Sometimes voicing what is happening in your head can help you realize how unrealistic or extreme it is. And saying phrases out loud to counteract the negative thought has been shown to be very effective.

5. **Set aside ample time to feel positive emotions.** Engage in gratitude exercises, savoring, laughing, enjoying beauty, helping others, using your hands and/or mind, and other positive things. Create specific spaces where you know negativity will not dwell.

6. **Once you think a negative thought, spend at least five minutes thinking good things about yourself.** Change those negative neural pathways.

7. **Visualize yourself** in a good way using the five senses.

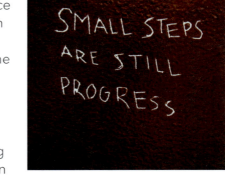

EXERCISE: What areas of your life are you most negative about? List three to five areas. For each area, think of three positive things to counter your negative thoughts.

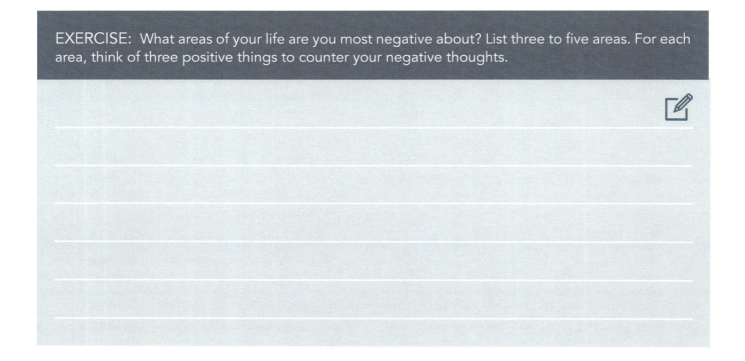

EXERCISE: Which ways of twisted thinking are you most likely to fall into? Choose two to three strategies to stop your addictive thinking this week.

KEY TAKEAWAYS

- Awareness of addictive thinking patterns is the first step to changing them.
- There are numerous forms of addictive thinking you may experience at any time.
- After awareness, addictive thinking can be unlearned or replaced through effort.
- Cognitive distortions are types of addictive thinking with many sub-types. These are inaccurate thought patterns that get in the way of how you process the world around you.
- Self-talk greatly impacts your mood. There are many strategies to combat negative self-talk.

MODULE 9
RELATIONSHIPS & COMMUNICATION

PRINCIPLE
SERVE OTHERS
Enrich Lives with Your Good Works

THOUGHT QUESTIONS

Do you have strong relationships that are supportive and uplifting?

How has loneliness played a part in your addiction?

Are you able to be assertive and set healthy boundaries?

Are you a pleaser? Do you have the skills to deal with difficult people?

Is it hard for you to give of yourself?

Some have proposed that the opposite of addiction is connection. The World Health Organization recently released results from a study where they found that more people die from loneliness than from smoking or drinking. When we're lonely, we do things we would never do otherwise: form harmful relationships, self-medicate with chemicals to get rid of that knot in our stomach, isolate, and become "me" centered instead of outwardly focused. Research is replete with examples of **how altruistic acts or serving others** creates not only a **love for others** but a **love for yourself**. And when you love yourself, you don't do harm or feel driven to engage in addictive behaviors. Your life becomes rich and full. And love always comes back to you.

A man was driving his car when he saw an older lady stranded on the side of the road. He saw that she needed help, so he stopped his Pontiac near her Mercedes and got out.

He smiled while approaching her, as he could tell she was worried. He was aware of his shabby and somewhat dirty appearance. He had just gotten off work. Trying to reassure her, he said, "Don't worry, I'm here to help you. My name is Bryan Anderson."

The woman's tire was flat so he had to crawl under the car, which only made his dirty appearance worse.

When the job was done, she asked how much she owed him for his help. Bryan smiled. He said, "If you really want to pay me back, the next time you see someone who needs help, give that person the needed assistance. And think of me."

On her way home, the lady stopped by a small cafe. Her waitress, nearly eight months pregnant, looked tired and somewhat bedraggled, but she was extremely helpful and friendly.

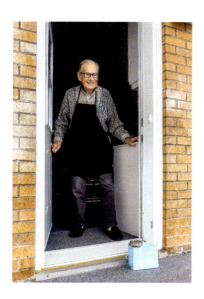

The lady wondered how someone in her condition could be so kind and giving to a stranger, especially at the end of the day. Then she remembered Bryan. She finished her meal and paid with a hundred-dollar bill. The waitress went to get change, and when she came back, the lady was gone. She had left a note on the napkin: "You don't owe me anything. Somebody once helped me, just like I'm helping you. If you really want to pay me back, do not let this chain of love end with you." The waitress found four more one-hundred-dollar bills under the napkin.

That night, the waitress went home early. She was thinking about the lady and the money she had left. She was wondering how the lady could know how much she and her husband needed help, especially now, when the baby would soon arrive. She knew that her husband worried about that, so she was glad to tell him the good news. Then she kissed him and whispered, "Now everything will be all right. I love you, Bryan Anderson."

Pay it forward. Love and service **always** come back around.

RELATIONSHIPS

Relationships are unavoidable. They start from birth and affect you throughout your life. Your relationships shape much of who you are and how you see the world. Connection impacts your sense of meaning and your self-regard, providing a means to cope and receive support through difficulties. Research has also found that connection has a tremendous impact on mental health, including the tendency toward addiction.

> EXERCISE: Consider who you are connected to. One way to do this is to think through various groups you are part of (whether by choice or default), including your family, your neighborhood, your work, community, and others. How have these various connections uplifted you in the past? How can you turn to them in the future?

MODULE 9

The first step in being able to form strong, healthy relationships is knowing yourself. You are half of the equation in any relationship and the only part over which you have any control. Do what you can to be a good half! Part of this comes through gaining awareness of how your experiences have shaped the ways you interact with the world. Also consider other areas of self-awareness discussed previously, including life vision, values, and self-defeating tendencies. Up to this point we've focused primarily on inner resources and tools. Relationships can provide external resources to aid in the recovery process as well as stave off monotony and depression.

You were earlier asked to recognize your inborn and developed strengths. Now you are asked to consider the strengths of others and your relationships.

EXERCISE: Write a list of your closest relationships, including family, friends, and community members. Spend some time pondering each name you write. Identify three to five top strengths of each person. Think about ways you may take notice of and express appreciation for these qualities. Perhaps you can make a phone call or write a brief note.

EXERCISE: Look at the many strengths you wrote in the exercise above. How can you invite these people and their strengths into your recovery process? How may some of their specific strengths become a help to you going forward?

ATTACHMENT

Our first formative relationships are with our caregivers from birth; the relationship dynamics within these early bonds are known as attachment. Attachment is formed based on how a caregiver or parental figure responds to the needs of an infant, and attachment style influences how we interact with people and respond to situations from early childhood through adulthood.

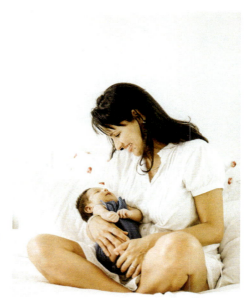

Below are the four attachment styles, their characteristics, and early caregivers' roles with each:

- **Secure attachment.** Parents of securely attached children respond quickly and appropriately to their children's needs and cues for attention, such as crying. Securely attached children are comfortable seeking comfort from their caregivers when upset or frightened. They prefer their parents over strangers, yet they can separate from parents to explore and learn. As adults, these children are able to form trusting relationships. They are comfortable sharing feelings with loved ones and easily seek social support when in need. They tend to have strong self-esteem. Approximately 56 percent of adult respondents self-identified with this attachment style.

- **Ambivalent attachment.** Ambivalently attached children have caregivers who are inconsistent with their attention, sometime smothering the child with attention and other times ignoring the child's emotional needs. Their engagement is dictated more by the parent's needs than the child's. Ambivalently attached children are suspicious of strangers. They become upset when their parents leave them but are not easily comforted by their parents' return. These children grow up to be clingy and dependent. As adults, they tend to feel insecure about their relationships and worry that affection is not being reciprocated. They may use their children as a sense of security. Nineteen percent of respondents identified as ambivalently attached.

- **Avoidant attachment.** Caregivers of avoidant children show little response when the child is distressed. They discourage displays of emotion and may interact with their child in low-quality play. Avoidantly attached children do not openly care for their parents; they show indifference in their caregivers' presence. They do not turn to caregivers for comfort. In adulthood, these individuals struggle to form close relationships. They are not open with thoughts or feelings and have difficulty showing empathy toward others' emotions. Around 25 percent of respondents identified with avoidant attachment.

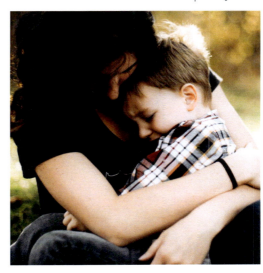

- **Disorganized attachment.** Children with disorganized attachment demonstrate a mixture of avoidant and ambivalent behaviors. Parents of these children are inconsistent and often put their children in the role of parent. Many individuals with disorganized attachment grew

MODULE 9

up with abuse and/or neglect. They may find themselves in a tug-of-war between a need for connection and belonging and a need to protect themselves at all costs. As adults, they may yearn for loving relationships but act erratically in a way that sabotages those connections.

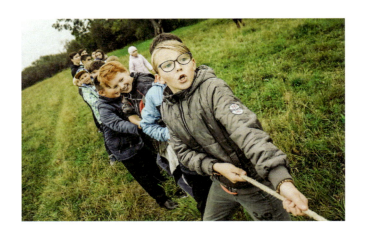

> EXERCISE: Based on these descriptions, which attachment style are you? How does your attachment style affect your life today and particularly your addictive behavior?

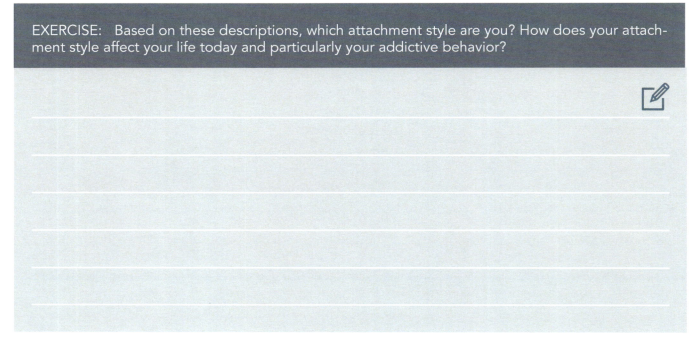

More current research has found that attachment is not as permanent as once thought. Attachment styles can change based on adult interactions and support from others. An avoidantly attached child can become securely attached through healthy relationships in adulthood. But early patterns of bonding do influence how you perceive and interact in situations throughout your life. Recognizing your attachment style can give you insights into some of your (possibly unconscious) beliefs and automatic reactions, especially in the context of experiencing and coping with emotions.

CONNECTION, LONELINESS, AND ADDICTION

Merlin and his wife, Leah, were inseparable. He was retired and they both enjoyed spending time together. Merlin always thought he would go first because of his work in the mines–his lungs were diseased. But Leah got sick and died quickly. He mourned for her.

He spent his days tinkering around the house and trying to keep himself busy. But nothing seemed to work. The pit in his stomach only increased with each passing day. His favorite pastime was looking out the window and dreaming of another life. He was really lonely. Merlin lived on a busy street and every time a car would go past, he'd wave. It helped his loneliness. It was hard for Merlin because he was so social and he missed Leah terribly. He had no one to talk to and so he just looked out the window and waved. He smiled and waved. People called him the "man in the window" and pretty soon people started waving back. Then they started stopping in for a visit. After school, kids would stop in and talk to Merlin. He loved it and they loved

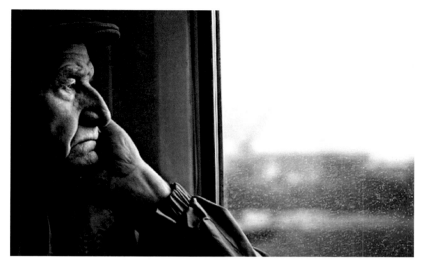

him. He was a kind, grandfatherly type. Teenagers found a friend in Merlin–they could talk about their problems and he would listen. He never nagged or lectured. What a relief this was for kids who just needed to talk to someone.

Soon, Merlin had so many visitors that he bought a guest book. At the end of two months that guest book was completely full. So, he got another one. He loved to look at the names in the book and try to put the names with faces. He loved the stories people would tell him and he loved to be loved. At Christmastime, his small house came alive with gifts and goodies. He missed Leah but he wasn't lonely anymore. He had hundreds of new friends. This went on for a few years–this give and take of caring humanity.

One day, passersby didn't see Merlin in the window. They worried wondering where he had gone. There was no smiling face to wave and greet them. He always wanted to die quickly and he did. His circle of influence was amazingly large, and people mourned his passing. They missed his face in the window, his listening ear, and most of all, his love. Posters with messages of love littered his yard for weeks and Paul Harvey talked about "the man in the window" on his radio show. Merlin had learned the secret to loneliness. It was just simply smiling, waving from the window, and loving. He wasn't the only one who was lonely.

Have you ever wondered why some people can use a drug without forming an addiction while others dabble a handful of times and quickly become hooked? As shown throughout this workbook, the answer to this question is complex. Brain chemistry, genetic predisposition, risk factors like trauma history, and more all come into play. Research gives another perspective: connection—or lack of it in the form of loneliness—is an important factor.

As social creatures, we have spent millennia building communities in the form of families, tribes, neighborhoods, and cities. We are wired to need each other, to socialize, and interact. But as technology advances, our lives are becoming more isolated, and connection gets lost in the busy-ness of day-to-day life and the static of digital communication. In fact, our time has been called **"the age of loneliness", which has produced, as some call them, the "diseases of despair," including addiction and suicide.** When we are unable to connect socially, we connect with other things, such as behaviors and substances. One way to look at an addiction is **a bond with something that is hurting you.**

MODULE 9

The role of connection in addiction makes sense when considering the impact of loneliness on mental and physical well-being. Lonely people, those lacking connection in their lives, report greater instances of depression and suicide, diminished brain functioning, and increased cardiovascular disease and stroke.

In addition, loneliness creates a longing in the brain that changes the reward system. The connections that once increased feel-good chemicals in the brain are no longer available, which causes depression and possibly a need for self-medication to relieve the negative mood states. These behaviors are perpetuated and intensified as addiction leads to greater secrecy and pulling away from existing supports. This can create a downward spiral as addiction deepens, isolation and loneliness grow. As loneliness deepens, addictive behaviors may be used for more comfort and numbing.

EXERCISE: For each item, write how often you agree with the statement: Never, Rarely, Sometimes, or Always.
1. I don't have anyone to turn to.
2. No one really knows me well.
3. I feel left out by others.
4. There are people around me but not with me.
5. I am isolated.
6. I don't have anyone close to me.
7. My relationships aren't meaningful.
8. Those around me don't share my interests.
9. I do things alone.
10. I feel unable to reach out to others.

Score your responses as follows: Never – 1, Rarely – 2, Sometimes – 3, Always
Now add up your total. Your score will fall between 10 and 40. Higher scores indicate greater loneliness.

Based on this scale,
- How lonely are you?
- Were there any statements that stood out to you?
- What do you think your score would have been at the peak of your addiction?

Whether you are addicted to something or just feeling stressed, lonely or down, connecting is a key to the way out. Connecting also means belonging. Remember from Module 5 that one of our major needs is to belong. If this need is not satisfied, your progression toward positive self-esteem and authenticity is halted and can result in negative behaviors.

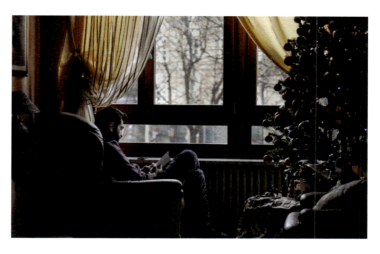

EXERCISE: Throughout your addiction, what are the parts of life that you have felt disconnected from?

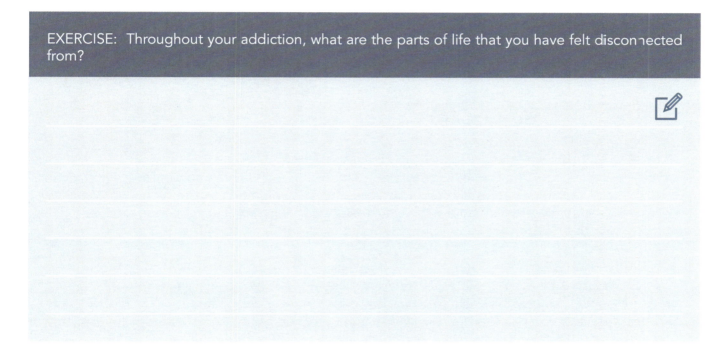

Reconnecting to yourself and others can be experienced in many ways through turning both outward and inward. The important thing is to **take whatever steps you can muster toward building greater connection with yourself and other people.** Try to catch yourself when you revert to "connecting" with a behavior or substance and replace it with one of the suggestions below.

RECONNECTING INWARD

- Define or revisit your values. Adjust your life to be more in line with what is most important to you.
- Come to know your strengths. Seek opportunities to use them daily.
- Feel your emotions and work through them.
- Practice self-compassion and develop self-love.
- Take steps to heal past wounds.
- Forgive yourself.
- Take care of your body.
- Engage in mindfulness.

MODULE 9

RECONNECTING OUTWARD

- Spend time with people you care about.
- Volunteer in your community.
- Explore your relationship with a higher power.
- Mentor others, such as students, others in recovery, or new employees.
- Meet new friends by doing something in which you are interested. Consider joining a group with similar hobbies.
- Introduce yourself to neighbors or others you see on a regular basis.

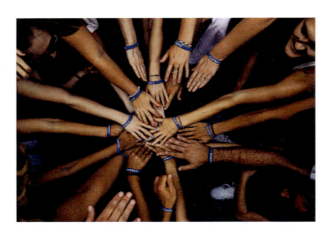

BOUNDARIES

Boundaries are the literal and figurative space between you and another person that define where you end and the other person begins. They can fall anywhere on a spectrum from loose to rigid. They are the emotional, mental, and physical limits that protect your well-being.

> "Setting boundaries is a way of caring for myself. It doesn't make me mean, selfish, or uncaring just because I don't do things your way. I care about me too." —Christine Morgan

During times of addiction, you may have struggled to maintain boundaries with others or with certain roles, such as a work position or family responsibilities. Perhaps you didn't say no to work or family demands were unrealistic or you didn't want to hurt feelings so you didn't stand up for yourself. **Maintaining healthy boundaries is an important part of caring for yourself and is crucial to recovery.**

One way to think about boundaries is to consider property demarcations. Imagine a neighborhood of homes surrounded by grassy lawns. Some property lines may be designated by a decorative wash of river rocks, easily stepped over from one yard to another. Others may be separated by fences or walls, whether waist-high wooden slats or ten-foot-tall stacked, solid, cinder block. Some properties may not be separated by lines or walls at all; homeowners just know or assume where their land ends and their neighbor's land begins. Boundaries you hold between you and others are like these property lines. Certain people, maybe a manipulative friend, require you to enforce strict boundaries like high walls to protect yourself. Other relationships may warrant more flexible boundaries. In reviewing your relationships past and present, you may think of times you had no boundaries at all. This is usually a hallmark of a lack of identity, a toxic relationship, or complete enmeshment in others' lives and tends to be a real problem for those with addictions.

Set boundaries to help with recovery in the following ways:

Identify boundaries. Start by identifying types of boundaries that will help facilitate your recovery. This requires self-awareness and a willingness to think about your feelings. When do you feel most pushed to act out? When do you feel shame or general emotional discomfort? These are likely places where setting a boundary would be appropriate.

You may want to think through the following types of boundaries:
- Physical boundaries, including your home, your belongings, your body
- Emotional and mental boundaries
- Sexual boundaries
- Relationship boundaries, including romantic partners, friends, acquaintances, strangers
- Spiritual boundaries
- Legal boundaries
- Work boundaries
- Financial boundaries

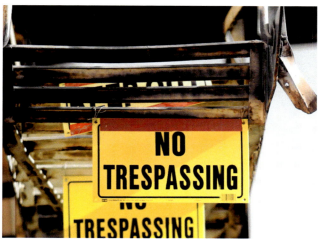

What are your needs in each of those areas? For example, a need for work-life balance can inform your work boundaries; a need for support rather than criticism may impact emotional and mental boundaries. Maintaining recovery may necessitate setting boundaries with family members and old friends.

EXERCISE: Complete the following sentences with at least eight items each.
People may not _____.
(Examples: invade my space, go through my things, berate, or yell at me)
I have the right to ask for _____.
(Examples: time to make difficult decisions, support, time to take care of myself)
To protect my time, energy and emotions, it is okay to _____.
(Examples: silence my phone, end a negative conversation, say no, change my mind)

Decide how you will set your boundaries. It is helpful to have some brief firm statements in mind when setting boundaries. You do not need to justify, be defensive about, or over-explain your boundaries. You may simply state your boundary or, if you anticipate it being violated, also name the consequence of it being disrespected. Be prepared to repeat your statement(s) more than once if you receive resistance. For example:

MODULE 9

- "You may not yell at me. If you continue, I will end the phone call."
- "I will not be doing any work over the weekend. If you email me, I will get back to you on Monday."
- "Do not touch me in that way."
- "I need to think about that before I make a decision."

Share and enforce your boundary. When appropriate, either with a planned conversation or as circumstances arise, state your boundaries in an assertive way. Remember that it's okay to practice being assertive, as discussed in Module 5. Take a few deep breaths to center yourself and prepare for the response you anticipate and for feelings that may arise within you. If you tend to feel guilty when you enforce boundaries, let the statements about your rights become affirmations that you practice each day to remind you that boundaries are okay. This is particularly true for those with addictions as you may not feel worthy to stand up for yourself.

Take care of yourself and bolster your internal boundaries. Engage in self-care and remind yourself that you are worthy of protecting through appropriate boundaries. When criticism is thrown at you, treat it similarly to cognitive distortions and self-talk (see Module 8). That is, ask yourself how much of the criticism is true and helpful and how much is about the criticizer. Use mindfulness and your other favorite coping skills to manage the discomfort of standing up for yourself.

> EXERCISE: Think of a person with whom you need to establish boundaries (maybe a codependent loved one or someone you used to use with) and walk through the steps just mentioned. Record the following:
>
> Person:
> Type(s) of boundaries:
> Associated needs:
> Statements to enforce:
> When will you share:
> How will you take care of yourself:

Here is an example:

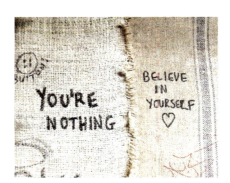

Person: Friend from work who I used to drink with after big meetings and when traveling.
Types of boundaries: Emotional and mental.
Associated needs: Avoid relapse, keep myself positive and grounded as I move forward in recovery, have the strength to face triggers.
Statements to enforce: "I'm not interested in visiting our usual bar but would be up for the coffee shop down the road." "I'm not drinking anymore. Please don't pressure me into 'just one beer.'" "I'll be heading straight to the hotel after the conference."
When you can share: Next time a meeting or any work travel comes up.
How will you take care of yourself: Remind myself of the strides I have made in recovery, focus on goals for the future, monitor my self-talk and keep it compassionate, connect with friends, family and coworkers that build me up, practice mindfulness and distraction to get through urges, find good replacement behavior for work trips such as exercising in the hotel gym.

CODEPENDENCY

One consequence of lacking boundaries can be codependency. Codependency can be thought of as a lopsided relationship in which one person relies on the other to meet all (or nearly all) of their needs. Codependent relationships can also be toxic and are common in addiction. Loved ones become caught up in the problems of the person with the substance or behavior abuse problem and believe they can fix the person. These types of dysfunctional relationships can result in unintended enabling, resentment, and deteriorating mental health. Sometimes codependent relationships result in addictive behaviors as one partner finds ways to escape from the toxicity of the relationship through addiction.

To assess whether any of your close relationships are codependent, ask yourself the following questions:
- Do I receive satisfaction and sense of purpose from means outside of my relationship?
- Do I ignore or write-off unhealthy behaviors?
- Do I have difficulty saying no to or maintaining boundaries with this person?
- Do I repeatedly sacrifice my own physical, emotional, or mental needs for this person?

To break the cycle of codependency in your relationship, start with simple but consistent boundaries. This may first require you to be in touch with your own needs and values. Do this by noticing ways you feel depleted or irritated by the relationship dynamics. What part of you is being pushed against or disregarded? As you begin to set better boundaries, expand your social support by reaching out to others from whom you may have isolated yourself. Turn to family, friends, and colleagues for support and connection then look inward for ways to connect with yourself. Seek opportunities to develop yourself through hobbies and interests and invest in quality self-care.

MODULE 9

COMMUNICATION

Communication is the foundation of relationships. Simply put, **communication is connection.** Whether it is verbal or nonverbal, it is what links us to those around us. As you have become disconnected through the course of your addiction, your communication skills may have deteriorated. Addictive thinking patterns and shame can promote a tendency to avoid honest or assertive communication or may result in being defensive or aggressive during interactions with others (especially loved ones). Cloudy or confused perceptions of reality may result in disjointed or "me" centered communication. But, there is good news. Good communication skills can be developed through awareness followed by practice.

> "Communication leads to community, that is, to understanding, intimacy and mutual valuing." —Rollo May

Communication is a two-way street; at any given time, you will be acting as sender or receiver. Both require a degree of competence. Skills in this area are important to review due to their far-reaching influence.

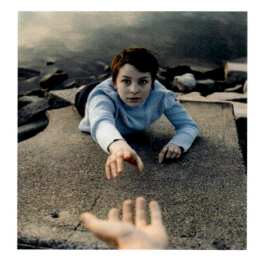

> "Good communication is the bridge between confusion and clarity." —Nat Turner

EXERCISE: To define how you would like to communicate with others, take a moment to ponder on great communicators you know. Think of one person who leaves you feeling understood and appreciated after you speak with them. Write a few of the specific behaviors and characteristics that contribute to this. Then, think of someone who gets their point across firmly but respectfully. Again, write down behaviors and characteristics you observe in them. The person who leaves you feeling understood more than likely has many "Receiver Skills", and the person who communicates their point well likely has many "Sender Skills."

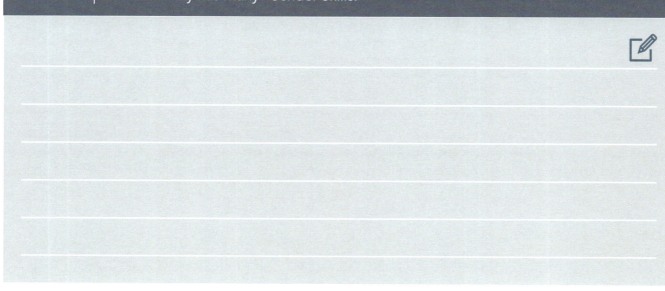

SENDER SKILLS

Good senders convey their point with assertiveness and respect. They make an effort to avoid heated conversations and think through what they would like to communicate. They balance sharing their stance and considering the perspectives of those to whom they are speaking. As a sender, your goal is getting the right message across. Do the following:

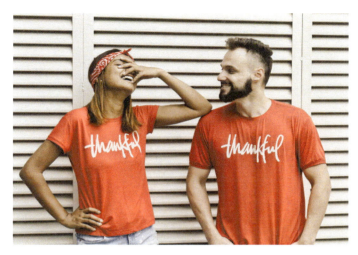

- Know your audience. Who are you speaking to and what is your relationship to them? Some audiences may require simpler words, some more tenderness, others more firmness. Choose words tailored to the people in front of you.
- Think before you speak, especially when conveying emotion-laden messages. When you are sharing something that will be or has been upsetting, it is easy to share things you would rather not or to speak in a manner you do not intend. Plan what you want to say. If it helps, write down a few bullet-points.
- Be open and honest. Everyone deserves respect and honesty. As you are forthright with others, you will gain their respect and trust and strengthen your relationship. People can see right through those who are dishonest.
- Be appropriately assertive. Being assertive means standing up for your personal rights. Start by remembering your value and recognizing what you need out of a given situation. Speak with confidence and firmness and rely on "I" statements to get your point across ("I need," "I feel," "I want").

RECEIVER SKILLS

Good receivers attend to the sender speaking to them. They listen without interrupting, correcting or becoming defensive. They make an effort to understand the things being communicated to them and allow the sender to feel heard and understood. As a receiver, your aim is to absorb the full message. Remember to:

- Make eye contact. Eye contact signals to the sender that you are ready to hear what s/he has to say. It is one of the simplest ways to show respect.
- As you listen, give encouragement by nodding your head and making simple sounds like, "Mmhmm." Your sender will know you are engaged and will continue to speak.
- Clarify what you are hearing. Do this by asking questions and by repeating simple versions of what you heard. This gives the sender an opportunity to correct and will ensure you understand the message s/he is trying to get across.
- Avoid thinking about what you would like to say in return. Instead of formulating a response as someone talks, fully listen to and hear what is being said to you. It is easy to miss nuances in the message if you are planning what you're going to say next.
- Suspend biases. Every message is filtered through your own beliefs and perceptions It takes effort to obtain a clear message. Consciously set aside your feelings about the message, and just focus on what is being said. Use the same challenging questions you use with your own self-talk to make sure you are receiving with clarity.

MODULE 9

One key to good communication, whether sending or receiving, is present-mindedness. Think of a time you knew someone was giving you only a portion of his or her attention as you tried to relay or receive a message. Half-minded conversations tend to do more harm than good. Make a habit of being fully present and engaged in the interactions you have with others. You will likely find yourself sending clearer messages and gaining a deeper understanding of what is shared with you. The other person will trust you and want to share with you more as well,

> EXERCISE: With a partner or friend, test out the opposite of a few of these sending and receiving skills. For example, listen to your friend speak without giving any eye contact. Try again without giving any encouragement. Ask the other person to do the same. How did you feel when you didn't receive any cues to continue? How much did you want to continue sharing?

EMPATHY

"Receiver skills" can contribute to a characteristic that is crucial to strong connection: Empathy. Empathy is the ability to understand how others feel and have compassion towards them.

> "Empathy is seeing with the eyes of another, listening with the ears of another and feeling with the heart of another." —Alfred Adler

It means putting yourself in someone else's shoes, working to understand their perspective and then acting based on that understanding. It is doing unto others as they would have you do. Playwright George Bernard Shaw put it well, "Do not do unto others as you would have them do unto you. They might have different tastes." Empathy contrasts the selfish, inward focus addiction promotes. It counters addictive thinking patterns such as manipulating others, projection, and denial.

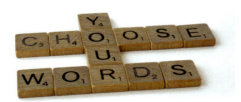

Family members and the loved ones of those suffering from addiction often complain that the addicted individual no longer cares about anything, even himself or others. Empathy is critical to moral development and is associated with service and caring for others. If you don't care about another person's feelings, you are not going to behave in a moral way towards them. Stealing from the family, lying, and aggressive behaviors are common as self-serving and "me" centered behaviors become more habitual. At this point, feelings of care have been overrun by addiction.

Over the course of addiction, drugs or addictive behaviors become more and more important and respect for the feelings of others becomes less and less as the brain only wants one thing: more substances or behaviors. And as cravings and withdrawal symptoms dominate the emotional state, the ability to relate to others becomes nonexistent. The diseased brain is just trying to survive.

Those with addiction issues struggle to identify their own feelings and so it is doubly hard to understand the emotions of others. Research has shown that alcoholics are uniquely challenged with empathy. Almost, 40 percent of them are unable to identify and describe their own feelings as compared with only 5 percent to 7 percent of the general population.

Though some people seem born with inherent empathy, research has found that it is a quality and skill that can be developed. What's more, social scientists are finding evidence that **cultivating empathy will improve the quality of your life!** In some senses, we are wired to benefit from giving and receiving empathy. We're made for connection, and how can we connect and commune without appreciation of each other's viewpoints. During the recovery process, increased empathy can help you consider ways your addiction may have impacted those close to you. In a safe and supportive environment, you can get honest about what the disease of addiction has taken from you and start on the road to healing. Empathy for others starts with experiencing it toward yourself. It is seeing yourself with compassion, forgiving the wrongs you committed while addicted, and releasing the shame that stands in your way of lasting recovery. Empathy for others can then result.

Empathy expert, Roman Krznaric, suggests the following practices to develop empathy:
- Cultivate curiosity about others, especially strangers. Empathy is difficult to grow without information to fodder it. Be curious about others around you and ask questions to know more. Aim for at least one conversation with a stranger each week. You'll be surprised what you learn and gain.
- Listen and share. Empathic conversations have two characteristics: radical listening and vulnerability. Radical listening is intent on staying in the present and understanding the feelings of the sender. Vulnerability, as introduced in Module 2, means opening up to share a part of yourself. Doing this opens the way for mutual understanding.
- Challenge prejudices. We each hold ideas and stereotypes about others that may or may not be based on pieces of truth or past experiences. Practice awareness of when these ideas pop up and influence your actions or thoughts. Take time to think about what people or groups you may hold biases against and then seek information to counter your prejudice.
- Find commonalities. Have you ever had the experience of getting to know someone different than you (maybe older, of a different ethnicity) and been struck by how many similarities you have? As you challenge your biases, look for ways you and others are the same rather than different. This will connect you and make understanding their perspectives feel more in reach.

George Orwell, acclaimed author of novels such as *Animal Farm* and *1984*, provides a prime example of seeking empathy. He set out to understand what life was like for those less fortunate than himself. He explained, "I wanted to submerge myself, to get right down among the oppressed.' To do so, he lived with beggars on the streets of London, dressed and acting to fit the part. Orwell had a transformative experience, challenging his preconceived notions and developing friendships.

MODULE 9

EXERCISE: Think of someone you may be able to get to know better and develop empathy towards. Write a plan for how you may do this. Think through the setting, time frame and what questions you may ask. A plan will provide you with greater courage and lessen the anxiety you may feel in discovering unfamiliar emotions for others.

COPING WITH DIFFICULT PEOPLE

"Feeling compassion toward a dangerous person will not lead you to submit to them or put yourself at risk or condone their actions. What it does simply is relieve your anxiety—which immediately makes you stronger and more resilient." —Laurie Perez

Regardless of how skilled you may be in listening to others and communicating your point, you will inevitably come across situations that require you to deal with a challenging or troublesome person. A comprehensive guide on how to manage communication with the many types of difficult people you may interact with regularly would be twice the thickness of this workbook. Whether facing someone prone to aggression, back-biting, people pleasing, or manipulating, the **COPE** framework can help you deal with challenging personalities.

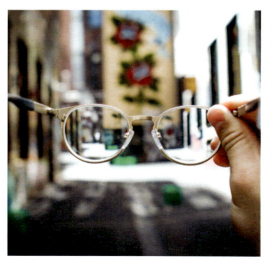

Center. Center yourself and relax. Centering is the first step in communicating under pressure. It is a process of maintaining psychological balance (staying relaxed but alert) under fire. Maintaining mental equilibrium is difficult in any situation that causes strong emotions but it is especially hard when you feel threatened or attacked. When upset or psychologically out-of-balance, it is difficult, if not impossible, to handle any situation effectively. In fact, the way you react to such situations may provoke and escalate the conflict further, and you may end up making matters worse.

141   Copyright © 2021 by Trish Barrus and Jade Ozawa-Kirk

The goal of centering is to not let the other person's attack upset you or to recover as quickly as possible. Here are some concepts and techniques that may help you learn how to center:
- Take a deep breath and exhale your excess negative energy. Visualize breathing in positivity and breathing out negativity. Repeat as necessary.
- Relax your muscles. Tell them to relax even if they resist. Intentionally tensing often helps release stubborn areas.
- Focus on process. Mentally describe what is happening as if you were an observer. For example:
  —See yourself about to become unglued.
  —Feel your muscles moving to a state of war alert.
  —Talk to yourself about what is happening: "My, how upset he is," or "Look how red her face is," or "I'll bet he has had a rough day."
- Ask yourself: Why is this person acting this way? Why is s/he telling me this? Does this person want sympathy? Help? Is s/he merely blowing off steam or does s/he really want information? Maybe this person is sharing an experience or just airing an anxiety.
- Count to ten. It usually helps to slow down the automatic knee-jerk reaction.

> As we go through the **COPE** framework, let's look at an example that may be relatable to many: a parent or family member is harping on you again for what he sees as poor choices. He's reminding you of past mistakes he can't seem to get over and he's nagging at you to change your ways.
>
> To center yourself, you might briefly close your eyes and take a deep breath. You can remind yourself that you've handled these conversations in the past and that you know your life is moving in the right direction even if his mind is stuck in the past.

Objectives. Identify your objectives. The difference between where you are and where you want to be is your objective. You can identify general (long-term) or specific (short-term) objectives. One of the general objectives of any conflict situation is to move into it with tact and grace and to blend into the encounter without making it worse. Additional general objectives can be stated as goals related to the specific encounter with the difficult person. For example, your objective might be to maintain a good relationship, to keep your job, or to learn from the experience so it doesn't happen again.

After selecting some general objectives, identify specific objectives for managing the situation and moving it in the direction you want it to go. For example, specific objectives relating to a single encounter might be to keep calm, to get the facts, to avoid making the situation worse, or to work out a win-win solution.

In most pressured situations, you don't have much time to stop and think about objectives or goals. But it is usually possible to quickly formulate some relevant short-term objectives that are appropriate for the situation. In the heat of the action, you don't have to stop and formulate general or long-term objectives—not because they are unimportant, but because they are often the same for most conflict situations. As you work through recovery, objectives may include avoiding relapse, managing stress and emotions, and enforcing boundaries.

Following the example of the petulant family member, your objectives may be as follows:
- General. Keep a decent relationship and get through the family gathering

MODULE 9

- Specific. Stay calm and remind the family member that you have apologized for past mistakes already, end the conversation quickly

Plan. Once you have thought through your objectives, plan how you will realize them. Remember the sender skills reviewed earlier in this module and add these tips:
- Be cool. If you flame, you'll put others on the defensive and consign your complaint to the trash. If you appear reasonable, the other person is more likely to respond in kind.
- Be fair in what you ask for. Let's say your baggage was torn by an airline. You demand first-class tickets to anywhere. You are angry when the airline doesn't respond. In a situation like that, you asked for too much. If you had requested $100 for new baggage or a voucher for that amount off on your next flight, you would have received it.
- Be precise. Ask for a deadline. Say something like, "I'll expect to hear from you by . . ." or "I'll expect this matter to be cleared up by . . ." Making a statement like that demonstrates that you are not going to just fade away. Your plan may be to stay calm as you make a few statements before asking that the topic be dropped.

Execute. Proceed according to your plan. Prepare to center and re-center yourself as needed throughout the encounter. Once the conversation has ended, review what went well and what you can learn from what happened. Note what you could do differently next time, whether keeping yourself calm or stating your need.

To execute the plan, you may say, "Dad, I know you care about me and want me to do well in life. I have apologized for those mistakes and am working to become a better person. Please stop bringing up the past. I will leave the room if this is what you continue to talk about."

> EXERCISE: What is a difficult conversation you have been putting off? Figure out how you will use the COPE procedure to address it.

C—

O—

P—

E—

143

Copyright © 2021 by Trish Barrus and Jade Ozawa-Kirk

ALTRUISM—SERVING OTHERS

Altruism is defined as a selfless act for the benefit of others or giving service. You might think that the recipient of altruism gets all the benefits but the benefits of the service to the giver are also great. Altruism has been found to be associated with:
- "Helper's high," a rush of endorphins released when you come to the aid of others
- Increased longevity
- Less chronic pain and improved immune functioning
- Increased sense of happiness and well-being
- Decreased psychological distress and depression
- Improved relationships and communication skills
- Deepened sense of meaning, purpose, and gratitude

In addition to the benefits listed above, **altruism builds connection** through a sense of community or greater good. Addiction tends to promote selfishness, as it is often focused on soothing the self through getting the next fix. Those with addictive thinking patterns and addictive behaviors tend to disregard the needs of others. Conscious acts of outreach and altruism are ways of combating loneliness as you look outward and focus on others. Perspective of your own problems change when you hear about the problems of others. Through this, connection is built and acts as a buffer against relapse.

> "Altruism is innate, but it's not instinctual. Everybody's wired for it, but a switch has to be flipped." —David Rakoff

A caveat about serving others: If you are already overwhelmed by what you have on your plate, pressuring yourself to make time to volunteer on top of everything else may lead to burnout. If this applies to your situation, focus on small instances to do for others rather than grand, time-consuming efforts. For example, open the door for a stranger, smile at a passerby, or help a family member with a quick chore.

Ways to incorporate service into your day-to-day life:
- Do random acts of kindness
- Participate in coordinated volunteer efforts
- Use one of your signature strengths to help others
- Serve individuals in your household
- Mentor or support someone else in recovery

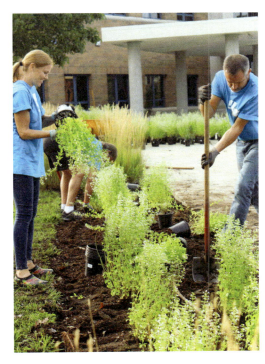

MODULE 9

EXERCISE: Return to the strengths you identified in Module 5. Choose one that may be helpful to someone close to you. Record some thoughts about how you might create an act of altruism using this strength.

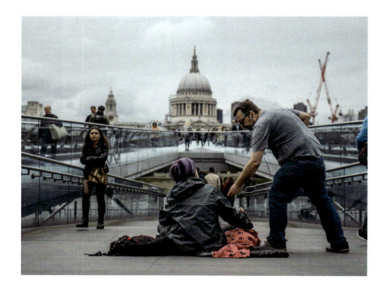

KEY TAKEAWAYS

- Relationships and connection are a crucial part of life satisfaction, well-being, and recovery.
- Attachment forms early in life. It shapes our interactions and perceptions.
- Emotions protect your emotional, mental, and physical well-being.
- Communication skills apply to both the sender and receiver and include verbal and nonverbal interaction.
- Altruism is a way to build connection and cultivate positive emotion.

MODULE 10
LIVING WITH INTEGRITY

PRINCIPLE
LIVE WITH INTEGRITY
Move Forward with Authenticity and Determination

THOUGHT QUESTIONS
Think back to your value exercise and the legacy you wrote. After working through the exercises in this workbook, are there things you would change?

Are you finally being honest with yourself?

What do you still need to change to move forward with authenticity?

Living with integrity means not only **living true to yourself and your beliefs** but also means engaging in self-care. Bring out the best in yourself by getting plenty of sleep, eating nutritious foods, setting goals, and practicing stress management skills. Science has shown that if you don't sleep or eat well, your mind and physical health will deteriorate. Suffering from addiction has probably taken a toll on your body. We hope you will rebuild and strengthen your physical and mental health, manage the stressors in your life, and center your goals around your defined purpose and meaning. But most importantly, we hope you will **move forward with authenticity and determination** as you strive for a wonderful life.

Bill's parents divorced when he was seven. His mother gave him away to a foster family when he was eight. She didn't abandon her other children, just him, because he reminded her too much of his dad. He was sexually abused from the time he was seven until he was twelve. No one cared for him or protected him. He didn't know why. He wondered if he was defective in some way. Being alone was to define his life.

Into his seventies, Bill had never received a Christmas or birthday present or card from a family member. Never in his life! He graduated with honors from both high school and a prestigious university. No one attended his graduations. Again, he was all alone.

Bill became a successful businessman. I asked him how. He explained that creating and building had given him a cause and a purpose. He thought that if he made something of himself and was successful, maybe he would be loved.

Bill's ability to love expanded. He became a light to all that know him. He encourages and loves because of the inner strength gained from his challenges. He understands pain and its awful grip on the soul. He knows the despair of loneliness. But he also knows what it means to not allow life or others to define or destroy who you are. He is the epitome of living with integrity.

Living true to yourself and who you are has been explored throughout this workbook. People love because they choose to love. And just because your love is not reciprocated doesn't mean that you should stop loving. Your ability to love is expanding.

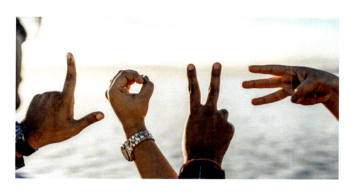

After going through the recovery process, you will find that much of your life will be the same. You may find yourself living within the same four walls. Your commute to work will feature the same oblivious drivers. Your family members might have aged slightly, but they will use the same tone of voice when talking to you. Your boss will continue to make the same demands on you. You will have the same annoyances in your marriage that you've always had.

Despite the sameness, everything may feel different because you are different. **We hope you find yourself walking (if not marching) into the next phase of your life with a new sense of identity and purpose.** We see you as a brave conqueror, and we hope you can view yourself with the same confidence and optimism. Recovery is not easy, and it is ongoing. There will surely be unexpected twists and turns on the path ahead. But your journey will be worthwhile.

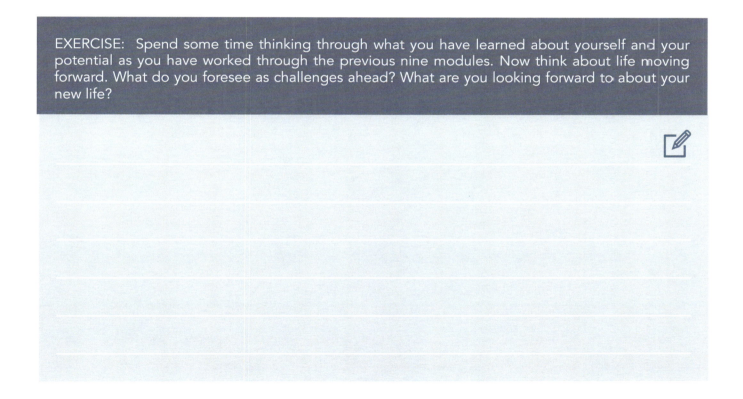

EXERCISE: Spend some time thinking through what you have learned about yourself and your potential as you have worked through the previous nine modules. Now think about life moving forward. What do you foresee as challenges ahead? What are you looking forward to about your new life?

As you move forward, it is important that you stay true to your values and continue to set and work toward specific goals that will guide you and keep you free from addiction. It will also be important that you engage in good self-care and stress management skills. The following sections will talk about these important life skills.

MODULE 10
SETTING AND ACHIEVING GOALS

If you hope to change in some way or increase your happiness, it is useful to start with a goal. Remember learning in Module 1 that happy people set goals. You might have a goal(s) in mind but it's very important to formally write it down and make a plan. According to research from Harvard, those who write down their goals are far more likely to accomplish them. Written goals are more concrete. Without having a plan of action, you may feel like you are going nowhere and accomplishing nothing. In contrast, setting firm, strengths-based goals and acting on your plan can provide a long-term vision as well as motivation in the present. The following activity will help you to consider your long-term vision.

EXERCISE: Read through the list of areas that research shows contribute to life satisfaction. Think about how you would like your future to look. What do you want your life to be like years and decades down the road? Ask yourself what areas are most important to you. What do you value most? Mark them. Of the areas you marked, which would you like to improve? Consider your ideal for this area. How would you like it to look in five, ten, or twenty years? Refer back to the Legacy that you wrote at the beginning of this program. Have your goals changed? You might want to rewrite your Legacy after going through the exercises in this workbook.

After identifying your priority areas, write a few long- and short-term goals. Don't overwhelm yourself with too many goals all at once. Start with a simple plan for one or two goals.

Long-term Vision of Yourself

- Love
- Career
- Financial
- Play
- Health
- Relationships
- Family
- Learning
- Service
- Creativity
- Spirituality
- Home
- Confidence
- Exercise
- Nutrition
- Hobbies

149

Copyright © 2021 by Trish Barrus and Jade Ozawa-Kirk

Goals should be SMART:
- Specific—Be as specific as possible. State with exactness what you would like to do. For example, if you want to be more creative, in which areas? What would you like to create?
- Measurable—Quantify your goal. This will allow you to see if you've hit the mark when you reach your deadline and will help you check in on progress. If you want to save more this year, how much more? How will you know when you've met the goal?

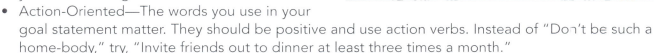

- Action-Oriented—The words you use in your goal statement matter. They should be positive and use action verbs. Instead of "Don't be such a home-body," try, "Invite friends out to dinner at least three times a month."
- Realistic—Goals should challenge you, but unrealistic and unachievable goals will just leave you disappointed. Stretch yourself within reason. If you're taking up running for the first time in your life, start with a lap around the block, maybe train for a 5k instead of a marathon.
- Time-Bound—Setting a date to accomplish your goal goes along with making it measurable. It allows you to check in with yourself as you work toward the end. It also motivates you and creates a sense of urgency.

Sharing your goal with others increases accountability and commitment. It isn't necessary to blast your Facebook wall with goal statements (unless you feel this will motivate you). Rather, choose one or two confidantes who you know will support and motivate you. Ask them to check in with you periodically about the goal. In addition, start working on your goal within two days. Research shows that if you don't take action within forty-eight hours of setting a goal, you probably won't do anything toward accomplishing that goal.

> **EXERCISE:** Using the outline below, take one of your short-term goals and make a specific plan.

STEP 1: What do I want to accomplish? (Write it down.)

STEP 2: When do I want to accomplish it? (Set a date.)

MODULE 10

STEP 3: I need to take these small steps in order to reach my goal. How will I do it? Remember to be "SMART" about it.

a)

b)

c)

STEP 4: I will tell the following person (or people) about this goal.

STEP 5: What will I do within 48 hours to start achieving this goal?

STRESS MANAGEMENT

A college psychology professor was lecturing about stress and its effect on happiness. As she raised a glass of water during her lecture, everyone expected they'd be asked the typical "glass half empty or glass half full" question. Instead, with a smile on her face, the professor asked, "How heavy is this glass of water I'm holding?" Students shouted out answers ranging from eight ounces to a couple of pounds.

> "What stress really does, though, is deplete willpower, which diminishes your ability to control those emotions."
> —Roy F. Baumeister

She replied, "From my perspective, the absolute weight of this glass doesn't matter. It all depends on how long I hold it. If I hold it for a minute or two, it's fairly light. If I hold it for an hour straight, its weight might make my arm ache a little. If I hold it for a day straight, my arm will likely cramp up and feel completely numb and paralyzed, forcing me to drop the glass to the floor. In each case, the weight of the glass doesn't change, but the longer I hold it, the heavier it feels to me."

As the class nodded their heads in agreement, she continued, "Your stresses and worries in life are very

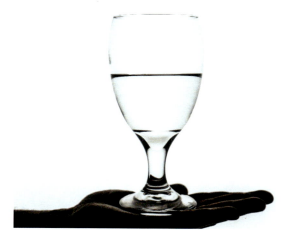

much like this glass of water. Think about them for a while and nothing happens. Think about them a bit longer, and you begin to feel anxiety. Think about them all day long, and you will feel completely numb and paralyzed—incapable of doing anything else until you drop them."

Stress is an expected part of life. It impacted you before and during your addiction, and it certainly will continue to impact you going forward. **Learning healthy and maintainable ways of managing your stress will prevent you from turning back to an addictive behavior.** Because of this, we'll look in-depth at ways to manage and cope with stress throughout recovery and sobriety.

There are three facets of or ways to approach the broad idea of stress management:
- Change your attitude and thoughts about stress.
- Adjust your life to minimize stress.
- Cope with stress in the moment and in general.

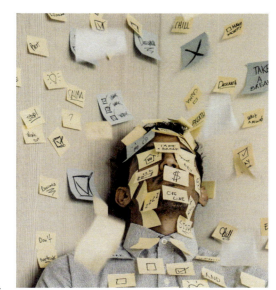

CHANGE YOUR THOUGHTS ABOUT STRESS

Think about the different ways stress affects your mind and body. Take a moment to consider a time when you felt very stressed. Close your eyes and mentally put yourself back into that stressful situation. Let your body follow. Stress has numerous physical symptoms that are known to negatively impact your health and well-being. But new research shows that the way you think about your stress and your body's reaction is more impactful than the physical symptoms themselves. Yes, regularly raised blood pressure caused by stress and anxiety can wear down the cardiovascular system. But, by thinking about this symptom differently, you can override its detrimental effects. Reframing your body's stress response can make stress reactions helpful rather than hurtful and can help you use your experience to strengthen your relationships and to learn new things.

Try these ways of reframing your thoughts about stress:

- Original Thought: "My breath is getting faster and faster. Am I hyperventilating? Am I getting enough air?"
  Reframe: "My lungs are signaling me to take a deep breath. I know fast breathing means oxygen is moving to my brain to help me think more clearly."

- Original Thought: "No one understands the stress I'm under! They don't get it!"
  Reframe: "Everyone experiences stress sometimes. Who do I know who has gone through something similar? Maybe we can support each other."

- Original Thought: "I don't know if I'll ever get through this. This week has been so awful."
  Reframe: "I am doing hard things and I can continue doing them. What lessons am I learning? How will I be stronger and wiser when this has passed?"

Changing your thinking this way takes time and practice. You may want to use some type of visual reminder in an area where you frequently experience or reflect on stress, such as your desk at work, the dashboard of your vehicle, or the wallpaper of your computer.

MODULE 10
ADJUST YOUR LIFE TO DECREASE/MINIMIZE STRESSORS

> EXERCISE: On a piece of paper, write the tasks you have currently in your various roles. Draw a circle around each one. These are the balls you are juggling. Examples may include nurture and care for family members, maintain a household, work as a caring partner, and prepare for the upcoming fiscal year. Roles to consider as you list tasks include your profession/occupation, your relationship/family/social life, your identity as an individual, your place within your community/society, your spiritual life, and so on. Once you have a fair number of "balls" on your page, think through the week or two ahead and ponder each task you've written. Label each task—or ball—as "glass" or "rubber." In other words, if this ball is dropped this week, will it recover and bounce back (rubber) or will it break (glass)? This activity is meant to help you gain perspective on what might be most important this week.

In his productivity-oriented book, *Essentialism*, author and business consultant Greg McKeown presents multiple ideas for decreasing stress. First, he uses the acronym WIN to ask, "What is important now?" One way to minimize stressful task-clutter in your mind and life is to focus on the most important items to do in any moment or day. Focus on just the most important task and allow the others to rest. If certain tasks or responsibilities are low on your priority list for several days or a couple of weeks in a row, consider delegating, outsourcing, or removing them. Let the essentials float to the top and all others to fall away.

Another way to decrease stress is to cut out stressors. Throughout this workbook we have discussed toxic relationships, triggers that lead to use, and other stressors in your life. Can any be removed or decreased from your schedule, or can adjustments be made to make them more tolerable? Remember you have to engage in self-care all of the time.

COPE WITH STRESS IN THE MOMENT AND OR IN GENERAL

There are two timeframes in which you may need to cope with stress:
- In the moment as you face specific stressors,
- in general, when stress is ongoing.

Think of it this way: There is the stress of walking into a notoriously tense year-end meeting with management (in the moment), and then there is the stress of finishing up end of the year tasks as a whole (in general).

TO FIGHT STRESS IN THE MOMENT:
- Clue into what your body is telling you. Recognize stress cues in your body (tightened neck or jaw, clenched fists, a knot in the pit of your stomach). These are your body's reaction to the release of stress hormones and they can provide you with useful information. These cues signal that it's time to engage in immediate stress reduction.

- Reframe and reassure. "This is helping me, and it will pass." Try some of the reframes listed previously. Engage in positive self-talk.
- Take slow, deep breaths. Give your brain oxygen and the vagus nerve down your spine a calming hug with deliberate breaths. Elongate your breath with each inhale and exhale, keeping your exhale longer than your inhale.
- Maintain composure as you speak to yourself and others with a calm, low, soft voice (probably the opposite of what you feel inclined to do). Gently reassure yourself and then focus on staying collected for the benefit of those around you. It's natural to mirror stress reactions, and the last thing you need is everyone else getting amped up as well.
- Practice mindfulness skills by tuning into your senses. Sensory information is grounding and centering. Notice what you hear, see, smell, feel, and taste. Focus on each sense for a moment.

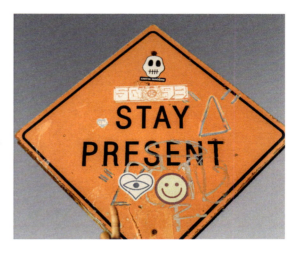

SELF-CARE

Regular self-care enhances physical and mental health and increases resilience against stress. It's your best defense against the ongoing, general stress mentioned above. Make plans to consistently incorporate the positive changes you have made throughout this workbook. You deserve to be happy and part of being happy is self-care. Instead of proactively tending to their needs, people caught up in addiction run themselves dry and then numb or avoid to get away from the bad feelings that accumulate. Self-care is key to staying addiction free!

As you think about healthy habits and self-care routines, consider various aspects of your well-being:
- Personal
- Social
- Physical
- Emotional
- Psychological
- Professional

Self-care and coping skills are two sides of the same coin. The difference is in intention/purpose. Coping skills are used to help you move through stress. Self-care is used to continually bolster mental health so internal stress does not pile up. The same strategies can be used for both! Your weekly self-care routine may be what you need to cope with the figurative year-end stress mentioned above.

Coping skills are many and varied. Anything you do to alleviate stress or pressure is a coping skill! For example, during an extremely stressful time, you can go on a walk outside or you can binge on a pint of Ben & Jerry's ice cream. Both may alleviate some stress, but one is more sustainable and has fewer negative side effects. Your addiction is probably a prime example of a coping skill that ended up being detrimental and unsustainable.

MODULE 10

EXERCISE: Look through this list of coping skills that can be used to relieve stressors. Which ones do you use regularly? Which have you tried occasionally or just once? Pick the ones that stand out to you and plan how you will use them. Consider which may be helpful to use in the moment or as a break from a stressful situation, and which could be worked into a self-care routine.

COPING SKILLS

- Listen to music
- Go for a walk
- Take a relaxing bath or shower
- Deep breathe (5 counts in, 5 counts out)
- Call/text a friend
- Meditate
- Stretch
- Think about something you are grateful for
- Make a list of things you are grateful for
- Watch a funny video
- Eat your favorite snack
- Write a thank-you card to someone
- Journal (write your thoughts/feelings)
- Focus on being in the present moment
- Read a book
- Cook or bake
- Dance
- Sing or play an instrument
- Hug someone
- Express yourself creatively through art
- Smile
- Use positive affirmations
- Plan something fun to look forward to
- Watch your favorite TV show
- Play a board game or cards
- Play video games
- Take pictures
- Exercise (for example, running or yoga)
- Set a positive intention for the day
- Take a moment to notice something beautiful
- Pray or contemplate your hope
- Write a letter (to yourself or someone else)
- Focus on self-compassion
- Name your emotion and allow yourself to observe the emotion without judgment
- Cry
- Clean or organize something
- Go to a park
- Compliment someone
- Express your thoughts/feelings to someone
- Review old photos of positive memories
- Paint your nails
- Spend time with a pet
- Do a relaxation exercise
- Redirect negative thoughts to more balanced thoughts
- Find the silver lining in a negative situation
- Help someone else
- Eat something healthy and refreshing
- Play a sport
- Brainstorm or problem solve
- Contemplate on your meaning/purpose/values
- Use guided imagery
- Collect rocks or shells
- Make a list of your choices
- Create a schedule for your day
- Spend time with someone positive
- Sit in a hot tub, sauna, or pool
- Read inspirational quotes
- Read self-help articles or books
- Name three or more of your positive attributes
- Take care of your physical appearance
- Take responsibility for your part of a problem
- Go for a drive
- Sew, knit, crochet, or cross-stitch
- Think of all the people who care about you
- Do a puzzle, word search, or sudoku
- Go out to eat
- Have a picnic
- Go to the library
- Squeeze a stress ball (or a pillow)
- Express your appreciation/gratitude to someone
- Read jokes, comics, or celebrity gossip
- Read a magazine
- Get a massage
- Be in nature
- Listen to an inspirational podcast or video
- Volunteer

Self-care can be confused with self-indulgence or pampering. Be careful of this. Self-care should be rejuvenating and recharging or protecting and fortifying. It should fill up a depleted area of your well-being or lessen a potential stressor. For example, "self-care" through binging on a whole package of chocolate almonds because you need to "decompress" or "zone out" may not be the healthiest solution. Watching a good documentary would be better. Good self-care may end up being less pleasurable than you may expect but can have long-term benefits. Examples of this kind of self-care include regular doctor's visits, exercising, and setting aside regular time to review your finances.

THE IMPORTANCE OF SLEEP

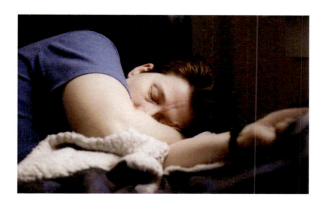

Sleep deficiency, or not getting the amount of sleep your body needs, is a common problem, especially among those suffering from addiction because their sleep patterns are so erratic. People across all ages and circumstances report getting poor quality or too little sleep, but often do not realize the implications. Sleep problems have been linked to serious chronic physical and mental health problems, including heart disease, stroke, diabetes, and depression. In the short-term, sleep deficiency can cause decreased short-term memory, irritability, and cognitive impairment with effects similar to drunkenness. Decision-making skills waver and risk-taking increases when sleep is lacking. Sleep-deprived people feel more stressed and struggle to control their emotions. When considered as a whole, the detrimental effects of poor sleep are a recipe for trouble in the recovery process and in living life in general.

Sleep also provides an important foundation for your personal, social, and career successes. You will experience a considerable return as you invest in your sleep. Research shows that you should get between 8-10 hours of sleep each night. At times, this may seem impossible, but it is important to try by incorporating sleep-care strategies:
- Prioritize your sleep. Sleep is often the first thing to be shaved down when life gets busy. Guard against that tendency.
- Establish sleep routines, including regular sleep and wake times each day and ritual activities to cue your mind to start to wind down. Begin your bedtime ritual at least thirty minutes before you would like to fall asleep.
- Avoid screens, bright lights, strenuous exercise, and alcohol for several hours before bedtime. Blue light from cell phones and computers has been shown to interrupt circadian rhythms and sleep patterns.
- Make time for physical activity and enjoying sunlight each day. Rays from the sun help trigger the brain to make chemicals that aid in sleep regulation.

MODULE 10

THE IMPORTANCE OF EXERCISE

Regular exercise is an important element in addiction recovery particularly because people with addictive habits are often very sedentary. An exercise regimen is good for anyone but is particularly valuable for someone recovering from addiction. Consider these benefits:

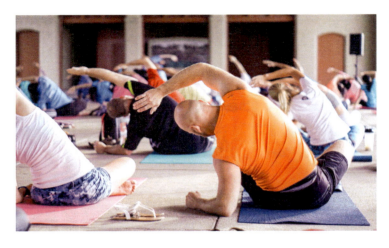

- Exercise can reduce drug-seeking behavior, as regular movement can actually prevent a return to alcohol or drug use. Some research suggests that regular physical activity can increase the abstinence rate for substance use by 95 percent.
- Exercise aids in the prevention of a large variety of diseases. This is especially important for those with substance use disorders because they experience significantly lower levels of physical and mental health and a greater prevalence of illness.
- Exercise improves cardiovascular fitness, strength, coordination, and flexibility. This is important because addictive patterns commonly lead to sedentary lifestyles, significantly lower levels of cardiovascular fitness, and increase in musculoskeletal degeneration as a result of substance use. Improved fitness also leads to increased energy.
- Those with substance misuse problems show much higher rates of depression and anxiety than the general population. Interestingly, there is growing evidence that exercise can be just as effective for treating these problems as psychotherapy!
- Substance abuse has also been shown to result in reduced blood flow, atrophy, and cell loss in the brain, which causes reduced mental functioning. On the other hand, exercise has been shown to have positive effects on mental activities. Those who regularly exercise often report experiencing a much clearer state of mind. This adds to the effectiveness of talk therapies for addiction.

Other benefits of exercise include:
- Exercise can help provide structure to your days.
- Exercise can fill up idle time in your day.
- When done with others, exercise can forge positive connections, especially in recovery.
- Exercise can serve as time for meditation and mindfulness.
- Exercise leads to better sleep.
- Exercise prevents weight gain.

Exercise can take many forms and intensities, as guided by your doctor. It's important to choose exercises you enjoy, whether walking the dog, hiking a beautiful local trail, or lifting weights in the gym. As your body and mind recover and you become more physically healthy, you'll find more options open to you, broadening the types of activities you can do and enjoy.

> **EXERCISE:** What type of exercise or physical activity have you enjoyed throughout your life, especially before your addiction? What can you do to prioritize adding exercise to your routine?

THE IMPORTANCE OF NUTRITION

Just like sleep and exercise, you may not have considered how your diet impacts recovery and sobriety, but the connection is clear. The main side effect of an unhealthy diet is malnutrition. Substance abuse actually increases the risk of malnutrition, not only because those with addictions tend to ignore their dietary needs, but because alcohol and other drugs actually inhibit the body's ability to absorb nutrients.

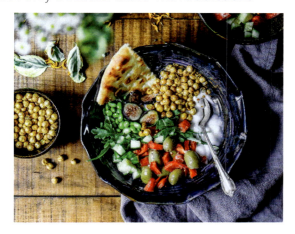

As you continue down your recovery road, try to eat more whole and less processed or fast foods. Essentially, whole food is any food that has a single ingredient, such as eggs, any fruit or vegetable, grains like oats and quinoa, milk or other dairy products, and meat. While any whole food is good for you, these examples of whole foods are particularly helpful for early recovery. The nutrients in them can boost brain health, improve mood, speed up the healing process, and even ease some of the mental and physical symptoms of withdrawal.

Nutrition throughout recovery (and beyond) should include healthy and complex carbohydrates, high-quality proteins, including lean meat, fish, and plant-based proteins, fresh fruits and vegetables, essential fats through fish and nuts, and ample hydration. Just as drug or alcohol withdrawal can cause headaches, drowsiness, and depression, malnutrition can cause the same symptoms, complicating recovery from addiction. Good nutrition rejuvenates your brain and body, promoting your well-being and health, and, hence, your sobriety.

MODULE 10

EXERCISE: Look back through the information presented within this module. Write one action you can do this week for each of the following areas:
- Stress management
- Sleep
- Exercise
- Nutrition

KEY TAKEAWAYS

- Life in recovery provides opportunities to prioritize your mental and physical well-being through the establishment of healthy habits.
- Effective goals are SMART (Specific, Measurable, Action-Oriented, Realistic, Time-bound), shared with others, and acted on within a day or two.
- Stress management includes minimizing, reframing, and coping with stress.
- Regular self-care bolsters resilience against anticipated and unanticipated stressors.
- Sleep, exercise, and nutrition play important, though sometimes overlooked, roles in successful recovery.

CONCLUSION

Once upon a time, a man discovered a butterfly that was starting to hatch from its cocoon. He sat down and watched for hours as the butterfly struggled to force itself through a tiny hole. Suddenly it stopped making progress and seemed to be stuck.

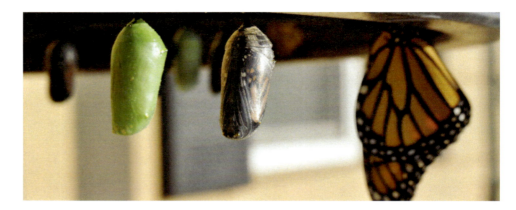

At that point, the man decided to help the butterfly out. He took a pair of scissors and cut off the remaining bit of the cocoon. The butterfly emerged easily, although it had a swollen body and small, shriveled wings.

The man thought nothing of it, and he sat waiting for the wings to enlarge enough to support the butterfly. However, that never happened. The butterfly spent the rest of its life unable to fly, crawling around with small wings and a swollen body.

Despite the man's kind heart, he didn't understand that restricting the cocoon and the struggle needed to get itself through the small hole were nature's way of forcing fluid from the body of the butterfly into its wings so it could eventually fly free.

It is like that in our lives; our struggles help make us strong enough to measure up to our potential. As your recovery process continues, authenticity and honesty with yourself are critical. Do not deny or rationalize your debilitating behaviors when they rear their ugly heads. Have the courage to go forward and create a wonderful and lasting life legacy.

The next stage of your recovery is a time to shape the many principles and skills you have been introduced to throughout this workbook into a personalized plan that will keep you living the good life. As you move forward with purpose, authenticity, and integrity, you will **flourish and thrive.**

AUTHENTICITY

The English word authentic originates from a Greek word, *authentikos,* which means "original or principal." It may seem ironic to talk about being "original" in the same breath as talking about change. But the kind of change we talk about in recovery is change that takes you back to your original, real, unhindered self: A self that lives with integrity and courage; A self that takes responsibility and is self-reliant; A self that doesn't use substances or addictive behaviors in order to feel whole and happy.

An authentic life is one that is congruent with one's beliefs and values. Authentic people are not an imitation of others nor do they allow others to define them. Further, they are not "pleasers" meaning they don't act in a way just to gain the approval of others.

When you are authentic, you become capable of real connection with others. This connection satisfies emotional and psychological needs, leaving little room or need for the substances or behaviors that you might otherwise turn toward to fill voids. When you are authentic, you will enjoy giving and receiving love, understanding, and acceptance.

Certainly, authenticity can be damaging to others if not filtered. There is something to be said for kindness, respect, and tact. Being respectfully authentic means being spontaneous, but appropriate. When you are respectfully authentic, you refrain from doing or saying anything that might be hurtful, and that is not dishonest. After all, as the old adage teaches, some things are better left unsaid.

How does authenticity impact your recovery? The opposite of authenticity, falsity, stems from self-doubt, and self-doubt in turn generates shame and even self-hatred. Very often, these negative emotions find their roots in past experiences with trauma, neglect, and abuse. These issues can blind you to the truth of who you are—a magnificent human being who is being damaged by self-loathing in the form of destructive thoughts and feelings.

In addition to awakening and gaining critical skills, the recovery process also includes developing confidence and learning to cherish yourself. At first, this might seem uncomfortable and undeserved. Make no mistake: It is deserved! You deserve self-love, self-appreciation, and self-confidence. Be gentle with yourself, whether your suffering was self-induced through patterns of addiction or brought on by the choices and acts of others out of your control. Cherishing yourself allows for authenticity, which in turn allows for healthy, loving connections with others, who can serve as valuable, supportive allies in your recovery. Practice cherishing yourself through mindfulness and self-compassion every day.

HONESTY

At times when you've struggled with addiction, you may have found it difficult to be honest with others. If that is the case, you certainly are not alone; addiction and deception commonly go hand in hand. Why is that? Research on the topic of honesty and addiction revealed that if people struggling with addiction feel their confidences will be kept and will not result in negative consequences, what they say to others tends to be reliable and valid. But if they feel that telling the truth about addictive behaviors is going to bring trouble, they are more inclined to be dishonest. In short, if people trust you, the evidence suggests they will be honest.

One study revealed that 60 percent of adults cannot even have a ten-minute conversation without lying at least once. Not only that, those in the study reported they told an average of two to three lies during the ten minutes! Even worse, participants stated they often weren't even aware they were lying and were surprised when they were shown recordings of conversations where they had lied.

Although most of the lies people tell are considered to be "harmless" (such as a lie told to make someone feel good), a habit of dishonesty is anything but harmless. The destructive element of most lies is not in the twisting of information, it is in the patterns formed by dishonesty. As you may have experienced, dishonest habits often hurt people. Further, dishonesty is very common due to feelings of shame and guilt. But as mentioned above, to become authentic and confident, it is imperative to be honest with yourself first and then with others.

You have probably worked very hard to get to this point in your life—a point of change, fresh perspective, renewed determination, and hopefully renewed meaning and purpose. After all of your

CONCLUSION

effort, the best thing you can do to stay your new course of clean and sober living is to adopt a pattern of honesty, or transparency, no matter the consequences. Even if you lapse or relapse, the people who have loved and supported you during your journey, those who know you and what you have gone through will be encouraged to stay the course with you if they know you are being honest both with them and with yourself. Sharing what is real about yourself or being vulnerable strengthens your chances of success and deepens connection in your relationship with others.

Dishonesty creates nothing but problems: it takes energy, generates anxiety and fear, produces loss of respect and self-respect, requires stressfully infallible memory, fosters guilt and shame, cheapens your brand, and opens the door for more poor choices to compensate for the lies. On the other hand, **patterns of honesty produce feelings of peace, wellness, and happiness. Consider these benefits of honesty:**

- Less stress and worry. Dishonesty requires high maintenance! With honesty, you never have to remember details or keep stories straight. You're better able to relax and feel at peace.
- Trust. Honest people are trusted by others.
- Self-confidence. It's a great feeling to trust yourself, isn't it?
- High-caliber friends. Integrity attracts integrity. People who are trustworthy and honest aren't that way by accident. They choose to be honest, and people who have made that choice, do so because they value it. And if they value it that highly, they'll likely look for that quality in others. Honest friends are the best friends to have! Also, when you're honest about yourself, you tend to choose people who accept you for who you are, and you tend to weed out those who are superficial, inconsistent, and fake.
- Closer friendships. Transparency is a necessary element for greater intimacy. Your friends and loved ones love the authentic you, not the one you've artificially created!
- Wellness. Research has found that lifestyle—especially stress and dishonesty—impacts the immune system. Being honest keeps you healthier
- Freedom. Every time you lie to someone, you're limiting your own options and enslaving yourself to the deception. Ayn Rand said, "People think that a liar gains a victory over his victim. A lie is an act of self-abdication, because one surrenders one's reality to the person to whom one lies. The man who lies to the world, is the world's slave from then on. . . . There are no white lies, there is only the blackest of destruction, and a white lie is the blackest of all."

Truth demands self-reflection. When you take truth-telling seriously, your responses in conversation will become less automatic. You will find yourself pausing more because what you are about to say is genuine, and therefore requires more thought. If you find yourself more self-reflective, take it as a good sign. Integrity at its core cannot exist without honesty.

COURAGE

Sometimes we have to step up and do the right thing even if it is dangerous or inconvenient to do so. That is courage.

This is the story of hundreds of people who were saved by the courage of one man who gave the order, "Mr. Dean, turn this ship around."

There were three ships in close proximity to the sinking ship when the distress signal was made. The first one, Sampson, was approximately seven miles away from the sinking ship. Only seven miles! They could see the sinking ship and the people on the deck. But they didn't answer the call. Why? Because the crew aboard the ship had been involved in illegal hunting of seals. They ignored the call to help because they didn't want to get caught.

Sometimes, courage is not about insane bravery. It's just simply about having the guts to do the right thing because someone is in dire need, even if it puts you at risk. Obviously, the crew of Sampson did not possess the integrity and courage to look beyond themselves.

There was another ship approximately fourteen miles away from the sinking ship. The Californian saw the distress signals as it was within eye shot but they were surrounded by ice and it was nighttime. They decided to wait till the morning for the conditions to improve. They listened as the distress signals came in and did nothing.

The third ship was about fifty-eight miles away and was already moving in the other direction but when they heard the cries over the radio, they decided to be the lifeboat. The captain of this ship just prayed to God for direction and turned his boat. They maneuvered around ice fields in the dark and narrowly missed crashing themselves, but they kept going.

The lifeboat was Carpathia. And the shipwreck it sailed to was none other than the Titanic. They saved 705 lives that night. Those 705 lives were saved because one man chose the right over the easy. He risked his own life and even through the fear he kept going. Captain Arthur Rostron was the man who was brave enough to turn the ship around.

Change requires courage. If you are reading this, you have already made changes (big and small). You're showing courage because you're working on further progress and change!

A misconception about courage is that it is the absence of fear. As a matter of fact, **courage is moving forward despite fear.** You may feel terribly afraid, but still choose to take chances like saying "I love you" first, asking for a raise, or moving to a new city. Those choices are courageous and create vulnerability. But that's okay; choose them anyway! As researcher Brené Brown puts it, "There's no courage without vulnerability." Brené Brown describes four pillars of courage:
- Vulnerability- Vulnerability is showing up when outcomes are uncertain. It is a strength, not a weakness.
- Clarity of Values- Values are at the core of our personal programming; they are what is most significant to you. They dictate how you spend your time and to what you devote your attention. It takes courage to identify and live your values.
- Trust- Trusting yourself first is necessary to being able to trust others. This is an important concept for those working on changing addictive behaviors. It takes courage to trust yourself and then others. You have to trust yourself enough to know that you can handle your emotions and thoughts even if someone lets you down or rejects you.
- Rising Skills- This means having the skills to pick yourself up and move on after "failing." People tend to stand in two general arenas of thought regarding making "mistakes": "I made a mistake, therefore I failed," or "I made a mistake, therefore I learned." It is our hope that you choose to see mistakes as opportunities for learning and improvement, not as cause to condemn or criticize yourself. Your rising skills come from the courage already in you, and with practice they will lead to more courage.

Courage is required every day. Choose to be brave, to know what your values are, and to have the

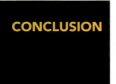

CONCLUSION

integrity to follow them. Choose to be vulnerable and emotionally available to others. Trust yourself; As you do, you will have the confidence to trust others. And finally, be resilient and bounce back when you make mistakes. Don't stay in a rut of negativity. Take one day at a time. Get out of your comfort zone and choose to be courageous. As you move forward with authenticity and integrity, you will call on your own courage and bravery to continue to change and persevere.

FINAL WORDS

In this workbook, you have been exposed to the latest research on the brain, addiction, and the steps to change. You have learned about positive psychology and how an emphasis on optimism, emotional exploration, hope, and gratitude impacts healing. Living consciously, being accountable, and being responsible are all important traits in overcoming addictive thinking patterns and being true to yourself. You have also seen how connection is important to the recovery process, including good communication skills, assertive behavior, boundary setting, and forgiving yourself and others. Good support systems have strengthened you in the past and will continue to do so in the future.

You have explored integrity and how it can impact you personally, emotionally, socially, psychologically, and relationally in drastically positive ways. You have learned skills and strategies that will help you to reengage in life with serenity and fullness as your choices are congruent with your values, as you set and work toward your goals, as you practice stress-reduction techniques, and as you move forward with honesty, authenticity, and courage.

We hope that through the exercises, activities, journaling, and introspective work you've done, you have found insight into your personal path and how to go forward with confidence. A strong belief in yourself is critical as you go forward with courage.

We hope the familiarity and sameness you may find in your home environment will serve as an anchor for you and your relationships will thrive there. We also hope that the sameness will feel different and new because the way you relate to it has changed.

We wish you all the best as you navigate the twists and turns of life, with all the challenge, joy, perspective, and meaning they will bring. Remember to focus on your strengths and not your weaknesses, who you are and not who you aren't, and what is grand and good in life instead of what is wrong. This is the way to fulfillment, contentment, and the good life.

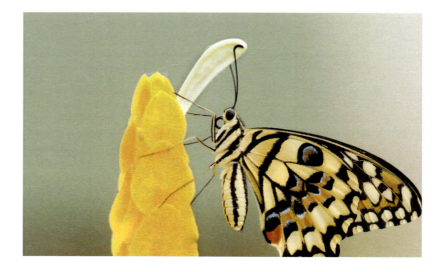

FINAL REFLECTION: Review the *10 Principles of Recovery*. What do they mean to you now? How do they fit into your life going forward?

RESOURCES

INTRODUCTION

Books
Dziurda, K. (2017). Gratitude Journal: A 52 Week Challenge to Mastering the Art of Gratitude and Positively Transforming Your Life. Scotts Valley, CA: CreateSpace.
Patel, M. L. (2015). Start Where You Are: A Journal for Self-Exploration. New York: TarcherPerigee.
Pennebaker, J.W., & Smyth, J.M. (2016). Opening Up by Writing It Down: How Expressive Writing Improves Health and Eases Emotional Pain. New York: Guilford Press.
Piccadilly Inc. (2017). 3000 Questions About Me. Del Mar, CA: Piccadilly.
Seligman, M. (2011). Flourish: A Visionary New Understanding of Happiness and Well-being. New York: Free Press.

Videos
PERMA explained by Martin Seligman - https://youtu.be/iK6K_N2qe9Y

Websites & Others
Center for Journal Therapy - https://journaltherapy.com/
PERMA Theory by UPenn's Positive Psychology Center - https://ppc.sas.upenn.edu/learn-more/perma-theory-well-being-and-perma-workshops
A Total Beginner's Guide to Keeping a Journal - https://www.thecut.com/2017/08/a-beginners-guide-to-keeping-a-journal.html
University of Pennsylvania's Authentic Happiness Website- https://www.authentichappiness.sas.upenn.edu/

MODULE 1 – HAPPINESS, VALUES & THE BRAIN

Books
Doidge, N. (2007). The Brain That Changes Itself: Stories of Personal Triumph from the Frontiers of Brain Science. New York: Viking.
Edelman, G. (1993). Bright Air, Brilliant Fire: On the Matter of the Mind. New York: BasicBooks.
Erikson, E.H., & Eriskon, J.M. (1998). Life Cycle Completed. New York: W.W. Norton & Company.

Videos
The Chemistry of Addiction - https://youtu.be/ukFjH9odsXw
Emily Esfahani Smith – There's More to Life than Being Happy TED Talk - https://youtu.be/y9Trdafp83U
Neuroplasticity in animation by Sentis - https://youtu.be/ELpfYCZa87g
Mechanisms of Drug Addiction and the Brain - https://youtu.be/NxHNxmJv2bQ
Robert Waldinger - What Makes a Good Life? Lessons from the longest study on happiness TED Talk - https://youtu.be/8KkKuTCFvzI
The Wall inspirational story - https://www.passiton.com/inspirational-stories-tv-spots/85-the-wall

Websites & Others
Brain Science Podcast – Episode #10 "Neuroplasticity: A Review of its Discovery"
Greater Good Magazine - https://greatergood.berkeley.edu/
The Science of Addiction: Genetics and the Brain by University of Utah's Genetic Science Learning Center - https://learn.genetics.utah.edu/content/addiction/
Substance Abuse and Mental Health Services Administration - https://www.samhsa.gov/

MODULE 2 – EMOTIONS

Books
Bariso, J. (2018). EQ, Applied: The Real-World Guide to Emotional Intelligence. Brooklyn, NY: Borough Hall.
Barrett, L.F. (2017). How Emotions Are Made: The Secret Life of the Brain. New York: Houghton Mifflin Harcourt.
Berger, A. (2011). Self-Regulation: Brain, Cognition, and Development. Washington, DC: APA Books.
Brackett, M. (2019). Permission to Feel: Unlocking the Power of Emotions to Help Our Kids, Ourselves, and Our Society Thrive. New York: Celadon Books.
Fredrickson, B.L. (2009). Positivity: Top-Notch Research Reveals the 3-to-1 Ratio That Will Change Your Life. New York: Three Rivers Press.
Goleman, D. (2012). Emotional Intelligence: Why it Can Matter More than IQ. New York: Random House.
McLaren, K. (2010). The Language of Emotions: What Your Feelings are Trying to Tell You. Boulder, CO: Sounds True.

Videos
Lisa Feldman Barrett – You Aren't at the Mercy of your Emotions TED Talk - https://youtu.be/0gks6ceq4eQ
PBS This Emotional Life - https://www.pbs.org/show/this-emotional-life/
Barbara Fredrickson – Positive Emotions Open Our Mind - https://youtu.be/Z7dFDHzV36g
Ryan Martin – Why We Get Mad—And Why It's Healthy TED Talk - https://youtu.be/0rAngiiXBAc
Tiffany Watt Smith – The History of Human Emotions TED Talk - https://youtu.be/S-3qnZrVy9o

Websites & Others
Atlas of Emotions - http://atlasofemotions.org/
Emotional Intelligence Consortium - http://www.eiconsortium.org/
Yale Center for Emotional Intelligence - http://ei.yale.edu/

MODULE 3 – THE PROCESS OF CHANGE

Books
Gawain, S. (2010). Creative Visualization: Use the Power of Your Imagination to Create What You Want in Your Life. Novato, CA: Nataraj Publishing.
Heath, C. & Heath, D. (2010). Switch: How to Change Things When Change is Hard. New York: Broadway Books.
Prochaska, J.O., Norcross, J., & DiClemente, C. (2007). Changing for Good: A Revolutionary

RESOURCES

Six-stage Program for Overcoming Bad Habits and Moving Your Life Positively Forward. New York: Quill.

Prochaska, J.O. & Prochaska, J.M. (2016). Changing to Thrive: Overcome the Top Risks to Lasting Health and Happiness. Center City, MN: Hazelden Publishing

Videos

Barbara Corcoran – Rethinking Failure TEDx Talk - https://youtu.be/kU1DI8HsYAg
Carol Dweck – The Power of Believing That You Can Improve TED Talk - https://youtu.be/_X0mgOOSpLU
Daniel Amen – Change Your Brain, Change Your Life TEDx Talk- https://youtu.be/MLKj1puoWCg
Daniel Amen – The Most Important Lesson From 83,000 Brain Scans TEDx Talk - https://youtu.be/esPRsT-lmw8
Michael Merzenich – Growing Evidence of Brain Plasticity TED Talk - https://youtu.be/Z41BTeAU7DI
Adam Leipzig – How to Know Your Life Purpose in 5 Minutes TEDx Talk - https://youtu.be/vVsXO9brK7M

Websites & Others

The Best Possible Self Exercise - https://blogs.psychcentral.com/character-strengths/2012/09/the-best-possible-self-exercise-boosts-hope/

MODULE 4 – POSITIVE PSYCHOLOGY & ADDICTION

Books

Ben-Shahar, T. (2007). Happier: Learn the Secrets to Daily Joy and Lasting Fulfillment. New York: McGraw-Hill.
Benard, B. (2004). Resiliency: What We Have Learned. San Francisco: WestEd.
Boniwell, I. (2012). Positive Psychology in a Nutshell: The Science of Happiness. New York: Open University Press.
Bryant, F.B., & Veroff, J. (2006). Savoring: A New Model of Positive Experience. Mahwah, NJ: Lawrence Erlbaum.
Csikszentmihalyi, M. (2008). Flow: The Psychology of Optimal Experience. New York: HarperCollins.
Dweck, C.S. (2007). Mindset: The New Psychology of Success. New York: Ballantine Books.
Edwards, H. (2019). The Daily Better: 365 Reasons for Optimism. Highlands Ranch, CO: Authors Place.
Emmons, R.A. (2008). Thanks!: How Practicing Gratitude Can Make You Happier. Boston: Houghton Mifflin.
Emmons, R.A. (2014). Gratitude Works!: A 21-Day Program for Creating Emotional Prosperity. San Francisco: Jossey-Bass.
Gillham, J.E. (2000). The Science of Optimism and Hope. Conshohocken, PA: Templeton Foundation.
Grazer, B., & Fishman, C. (2016). A Curious Mind: The Secret to a Bigger Life. New York: Simon & Schuster.
Kabat-Zinn, J. (2005). Wherever You Go, There You Are: Mindfulness Meditation in Everyday Life. New York: Hachette Books.

Kashdan, T.B. (2010). Curious?: Discover the Missing Ingredient to a Fulfilling Life. New York: HarperCollins.

Leslie, I. (2015). Curious: The Desire to Know and Why Your Future Depends On It. New York: Basic Books.

Lopez, S.J. (2014). Making Hope Happen: Create the Future You Want for Yourself and Others. New York: Atria.

Lyubomirsky, S. (2008). The How of Happiness: A New Approach to Getting the Life You Want. New York: Penguin Press.

Seligman, M.E. (1990). Learned Optimism: How to Change Your Mind and Your Life. New York: Free Press.

Seligman, M.E. (2018). The Hope Circuit: A Psychologist's Journey from Helplessness to Optimism. New York: Hachette Books.

Sharot, T. (2012). The Optimism Bias: A Tour of the Irrationally Positive Brain. New York: Vintage Books.

Snyder, C.R. (2003). The Psychology of Hope: You Can Get Here from There. New York: Free Press.

Watkins, P. (2013). Gratitude and the Good Life: Toward a Psychology of Appreciation. New York: Springer.

Williams, M., Teasdale, J., Segal, Z., & Kabat-Zinn, J. (2007). The Mindful Way Through Depression: Freeing Yourself from Chronic Unhappiness. New York: Guilford Press.

Videos

Andy Puddicombe – All It Takes Is 10 Mindful Minutes TED Talk - https://youtu.be/qzR62JJCMBQ

The Benefits of Gratitude lecture by Robert Emmons - https://youtu.be/RRrnfGf5aWE

Carol Dweck – Developing a Growth Mindset - https://youtu.be/hiiEeMN7vbQ

Daron Larson – Don't Try to Be Mindful - https://youtu.be/Ze6t34_p-84

David Steindl-Rast – Want to Be Happy? Be Grateful TED Talk - https://youtu.be/UtBsl3j0YRQ

Fixed vs Growth Mindset - https://youtu.be/KUWn_TJTrnU

Martin Seligman – The New Era of Positive Psychology TED Talk - https://youtu.be/9FBxfd7DL3E

Mihaly Csikszentmihalyi – Flow, the Secret to Happiness TED Talk - https://youtu.be/fXIeFJCqsPs

Neil Pasricha – The 3 A's of Awesome TED Talk - https://youtu.be/uPE0G00XFV0

Robert Emmons – Cultivating Gratitude - https://youtu.be/8964envYh58

Shauna Shapiro – The Power of Mindfulness: What You Practice Grows Stronger TEDx Talk - https://youtu.be/IeblJdB2-Vo

Tali Sharot – The Optimism Bias TED Talk - https://youtu.be/B8rmi95pYL0

Websites & Others

365 Grateful - https://365grateful.com/

American Psychologist, Volume 55, Issue 1 (January 2000)

Big Life Journal - https://biglifejournal.com/

Gratitude by Greater Good Magazine - https://greatergood.berkeley.edu/topic/gratitude/definition

Gratitude Works, Dr. Robert Emmons' lab - https://emmons.faculty.ucdavis.edu/

Guided Meditations provided by UCLA Health - https://www.uclahealth.org/marc/mindful-meditations

RESOURCES

Just One Thing: Be Mindful of the Good - https://greatergood.berkeley.edu/article/item/just_one_thing_be_mind_full_of_good
Mindful Magazine - https://www.mindful.org/
Mindfulness and Positive Thinking - https://www.pursuit-of-happiness.org/science-of-happiness/positive-thinking/
Mindfulness Apps: 10% Happier, Calm, Headspace, Insight Timer
Mindfulness Exercises - https://mindfulnessexercises.com/
Positive Psychology Center at University of Pennsylvania - https://ppc.sas.upenn.edu/
The Positive Psychology People - https://www.thepositivepsychologypeople.com/
Resilience by American Psychological Association - https://www.apa.org/topics/resilience

MODULE 5 – SELF-ESTEEM

Books
Branden, N. (1985). Honoring the Self: Self-Esteem and Personal Transformation. New York: Bantam Books.
Branden, N. (1994). The Six Pillars of Self-Esteem. New York: Bantam Books.
Brown, B. (2010). The Gifts of Imperfection: Let Go of Who You Think You're Supposed to Be and Embrace Who You Are. Center City, MN: Hazelden.
Kay, K., & Shipman, C. (2014). The Confidence Code: The Science and Art of Self-Assurance—What Women Should Know. New York: HarperCollins.
Peterson, C., & Seligman, M.E. (2004). Character Strengths and Virtues: A Handbook and Classification. Oxford: Oxford University Press.

Videos
Brené Brown – Are People Doing the Best They Can? - https://youtu.be/zas2oJJS2qY
Brené Brown on Faking It, Perfectionism and Living Wholeheartedly - https://youtu.be/_YeulUgWNp8
Self-Esteem - https://youtu.be/wC9S_fFMnaU
Thomas Curran – Our Dangerous Obsession with Perfectionism is Getting Worse TED Talk - https://youtu.be/lFG1b1-EsW8

Websites & Others
Perfectionism Is a Disease - https://greatergood.berkeley.edu/article/item/perfectionism_is_a_disease

MODULE 6 – SELF-COMPASSION, CONFIDENCE, & SPIRITUALITY

Books
Brach, T. (2003). Radical Acceptance: Embracing your life with the heart of a Buddha. New York: Bantam.
Bloom, W. (2011). Power of Modern Spirituality: Your Guide to a Life of Compassion and Personal Fulfilment. London: Piatkus Books.
Brown, B. (2007). I Thought It Was Just Me (but it isn't): Making the Journey from "What Will People Think?" to "I Am Enough". New York: Avery.
Frankl, V.E. (2006). Man's Search for Meaning. Boston: Beacon Press.

Linley, A., Willars, J., & Biswas-Diener, R. (2010). The Strengths Book: Be Confident, Be Successful, and Enjoy Better Relationships by Realising the Best of You. Coventry, UK: CAPP Press.
Neff, K. (2015). Self-Compassion: The Proven Power of Being Kind to Yourself. New York: HarperCollins.
Newberg, A., & Waldman, M.R. (2006). Why We Believe What We Believe: Uncovering Our Biological Need for Meaning, Spirituality, and Truth. New York: Free Press.
Polly, S., & Britton, K.H. (Eds.) (2015). Character Strengths Matter: How to Live a Full Life. Philadelphia: Positive Psychology News.
Salzberg, S. (2002). Lovingkindness: The Revolutionary Art of Happiness. Boston, Shambhala Publications.
Vaillant, G. (2009). Spiritual Evolution: How We Are Wired for Faith, Hope, and Love. New York: Broadway Books.

Videos
Radhanath Swami – How to Find a Spiritual Connection TEDx Talk- https://youtu.be/zPB2EC0Z9z4
The Science of Character - https://vimeo.com/79444520
Tim Ferriss – Why You Should Define Your Fears Instead of Your Goals TED Talk - https://youtu.be/5J6jAC6XxAI
Tracy Thomson – The Human Brain: Hardwired for Spirituality TEDx Talk -https://youtu.be/nCeOBu6g8Kg
Why Maslow's Hierarchy of Need Matters - https://youtu.be/L0PKWTta7lU

Websites & Others
Beliefnet - https://www.beliefnet.com/
Centre for Confidence - http://www.centreforconfidence.co.uk/
Eckhart Tolle - https://www.eckharttolle.com/
Fetzer Insitute - https://fetzer.org/
Kristen Neff's Self-Compassion Website - https://self-compassion.org/
Mind & Life Institute - https://www.mindandlife.org/

MODULE 7 – BARRIERS TO CHANGE
Books
Enright, R.D. (2012). The Forgiving Life; A Pathway to Overcoming Resentment and Creating a Legacy of Love. Washington, DC: American Psychological Association.
Herman. J. (2015). Trauma and Recovery: The Aftermath of Violence—From Domestic Abuse to Political Terror. New York: Basic Books.
Joseph, S. (2013). What Doesn't Kill Us; The New Psychology of Posttraumatic Growth. New York: Basic Books.
Luskin, F. (2003). Forgive for Good. New York: HarperSanFrancisco.
McCullough, M.E. (2008). Beyond Revenge: The Evolution of the Forgiveness Instinct. San Francisco: Jossey-Bass.
McGonigal, K. (2013). The Willpower Instinct: How Self-Control Works, Why It Matters, and What You Can Do to Get More of It. New York: Avery.
Nussbaum, M.C. (2018). Anger and Forgiveness: Resentment, Generosity, Justice. New York: Oxford University Press.

RESOURCES

Pennebaker, J.W. (2004). Writing to Heal: A Guided Journal for Recovering from Trauma and Emotional Upheaval. Oakland: Raincoast Books.
Tedeschi, R.G., & Moore, B.A. (2016). The Posttraumatic Growth Workbook: Coming Through Trauma Wiser, Stronger, and More Resilient. Oakland: New Harbinger.
Tutu, D., & Tutu, M. (2014). The Book of Forgiving: The Fourfold Path for Healing Ourselves and Our World. New York: HarperOne.
Van der Kolk, B. (2015). The Body Keeps the Score: Brain, Mind, and Body in the Healing of Trauma. New York: Penguin Books.
Viscott, D. (1997). Emotional Resilience: Simple Truths for Dealing with the Unfinished Business of Your Past. New York: Three Rivers Press.
Williams, M.B., & Poijula, S. (2016). The PTSD Workbook: Simple, Effective Techniques for Overcoming Traumatic Stress Symptoms. Oakland: New Harbinger.
Worthington, E.L. (2013). Moving Forward: Six Steps to Forgiving Yourself and Breaking Free from the Past. Colorado Springs, CO: WaterBrook Press.

Videos
Aicha el-Wafi + Phyllis Rodriguez – The Mothers Who Found Forgiveness and Friendship TED Talk - https://youtu.be/bKQA6I4BA7o
Barry Schwartz – The Paradox of Choice TED Talk - https://youtu.be/VO6XEQIsCoM
Brené Brown – Listening to Shame TED Talk - https://youtu.be/psN1DORYYV0
John Rigg – The Effect of Trauma on the Brain and How it Affects Behaviors TEDx Talk - https://youtu.be/m9Pg4K1ZKws
Joshua Prager – In Search of the Man Who Broke My Neck TED Talk - https://youtu.be/3Z6x5t5A9so
The Link Between Trauma & Substance Abuse - https://youtu.be/aj4RCxjQIkY
Maximizers vs. Satisficers - https://youtu.be/9FshTCGZy-A
The Paradox of Trauma-Informed Care - https://youtu.be/jFdn9479U3s
Shaka Senghor – Why Your Worst Deeds Don't Define You TED Talk - https://youtu.be/GtXyGFMBWBs

Websites & Others
10 Extraordinary Examples of Forgiveness - https://listverse.com/2013/10/31/10-extraordinary-examples-of-forgiveness/
10 Great Moments in Forgiveness History - http://incharacter.org/archives/forgiveness/ten-great-moments-in-forgiveness-history/
Black Dog Institute - https://www.blackdoginstitute.org.au/
Brené Brown - https://brenebrown.com/
Everett Worthington - http://www.evworthington-forgiveness.com/
International Forgiveness Institute - https://internationalforgiveness.com/
Repairng Bad Memories by MIT Technology Review - https://www.technologyreview.com/2013/06/17/177763/repairing-bad-memories/
VA Approved PTSD Apps - https://www.ptsd.va.gov/appvid/mobile/index.asp

MODULE 8 – ADDICTIVE THINKING

Books
Burns, D.D. (1999). The Feeling Good Handbook. New York: Plume.

Chamberlain, M. (2000). Wanting More: The Challenge of Enjoyment in the Age of Addiction. Salt Lake City, UT: Shadow Mountain.
Clark, D.A., & Beck, A.T. (2011): The Anxiety and Worry Workbook: The Cognitive Behavioral Solution. New York: Guilford Press.
Hariman, R. (Ed.) (2003). Prudence: Classical Virtue, Postmodern Practice. University Park, PA: Pennsylvania State University Press.
Helmstetter, S. (2017). What to Say When You Talk to Your Self. New York: Gallery Books.
Hess, E.D., & Ludwig, K. (2017). Humility Is the New Smart: Rethinking Human Excellence in the Smart Machine Age. Oakland: Berrett-Koehler Publishers.
Twerski, A.J. (1997). Addictive Thinking: Understanding Self-Deception. Center City, MN: Hazelden.
Worthington, E.L. (2007). Humility: The Quiet Virtue. Philadelphia: Templeton Foundation.

Videos
Brené Brown on Blame - https://youtu.be/RZWf2_2L2v8
David Burns – Feeling Good TEDx Talk - https://youtu.be/H1T5uMeYv9Q
How Denial Works: Inside the Mind of an Addict - https://youtu.be/PDJAcvquL-g
Michael Shermer – The Pattern Behind Self-Deception TED Talk - https://youtu.be/ODKUnO7aZ8k
The Psychology of Self-Deception - https://youtu.be/Uig8Lw7ixI0
Rory Sutherland – Perspective is Everything TED Talk - https://youtu.be/iueVZJVEmEs

Websites & Others
Beck Institute for Cognitive Behavioral Therapy - https://beckinstitute.org/
David Burns - https://feelinggood.com/
Why Saying Is Believing – The Science of Self-Talk - https://www.npr.org/sections/health-shots/2014/10/07/353292408/why-saying-is-believing-the-science-of-self-talk

MODULE 9 – RELATIONSHIPS & COMMUNICATION

Books
Arbinger Institute (2015). The Anatomy of Peace: Resolving the Heart of Conflict. Oakland, CA: Berrett-Koehler Publishers.
Beattie, M. (1986). Codependent No More: How to Stop Controlling Others and Start Caring for Yourself. Center City, MN: Hazelden
Cloud, H., & Townsend, J. (2017). Boundaries: When to Say Yes, How to Say No To Take Control of Your Life. Grand Rapids, MI: Zondervan.
Ferrucci, P. (2007). The Power of Kindness: The Unexpected Benefits of Leading a Compassionate Life. New York: Tarcher/Penguin.
Fredrickson, B.L. (2013). Love 2.0: Finding Happiness and Health in Moments of Connection. New York: Hudson Street Press.
Gottman, J.M., & Silver, N. (2000). Seven Principles for Making Marriage Work: A Practical Guide from the Country's Foremost Relationship Expert. New York: Three Rivers Press
Hendrix, H. (2007). Getting the Love You Want: A Guide for Couples. New York: Holt.
Johnson, S. (2008). Hold Me Tight: Seven Conversations for a Lifetime of Love. New York: Hachette Book Group.
Keltner, D., Marsh, J., & Smith, J.A. (Eds.) (2010). The Compassionate Instinct: The Science of Human Goodness. Berkeley, CA: Greater Good Science Center.

RESOURCES

Krznaric, R. (2015). Empathy: Why It Matters, and How to Get It. New York: Perigee.
Levine, A., & Heller, R.S.F. (2012). Attached: The New Science of Adult Attachment and How It Can Help You Find—and Keep—Love. New York: TarcherPerigee.
Lieberman, M.D. (2013). Social: Why Our Brains Are Wired to Connect. New York: Crown Publishers.
Markova, D. (1996). Open Mind: Discovering the Six Patterns of Natural Intelligence. Boston: Red Wheel/Weiser.
McLaren, K. (2013): The Art of Empathy: A Complete Guide to Life's Most Essential Skill. Boulder, CA: Sounds True.
Mirivel, J.C. (2014). The Art of Positive Communication: Theory and Practice. New York: Peter Lang.
Pileggi Pawelski, S., & Pawelski, J.O. (2018). Happy Together: Using the Science of Positive Psychology to Build Love That Lasts. New York: Tarcher and Perigee.
Putnam, R.D., & Feldstein, L. (2004). Better Together: Restoring the American Community. New York: Simon & Schuster.
Rosenberg, M.B. (2015). Nonviolent Communication: A Language of Life, Life-Changing Tools for Healthy Relationships. Encinitas, CA: PuddleDancer Press.
Ruiz, D.M. (1999). The Mastery of Love: A Practical Guide to the Art of Relationship. San Rafael, CA: Amber-Allen.
Siegel, D.J. (2011). Mindsight: Transform Your Brain with the New Science of Empathy. New York: Bantam Books.
Socha, T.J., & Pitts, M.J. (Eds.) (2012). The Positive Side of Interpersonal Communication. New York: Peter Lang.
Stone, D., Patton, B., & Heen, S. (2010). Difficult Conversations: How to Discuss What Matters Most. New York: Penguin Books.

Videos

Brené Brown on Empathy - https://youtu.be/1Evwgu369Jw
Celeste Headlee – 10 Ways to Have a Better Conversation TED Talk - https://youtu.be/R1vskiVDwl4
David Brooks – The Social Animal TED Talk - https://youtu.be/rGfhahVBIQw
Four Horsemen of the Apocalypse by The Gottman Institute - https://youtu.be/1o30Ps-_8is
It's Not About the Nail - https://youtu.be/-4EDhdAHrOg
Joan Halifax – Compassion and the True Meaning of Empathy TED Talk - https://youtu.be/dQijrruP9c4
Johann Hari – Everything You Think You Know About Addiction Is Wrong TED Talk - https://youtu.be/PY9DcIMGxMs
Julian Treasure – 5 Ways to Listen Better TED Talk - https://youtu.be/cSohjlYQI2A
Katie Hood – The Difference Between Healthy and Unhealthy Love TED Talk - https://youtu.be/ON4iy8hq2hM
Kio Stark – Why You Should Talk to Strangers TED Talk - https://youtu.be/rFpDK2KhAgw
Laura Trice – Remember to Say Thank You TED Talk - https://youtu.be/ag-Oyn8vIPE
Mandy Len Catron – Falling in Love Is the Easy Part TED Talk - https://youtu.be/3aYWvujaT6M
Roman Krznaric – How to Start and Empathy Revolution TEDx Talk - https://www.youtube.com/watch?v=RT5X6NIJR88
Sherry Turkle – Connected, But Alone? TED Talk - https://youtu.be/t7Xr3AsBEK4
Yann Dall'Aglio – Love –You're Doing It Wrong TED Talk- https://youtu.be/dJgiYBdD2VA

Websites & Others
35 Little Acts of Kindness - http://www.oprah.com/spirit/35-little-acts-of-kindness/all
36 Questions to Fall in Love - http://36questionsinlove.com/
Center for Nonviolent Communication - https://www.cnvc.org/
Centre for Family Research at Cambridge - https://www.cfr.cam.ac.uk/
The Gottman Institute - https://www.gottman.com/
Random Acts of Kindness - https://www.randomactsofkindness.org/
What Is Attachment Theory? - https://www.verywellmind.com/what-is-attachment-theory-279533

MODULE 10 – LIVING WITH INTEGRITY

Books
Brown, B. (2017). Rising Strong: How the Ability to Reset Transforms the Way We Live, Love, Parent, and Lead. New York: Random House.
Cloud, H. (2009). Integrity: The Courage to Meet the Demands of Reality. New York: Collins.
Covey, S.R. (2004). The 7 Habits of Highly Effective People: Powerful Habits in Personal Change. New York: Free Press.
Covey, S.R., Merrill, A.R., & Merrill, R.R. (1996). First Things First. New York: Free Press.
Mayer, E. (2016). The Mind-Gut Connection: How the Hidden Conversation Within Our Bodies Impacts Our Mood, Our Choices, and Our Overall Health. New York: Haper Wave.
McGonigal, K. (2016). The Upside of Stress: Why Stress Is Good for You, and How to Get Good at It. New York: Avery.
McGonigal, K. (2019). The Joy of Movement: How Exercise Helps Us Find Happiness, Hope, Connection, and Courage. New York: Penguin Random House.
McKeown, G. (2014). Essentialism: The Disciplined Pursuit of Less. New York: Crown Business.
Nagoski, E., & Nagoski, A. (2019). Burnout: The Secret to Unlocking the Stress Cycle. New York: Ballentine Books.
Pollan, M. (2008). In Defense of Food: An Eater's Manifesto. New York: Penguin Press.
Ratey, J.J., & Hagerman, E. (2013). Spark: The Revolutionary New Science of Exercise and the Brain. New York: Little, Brown and Company.
Sapolsky, R.M. (2004). Why Zebras Don't Get Ulcers, Third Edition. New York: Henry Holt and Company.
Simons, T. (2008). The Integrity Dividend: Leading by the Power of Your Word. San Francisco: Jossey-Bass.
Tribole, E., & Resch, E. (2020). Intuitive Eating, 4th Edition: A Revolutionary Anti-Diet Approach. New York: St. Martin's Griffin.
Vaillant, G.E. (2003). Aging Well: Surprising Guideposts to a Happier Life from the Landmark Harvard Study of Adult Development. New York: Little, Brown and Company.

Videos
Arianna Huffington – How to Succeed? Get More Sleep TED Talk - https://youtu.be/nncY-MA1lu8
A Complete Guide to Goal Setting - https://youtu.be/XpKvs-apvOs
Kelly McGonigal – How to Make Stress Your Friend TED Talk - https://youtu.be/RcGyVTAoXEL
Patti Dobrowolski – Draw Your Future TEDx Talk - https://youtu.be/zESeeaFDVSw
A Proven Way to Handle Stress - https://youtu.be/VFFp8GyQM00
Russell Foster – Why Do We Sleep? TED Talk - https://youtu.be/LWULB9Aoopc

RESOURCES

Websites & Others
Intuitive Eating - https://www.intuitiveeating.org/
Life Kits Podcast by NPR – Do This Today to Sleep Well Tonight - https://www.npr.org/2019/03/20/705224359/do-this-today-to-sleep-well-tonight
Life Kits Podcast by NPR - Get Started Exercising - https://www.npr.org/2018/12/12/676129459/get-started-exercising
Life Kits Podcast by NPR - Trust Your Gut: A Beginner's Guide to Intuitive Eating - https://www.npr.org/2019/05/23/726236988/trust-your-gut-a-beginners-guide-to-intuitive-eating
How to Sleep Better - https://www.headspace.com/sleep/how-to-sleep-better
Sleep Foundation - https://www.sleepfoundation.org/
Transparency International - https://www.transparency.org/

CONCLUSION

Books
Biswas-Diener, R. (2012). The Courage Quotient: How Science Can Make You Braver. San Francisco: Jossey-Bass.
Brown, B. (2015). Daring Greatly: How the Courage to Be Vulnerable Transforms the Way We Live, Love, Parent, and Lead. New York: Avery.
Keltner, D. (2009). Born to Be Good: The Science of a Meaningful Life. New York: W.W. Norton & Company.
Post, S., & Neimark, J. (2008). Why Good Things Happen to Good People: How to Live a Longer, Healthier, Happier Life by the Simple Act of Giving. New York: Broadway Books.
Schwartz, B., & Sharpe, K. (2011). Practical Wisdom: The Right Way to Do the Right Thing. New York: Riverhead Books.
Sheldon, K.M. (2014). Optimal Human Being: An Integrated Multi-level Perspective. New York: Routledge.

Videos
Anthony Cheam – You 2.0: What It Really Takes to Be the Best Version of Yourself TEDx Talk - https://youtu.be/M45HDbaW1DI
Angela Duckworth – Grit: The Power of Passion TED Talk - https://youtu.be/H14bBuluwB8
Call to Courage – Brené Brown Netflix Special
Discussion of The Four Agreements by Don Miguil Ruiz - https://youtu.be/ZBwY1YHMZr4
Matt Cutts – Try Something New for 30 Days TED Talk - https://youtu.be/UNP03fDSj1U
Randy Pausch Last Lecture: Achieving Your Childhood Dreams - https://youtu.be/ji5_MqicxSo

Websites & Others
Self-Determination Theory - http://selfdeterminationtheory.org/

MY NOTES:

REFERENCES

Akhtar, M., & Boniwell, I. (2010). Applying Positive Psychology to Alcohol-Misusing Adolescents: A group intervention. *Groupwork: An Interdisciplinary Journal for Working with Groups, 20(3)*, 6–31. https://doi.org/10.1921/095182410x576831.

Allen, T. M., & Lo, C. C. (2010). Religiosity, Spirituality, and Substance Abuse. *Journal of Drug Issues, 40(2)*, 433–459. https://doi.org/10.1177/002204261004000208.

Amenta, S., Noël, X., Verbanck, P., & Campanella, S. (2012). Decoding of emotional components in complex communicative situations (irony) and its relation to empathic abilities in male chronic alcoholics: *An issue for treatment. Alcoholism: Clinical and Experimental Research, 37(2)*, 339–347. https://doi.org/10.1111/j.1530-0277.2012.01909.x

Angelo, F. N., Miller, H. E., Zoellner, L. A., & Feeny, N. C. (2008). "I need to talk about it": A *Qualitative Analysis of Trauma-exposed Women's Reasons for Treatment Choice.* Behavior Therapy, 39(1), 13–21. https://doi.org/10.1016/j.beth.2007.02.002.

Beattie, M. L. (1987). *Codependent No More: Stop controlling Others and Start Caring for Yourself.* Hazelden.

Beck, A. T. (1976). Cognitive Therapies and Emotional Disorders. New American Library.

Beck, J. S. (2011). *Cognitive Behavior Therapy: Basics and Beyond.* Guilford Press.

Ben-Shahar, T. (2008). Happier: *Learn the Secrets to Daily Joy and Lasting Fulfillment.* McGraw-Hill.

Benard, B. (2004). Resiliency: *What We Have Learned.* WestEd.

Bennett E. L., Diamond M. C., Krech D., & Rosenzweig M. R. (1964). *Chemical and Anatomical Plasticity of the Brain.* Science, 146 (3644), 610-619. doi:10.1126/science.146.3644.610.

Bolier, L., Haverman, M., Westerhof, G. J., Riper, H., Smit, F., & Bohlmeijer, E. (2013). Positive Psychology Interventions: *A Meta-Analysis of Randomized Controlled Studies.* BMC Public Health, 13(1). https://doi.org/10.1186/1471-2458-13-119.

Boniwell, I. (2012). Positive *Psychology* in a Nutshell: The Science of Happiness. Open University Press.

Borrell-Carrió, F., Suchman, A. L., & Epstein, R. M. (2004). *The Biopsychosocial Model 25 Years later: Principles, Practice, and Scientific Inquiry.* Annals of Family Medicine, 2(6), 576–582. doi:10.1370/afm.245.

Bowlby, J. (1984). *Attachment*. Penguin.

Branden, N. (1994). *The Six Pillars of Self-esteem*. Bantam.

Branden, N. (2004). *Honoring the Self: Self-esteem and Personal Transformation*. Bantam.

Bremner J. D. (2006). T*raumatic Stress: Effects on the Brain. Dialogues in Clinical Neuroscience,* 8(4), 445–461.

Bretherton, I. (1992). *The Origins of Attachment Theory:* John Bowlby and Mary Ainsworth. Developmental Psychology, 28(5), 759–775. https://doi.org/10.1037/0012-1649.28.5.759.

Brown, B. (2007). I Thought It Was Just Me (but it isn't): *Making the Journey from "What Will People Think?" to "I Am Enough"*. Avery.

Brown, B. (2010). The gift of imperfection: *Let Go of Who You Think You're Supposed to Be and Embrace Who You Are*. Hazelden.

Brown, B. (2019). *Dare to lead: Brave Work, Tough Conversations, Whole Hearts.* Random House.

Bryant, F. B., & Veroff, J. (2007). *Savoring A New Model of Positive Experience*. Lawrence Erlbaum Associates.

Burke, D. (2006, October 5). *Amish Search for Healing, Forgiveness After 'The Amish 9/11'*. Religion News Service. https://web.archive.org/web/20061021051654/http://www.religionnews.com/ArticleofWeek100506.html.

Burns, D. D. (2012). *Feeling Good: The New Mood Therapy*. New American Library.

Buss, D. M. (1990). *The Evolution of Anxiety and Social Exclusion*. Journal of Social and Clinical Psychology, 9(2), 196–201. https://doi.org/10.1521/jscp.1990.9.2.196.

Cabanac, M. (2002). *What is Emotion?*. Behavioural Processes, 60(2), 69–83. https://doi.org/10.1016/s0376-6357(02)00078-5.

Calhoun, L. G., & Tedeschi, R. G. (Eds.). (2006). *Handbook of Posttraumatic Growth*: Research and practice. Routledge.

Carskadon, M., & Dement, W. (2005). *Normal Human Sleep: An Overview*. In M. H. Kryger, T. Roth, & W. C. Dement (Eds.), Principles and Practice of Sleep Medicine (4th ed.). Elsevier/Saunders.

Conti, R. (2000). *College goals: Do Self-Determined and Carefully Considered Goals Predict Intrinsic Motivation, Academic Performance, and Adjustment During the First Semester? Social Psychology of Education*, 4, 189–211. doi:10.1023/A:1009607907509.

REFERENCES

Covey, S. R., Merrill, A. R., & Merrill, R. R. (2017). *First Things First*. Simon & Schuster.

Csikszentmihalyi, M. (2000). *The Contribution of Flow to Positive Psychology*. In J. E. Gillham (Ed.), Laws of Life Symposia Series. The Science of Optimism and Hope: Research essays in honor of Martin E. P. Seligman (p. 387–395). Templeton Foundation Press.

Csikszentmihalyi, M. (2009). Flow: *The Psychology of Optimal Experience*. Harper & Row.

David, D., Cristea, I., & Hofmann, S. G. (2018). *Why Cognitive Behavioral Therapy is the Current Gold Standard of Psychotherapy*. Frontiers in Psychiatry, 9. https://doi.org/10.3389/fpsyt.2018.00004.

Diener, E., & Seligman, M. E. P. (2002). *Very Happy People*. Psychological Science, 13(1), 81–84. https://doi.org/10.1111/1467-9280.00415.

Doidge, N. (2007). *The Brain that Changes Itself: Stories of Personal Triumph From the Frontiers of Brain Science*. Viking.

Doran, G. T. (1981). *There's a S.M.A.R.T. way to write management's goals and objectives* Management Review, 70(11), 35-36.

Dunn, D. S., & Dougherty, S. B. (2008). *Flourishing: Mental health as Living Life Well*. Journal of Social and Clinical Psychology, 27(3), 314–316. https://doi.org/10.1521/jscp.2008.27.3.314.

Dweck, C. S. (2017). *Mindset: Changing the Way You Think to Fulfill Your Potential*. Random House.

Edelman, G. M. (1992). *Bright Air, Brilliant Fire: On the Matter of the Mind*. BasicBooks.

Ekman, P., & Cordaro, D. (2011). *What is Meant by Calling Emotions Basic*. Emotion Review, 3(4), 364–370. https://doi.org/10.1177/1754073911410740.

Emmons, R. A. (2007). *Thanks!: How the New Science of Gratitude Can Make You Happier*. Houghton Mifflin.

Emmons, R. A., & McCullough, M. E. (2003). *Counting Blessings Versus Burdens: An Experimental Investigation of Gratitude and Subjective Well-being in Daily Life*. Journal of Personality and Social Psychology, 84(2), 377-389. doi: 10.1037//0022-3514.84.2.377.

Emmons, R. A., & Mishra, A. (2011). *Why Gratitude Enhances Well-Being: What We Know, What We Need to Know*. In K. M. Sheldon, T. B. Kashdan, & M. F. Steger (Eds.), Series in positive psychology. Designing positive psychology: Taking stock and moving forward (p. 248–262). Oxford University Press. https://doi.org/10.1093/acprof:oso/9780195373585.003.0016.

Emmons, R. A., & Stern, R. (2013). *Gratitude as a Psychotherapeutic Intervention*. Journal of Clinical Psychology, 69(8), 846–855. https://doi.org/10.1002/jclp.22020.

Erikson, E. H., & Erikson, J. M. (1998). *The Life Cycle Completed.* W.W. Norton.

Frankl, V. E. (2006). *Man's Search for Meaning.* Beacon Books.

Fredrickson, B. L. (1998). *What Good Are Positive Emotions?* Review of General Psychology, 2(3), 300–319. https://doi.org/10.1037/1089-2680.2.3.300.

Fredrickson, B. L. (2005). *The Broaden-and-Build Theory of Positive Emotions.* The Science of Well-Being, 216–239. https://doi.org/10.1093/acprof:oso/9780198567523.003.0008.

Fredrickson, B. L., & Branigan, C. (2005). *Positive Emotions Broaden the Scope of Attention and Thought‐Action Repertoires.* Cognition & Emotion, 19(3), 313–332. https://doi.org/10.1080/02699930441000238.

Fredrickson, B. L., & Cohn, M. A. (2008). *Positive Emotions.* In M. Lewis, J. M. Haviland-Jones, & L. F. Barrett (Eds.), Handbook of Emotions (pp. 777–796)., Guilford Press.

Fredrickson, B. L., & Losada, M. F. (2005). *Positive Affect and the Complex Dynamics of Human Flourishing.* American Psychologist, 60(7), 678–686. https://doi.org/10.1037/0003-066x.60.7.678.

Fredrickson, B. L., & Losada, M. F. (2013). *"Positive Affect and the Complex Dynamics of Human flourishing":* Correction to Fredrickson and Losada (2005). American Psychologist, 68(9), 822–822. https://doi.org/10.1037/a0034435.

Fuchs, E., & Flügge, G. (2014). *Adult Neuroplasticity: More than 40 years of research.* Neural Plasticity, 2014 (5). doi:10.1155/2014/541870.

Galanter M., & Kaskutas L.A. (Ed.). (2008). *Recent Developments in Alcoholism* (Vol. 18). Springer.

Gawain, S. (2016). *Creative Visualization: Use the Power of Your Imagination to Create What You Want In Your Life.* New World Library.

Gomez-Pinilla, F., & Hillman, C. (2013). *The Influence of Exercise on Cognitive Abilities.* Comprehensive Physiology. https://doi.org/10.1002/cphy.c110063.

Grotzkyj-Giorgi, M. (2009). *Nutrition and Addiction: Can Dietary Changes Assist with Recovery?* Drugs and Alcohol Today, 9(2), 24–28. https://doi.org/10.1108/17459265200900016.

Harris, A. H., Luskin, F. M., Benisovich, S. V., Standard, S., Bruning, J., Evans, S. & Thoresen, C. (2006). *Effects of a Group Forgiveness Intervention on Forgiveness, Perceived Stress and Trait Anger: A Randomized Trial,* Journal of Clinical Psychology, 62(6) 715-733. doi: 10.1002/jclp.20264.

Hayes, S. C., & Hofmann, S. G. (2017). *The Third Wave of Cognitive Behavioral Therapy and the Rise of Process-Based Care.* World Psychiatry, 16(3), 245–246. https://doi.org/10.1002/wps.20442.

REFERENCES

Helliwell, J., Layard, R., & Sachs, J. (2019). World Happiness Report 2019, Sustainable Development Solutions Network.

Holmes, E. A., Coughtrey, A. E., & Connor, A. (2008). *Looking at or Through Rose-Tinted Glasses? Imagery Perspective and Positive Mood*. Emotion, 8(6), 875–879. https://doi.org/10.1037/a0013617.

Jose, P. E., Lim, B. T., & Bryant, F. B. (2012). *Does Savoring Increase Happiness? A daily diary study*. The Journal of Positive Psychology, 7(3), 176–187. https://doi.org/10.1080/17439760.2012.671345.

Joseph, S. (Ed.). (2015). *Positive Psychology in Practice: Promoting Human Flourishing in Work, Health, Education and Everyday Life* (2nd ed.). John Wiley & Sons.

Kahler, C. W., Spillane, N. S., Day, A., Clerkin, E. M., Parks, A., Leventhal, A. M., & Brown, R. A. (2013). *Positive Psychotherapy for Smoking Cessation: Treatment Development, Feasibility, and Preliminary Results*. The Journal of Positive Psychology, 9(1), 19–29. https://doi.org/10.1080/17439760.2013.826716.

Keyes, C. L. M. (2002). *The Mental Health Continuum: From Languishing to Flourishing in Life*. Journal of Health and Social Behavior, 43(2), 207–222. https://doi.org/10.2307/3090197.

Knüppel, A., Shipley, M. J., Llewellyn, C. H., & Brunner, E. J. (2017). *Sugar Intake From Sweet Food and Beverages, Common Mental Disorder and Depression: Prospective Findings From the Whitehall II study*. Scientific Reports, 7(1), 6287. doi:10.1038/s41598-017-05649-7.

Koltko-Rivera, M. E. (2006). *Rediscovering the Later Version of Maslow's Hierarchy of Needs: Self-Transcendence and Opportunities for Theory, Research, and Unification*. Review of General Psychology, 10(4), 302–317. https://doi.org/10.1037/1089-2680.10.4.302.

Koob G. F. (2015). *The Dark Side of Emotion: The Addiction Perspective*. European Journal of Pharmacology, 753, 73–87. doi:10.1016/j.ejphar.2014.11.044.

Krentzman, A. R. (2013). *Review of the Application of Positive Psychology to Substance Use, Addiction, and Recovery Research*. Psychology of Addictive Behaviors, 27(1), 151–165. https://doi.org/10.1037/a0029897.

Krznaric, R. (2015). *Empathy: Why it Matters, and How to Get It*. Rider Books.

Kunc, N. (1992). *The Need to Belong: Rediscovering Maslow's Hierarchy of Needs*. In R. A. Villa, J. S. Thousand, W. Stainback, & S. Stainback (Eds.), Restructuring for Caring and Effective Education: An Administrative Guide to Creating Heterogeneous Schools (p. 25–39). Paul H. Brookes Publishing.

Kvam, S., Kleppe, C. L., Nordhus, I. H., & Hovland, A. (2016). *Exercise as a Treatment for Depression: A meta-analysis*. Journal of Affective Disorders, 202, 67–86. https://doi.org/10.1016/j.jad.2016.03.063.

Laursen, E. K. (2003). *Frontiers in Strength-Based Treatment. Reclaiming Children and Youth*: The Journal of Strength-Based Interventions, 12(1), 12–17.

Lazar, S. W., Kerr, C. E., Wasserman, R. H., Gray, J. R., Greve, D. N., Treadway, M. T., … Fischl, B. (2005). *Meditation Experience is Associated with Increased Cortical Thickness.* NeuroReport, 16(17), 1893–1897. https://doi.org/10.1097/01.wnr.0000186598.66243.19.

Leahy, R. L. (2017). *Cognitive Therapy Techniques: A Practitioner's Guide* (2nd ed.). The Guilford Press.

Leung, P. W. L., & Poon, M. W. L. (2001). *Dysfunctional Schemas and Cognitive Distortions in Psychopathology: A Test of the Specificity Hypothesis.* Journal of Child Psychology and Psychiatry, 42(6), 755–765. https://doi.org/10.1111/1469-7610.00772.

Luders, E., Toga, A. W., Lepore, N., & Gaser, C. (2009). *The Underlying Anatomical Correlates of Long-Term Meditation: Larger Hippocampal and Frontal Volumes of Gray Matter.* NeuroImage, 45(3), 672–678. https://doi.org/10.1016/j.neuroimage.2008.12.061.

Luskin, F. M. (2010). *Forgive For Good: A Proven Prescription for Health and Happiness.* HarperCollins.

Luskin, F. M., Ginzburg, K & Thoresen, C. E. (2005). *The Effect of Forgiveness Training on Psychosocial Factors in College Age Adults, Humboldt Journal of Social Relations.* Special Issue: Altruism, Intergroup Apology and Forgiveness: Antidote for a Diviced World, 29(2) 163-184.

Lyons, G. C. B., Deane, F. P., & Kelly, P. J. (2010). *Forgiveness and Purpose in Life as Spiritual Mechanisms of Recovery from Substance Use Disorders.* Addiction Research & Theory, 18(5), 528–543. https://doi.org/10.3109/16066351003660619.

Lyubomirsky, S. (2013). *The How of Happiness: A Practical Guide to Getting the Life You Want.* Piatkus.

Lyubomirsky, S., King, L., & Diener, E. (2005). *The Benefits of Frequent Positive Affect: Does Happiness Lead to Success?* Psychological Bulletin, 131(6), 803–855. https://doi.org/10.1037/0033-2909.131.6.803.

Lyubomirsky, S., Sheldon, K. M., & Schkade, D. (2005). *Pursuing happiness: The Architecture of Sustainable Change.* Review of General Psychology, 9(2), 111–131. https://doi.org/10.1037/1089-2680.9.2.111.

Martin, R. A., Ellingsen, V. J., Tzilos, G. K., & Rohsenow, D. J. (2015). *General and Religious Coping Predict Drinking Outcomes for Alcohol Dependent Adults in Treatment.* The American Journal on Addictions, 24(3), 240–245. https://doi.org/10.1111/ajad.12181.

Martin, R. A., Mackinnon, S., Johnson, J., & Rohsenow, D. J. (2011). *Purpose in Life Predicts Treatment Outcome Among Adult Cocaine Abusers in Treatment.* Journal of Substance Abuse Treatment, 40(2), 183–188. https://doi.org/10.1016/j.jsat.2010.10.002.

REFERENCES

Maslow, A. H. (1970). *Motivation and Personality* (2nd ed.). Harper & Row.

Maslow, A. H. (1999). *Towards a Psychology of Being*. John Wiley and Sons.

Matthews, G. A., Nieh, E. H., Vander Weele, C.,M., Halbert, S. A., Pradhan, R. V., Yosafat, A. S., . . . Tye, K. M. (2016). *Dorsal Raphe dopamine Neurons Represent the Experience of Social iIolation. Cell,* 164(4), 617-631. doi:http://dx.doi.org/10.1016/j.cell.2015.12.040.

McCashen, W. (2005). *The Strengths Approach: Sharing Power, Building Hope, Creating Change*. Innovative Resources.

McCoy, K. K. (2009). *Flow and Spiritual Transcendence: The Conditions of Positive Experience and Usefulness for Therapeutic Outcome in Substance Abuse Recovery.* Dissertation Abstracts International: Section B: The Sciences and Engineering, 69(8-B), 5040.

McGaffin, B. J., Lyons, G. C. B., & Deane, F. P. (2013). *Self-Forgiveness, Shame, and Guilt In Recovery From Drug and Alcohol Problems. Substance Abuse,* 34(4), 396–404. https://doi.org/10.1080/08897077.2013.781564.

McKay, M., & Fanning, P. (2016). *Self-esteem: A Proven Program of Cognitive Techniques for Assessing, Improving, & Maintaining Your Self-Esteem*. New Harbinger.

Meyer, R. P., & Schuyler, D. (2011). *Old Age and Loneliness.* The Primary Care Companion for CNS Disorders, 13(2), e1–e2. https://doi.org/10.4088/PCC.11f01172.

Miller W. (2002). *Spirituality, Treatment, and Recovery. In Galanter M. (Ed.), Recent Developments in Alcoholism*: Research on Alcoholism Treatment (pp. 391-404) (Vol. 16). Kluwer.

Mruk, C. J. (2008). *The Psychology of Self-Esteem: A Potential Common Ground for Humanistic Positive Psychology and Positivistic Positive Psychology.* The Humanistic Psychologist, 36(2), 143–158. https://doi.org/10.1080/08873260802111176.

Nakamura J., & Csikszentmihalyi M. (2014) *The Concept of Flow. In Flow and the Foundations of Positive Psychology*. Springer, Dordrecht.

Neff, K. (2003). Self-compassion: *An Alternative Conceptualization of a Healthy Attitude Toward Oneself. Self and Identity,* 2(2), 85–101. https://doi.org/10.1080/15298860309032.

Norcross, J. C., Krebs, P. M., & Prochaska, J. O. (2011). *Stages of Change*. Journal of Clinical Psychology, 67(2), p. 143-154. doi: 10.1002/jclp.20758.

Panksepp, J. (1998). *Affective Neuroscience: The Foundations of Human and Animal Emotions*. Oxford University Press.

Park, N., Peterson, C., & Seligman, M. E. P. (2004). *Strengths of Character and Well-Being*. Journal of Social and Clinical Psychology, 23(5), 603–619. https://doi.org/10.1521/jscp.23.5.603.50748.

Pennebaker, J. W. (2013). *Writing to Heal: A Guided Journal for Recovering From Trauma and Emotional Upheaval*. Center for Journal Therapy, Inc.

Pennebaker, J. W. (2017). *Expressive Writing in Psychological Science*. Perspectives on Psychological Science, 13(2), 226–229. https://doi.org/10.1177/1745691617707315.

Pennebaker, J. W., Kiecolt-Glaser, J. K., & Glaser, R. (1988). *Disclosure of Traumas and Immune Function: Health Implications for Psychotherapy*. Journal of Consulting and Clinical Psychology, 56(2), 239–245. https://doi.org/10.1037/0022-006x.56.2.239.

Peterson, C. (2006). *A Primer in Positive Psychology*. Oxford University Press.

Peterson, C., & Seligman, M. E. P. (2004). *Character Strengths and Virtues: A Handbook and Classification*. Oxford University Press.

Piliavin, J. A. (2003). *Doing Well by Doing Good: Benefits for the Benefactor*. In C. L. M. Keyes & J. Haidt (Eds.), Flourishing: *Positive Psychology and the Life Well-Lived* (p. 227–247). American Psychological Association. https://doi.org/10.1037/10594-010.

Post, S. G. (2005). *Altruism, Happiness, and Health: It's Good to Be Good*. International Journal of Behavioral Medicine, 12(2), 66–77. https://doi.org/10.1207/s15327558ijbm1202_4.

Poulin, M. J., Brown, S. L., Dillard, A. J., & Smith, D. M. (2013). *Giving to Others and the Association Between Stress and Mortality*. American journal of public health, 103(9), 1649–1655. https://doi.org/10.2105/AJPH.2012.300876.

Prochaska, J. O., Norcross, J., & DiClemente, C. (1994). *Changing for Good: A Revolutionary Six-stage Program for Overcoming Bad Habits and Moving Your Life Positively Forward*, Quill.

Rand, A. (2018). *Atlas Shrugged*. New American Library.

Rees, B. L. (1993). *An Exploratory Study of the Effectiveness of a Relaxation with Guided Imagery Protocol*. Journal of Holistic Nursing, 11(3), 271–276. https://doi.org/10.1177/089801019301100306.

Rideout, E., & Montemuro, M. (1986). *Hope, Morale and Adaptation in Patients with Chronic Heart Failure*. Journal of Advanced Nursing, 11(4), 429–438. https://doi.org/10.1111/j.1365-2648.1986.tb01270.x.

Roesch, S. C., Duangado, K. M., Vaughn, A. A., Aldridge, A. A., & Villodas, F. (2010). *Dispositional Hope and the Propensity to Cope: A Daily Diary Assessment of Minority Adolescents*. Cultural Diversity and Ethnic Minority Psychology, 16(2), 191–198. https://doi.org/10.1037/a0016114.

REFERENCES

Salovey, P. & Mayer, J. D. (1990). *Emotional Intelligence. Imagination, Cognition, and Personality*, 9, 185-211. doi:0.2190/DUGG-P24E-52WK-6CDG.

Salzberg, S. (2018). *Lovingkindness: The Revolutionary Art of Happiness.* Shambhala.

Sarason, I. G., Spielberger, C. D., & Brebner, J. M. T. (Eds.). (2005). *Stress and Emotion: Anxiety, Anger, and Curiosity* (Vol. 17). Taylor & Francis.

Sasmita A. O., Kuruvilla J., & Ling A. P. (2018). *Harnessing Neuroplasticity: Modern Approaches and Clinical Future.* The International Journal of Neuroscience, 128 (11): 1061–1077. doi:10.1080/00207454.2018.1466781.

Scherer, M., Worthington, E. L., Hook, J. N., & Campana, K. L. (2011). *Forgiveness and the bottle: Promoting Self-Forgiveness in Individuals Who Abuse Alcohol.* Journal of Addictive Diseases, 30(4), 382–395. https://doi.org/10.1080/10550887.2011.609804.

Schwartz, C., Meisenhelder, J. B., Ma, Y. & Reed, G. (2003). *Altruistic Social Interest Behaviors are Associated With Better Mental Health.* Psychosomatic Medicine, 65(5), 778-785. doi: 10.1097/01.PSY.0000079378.39062.D4.

Seligman, M. E. P. (1990). *Learned Optimism: How to Change Your Mind and Your Life.* Free Press.

Seligman, M. E. P. (2011). *Flourish: A Visionary New Understanding of Happiness and Well-Being, and How to Achieve Them.* Free Press.

Seligman, M. E. P., & Csikszentmihalyi, M. (2000). *Positive Psychology: An Introduction.* American Psychologist, 55(1), 5–14. https://doi.org/10.1037/0003-066x.55.1.5.

Seligman, M. E. P., Rashid, T., & Parks, A. C. (2006). *Positive Psychotherapy.* The American Psychologist, 61(8), 774–788. https://doi.org/10.1037/0003-066X.61.8.774.

Seligman, M. E. P., Schulman, P., Derubeis, R. J., & Hollon, S. D. (1999). *The Prevention of Depression and Anxiety.* Prevention & Treatment, 2(1). https://doi.org/10.1037/1522-3736.2.1.28a.

Seuss, D. (1960). *Oh, The Places You'll Go!* Random House.

Snyder, C. R. (2000). *Handbook of hope: Theory, Measures & Applications* (1st ed.). Elsevier. Snyder, C. R., Harris, C., Anderson, J. R., Holleran, S. A., Irving, L. M., Sigmon, S. T.

Snyder, C. R., & Lopez, S. J. (2020). *The Oxford Handbook of Positive Psychology.* Oxford University Press.

Sobell, L. C., Ellingstad, T. P., & Sobell, M. B. (2000). *Natural Recovery from Alcohol and Drug Problems:* [Methodological Review of the Research with Suggestions for Future Directions.] Addiction, 95(5), 749-764. doi:10.1046/j.1360-0443.2000.95574911.x.

Tabassum, F., Mohan, J., & Smith, P. (2016). *Association of Volunteering with Mental Well-*

Being: A Lifecourse Analysis of a National Population-Based Longitudinal Study in the UK*. BMJ Open, 6(8). https://doi.org/10.1136/bmjopen-2016-011327.

Tedeschi, R. G., & Calhoun, L. G. (2004). *TARGET ARTICLE: "Posttraumatic growth*: [Conceptual Foundations and Empirical Evidence."] Psychological Inquiry, 15(1), 1–18. https://doi.org/10.1207/s15327965pli1501_01.

Teeters, J. B., Lancaster, C. L., Brown, D. G., & Back, S. E. (2017). *Substance Use Disorders in Military Veterans: Prevalence and Treatment Challenges*. Substance Abuse and Rehabilitation, 8, 69–77. https://doi.org/10.2147/SAR.S116720.

Tod, D., Hardy, J., & Oliver, E. J. (2011). *Effects of Self-Talk: A Systematic Review*. Journal of Sport and Exercise Psychology, 33(5), 666–687. https://doi.org/10.1123/jsep.33.5.666.

Tsuno, N., Besset, A., & Ritchie, K. (2005). *Sleep and Depression*. The Journal of Clinical Psychiatry, 66(10), 1254–1269. https://doi.org/10.4088/JCP.v66n1008.

Twerski, A. (1997). *Addictive Thinking: Understanding Self-Deception*. Hazelden.

UMass. *Amherst Researcher Finds Most People Lie in Everyday Conversation*. (2002, June 10). Retrieved from https://www.umass.edu/newsoffice/article/umass-amherst-researcher-finds-most-people-lie-everyday-conversation.

US Department of Veteran Affairs. (2007, January 1). *PTSD and Problems with Alcohol use*. https://www.ptsd.va.gov/understand/related/problem_alcohol_use.asp. van der Kolk, B. (2014). [The Body Keeps the Score: Brain, Mind and Body in the Healing of Trauma.] Penguin Books.

Waisberg, J. L., & Porter, J. E. (1994). *Purpose in Life and Outcome of Treatment for Alcohol Dependence*. British Journal of Clinical Psychology, 33(1), 49–63. https://doi.org/10.1111/j.2044-8260.1994.tb01093.x.

Walton, M.A., Castro, F.G., & Barrington, E.H. (1994). *The Role of Attributions in Abstinence, Lapse, and Relapse Following Substance Abuse Treatment*. Addictive Behavior, (19)3, 319-331. doi: 10.1016/0306-4603(94)90033-7.

Wang, D., Wang, Y., Wang, Y., Li, R., & Zhou, C. (2014). *Impact of Physical Exercise on Substance Use Disorders: A Meta-Analysis*. PLoS ONE, 9(10). https://doi.org/10.1371/journal.pone.0110728.

Waterman, A. (1993). *Two Conceptions of Happiness: Contrasts of Personal Expressiveness (Eudaimonia) and Hedonic Enjoyment*. Journal of Personality and Social Psychology, 64. doi: 10.1037/0022-3514.64.4.678.

Webb, J. R., & Jeter, B. R. (2015). *Forgiveness and Problematic Substance Use*. In L. L. Toussaint, E. L. Worthington, Jr., & D. R. Williams (Eds.), Forgiveness and Health: Scientific Evidence and Theories Relating Forgiveness To Better Health (p. 139–154). Springer Science + Business Media. https://doi.org/10.1007/978-94-017-9993-5_10.

REFERENCES

Webb, J. R., Hirsch, J. K., & Toussaint, L. (2015). *Forgiveness as a Positive Psychotherapy for Addiction and Suicide:* Theory, research, and practice. Spirituality in Clinical Practice, 2(1), 48–60. https://doi.org/10.1037/scp0000054.

Wilson, N., Syme, S. L., Boyce, W. T., Battistich, V. A., & Selvin, S. (2005). *Adolescent Alcohol, Tobacco, and Marijuana Use: The Influence of Neighborhood Disorder and Hope.* American Journal of Health Promotion, 20(1), 11–19. https://doi.org/10.4278/0890-1171-20.1.11.

Wilt, J. A., Stauner, N., Lindberg, M. J., Grubbs, J. B., Exline, J. J., & Pargament, K. I. (2017). *Struggle with Ultimate Meaning: Nuanced Associations with Search for Meaning, Presence of Meaning, and Mental Health.* The Journal of Positive Psychology, 13(3), 240–251. https://doi.org/10.1080/17439760.2017.1279208.

Yoshinobu, L., Gibb, J., Langelle, C., & Harney, P. (1991). *The Will and The Ways: Development and Validation of an Individual-Differences Measure of Hope.* Journal of Personality and Social Psychology, 60(4), 570–585. https://doi.org/10.1037/0022-3514.60.4.570.

Zangeneh, M., Barmaki, R., Ala-Leppilampi, K., & Peric, T. (2007). Commentary. International Journal of Mental Health and Addiction, 5(3), 210–218. doi: 10.1007/s11469-007-9111-7.

Zemore, S. E., & Pagano, M. E. (2008). *Kickbacks from helping others: Health and recovery.* In L. Kaskutas & M. Galanter (Eds.), Recent developments in alcoholism (Vol. 18). Springer.

Parenting with Wisdom

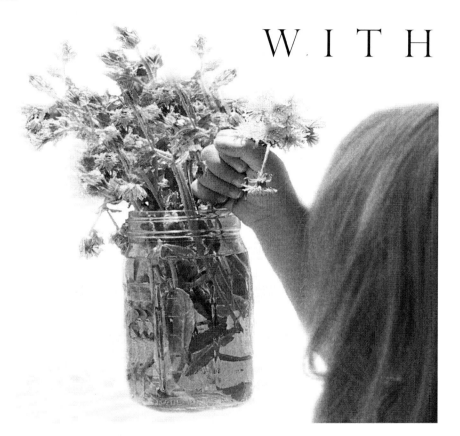

Debi Pryde

Iron Sharpeneth Iron Publications

A Ministry of Ironwood

Newberry Springs, California

TITUS 2 SERIES

Titus 2:4-8

> That they may teach the young women to be sober, to love their husbands, to love their children, to be discreet, chaste, keepers at home, good, obedient to their own husbands, that the word of God be not blasphemed. Young men likewise exhort to be sober minded. In all things showing thyself a pattern of good works: in doctrine *showing* uncorruptness, gravity, sincerity, sound speech, that cannot be condemned; that he that is of the contrary part may be ashamed, having no evil thing to say of you.

Copyright 2004 by Debi Pryde

ISBN 1-931787-12-3

LOC 2004106490

All rights reserved. No part of this book may be reproduced in any form or by any means, electronic or mechanical, or by any information storage and retrieval system, without written permission from the publisher. The only exception to this prohibition is "fair use" as defined by U.S. copyright law. All inquiries should be addressed to Iron Sharpeneth Iron Publications, 49191 Cherokee Road, Newberry Springs, CA 92365.

Unless otherwise noted, Scripture quotations are from the *King James Version*.

Managing Editor, Shannon B. Steuerwald

Photography and layout design, Susanna I. Capetz

Content layout, Allison F. Pust

Iron Sharpeneth Iron Publications

A Ministry of Ironwood

Newberry Springs, California

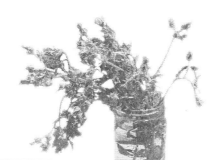

TABLE OF CONTENTS

LESSON 1
What Makes Christian Parenting Different 11

LESSON 2
The Successful Christian Parent's Secret Ingredient 27

LESSON 3
How to Really Love Your Child 41

LESSON 4
Understanding Your Child's Unique Personality 57

LESSON 5
Getting through the Bumpy Stages 85

LESSON 6
Discipline That Works, Part One 109

LESSON 7
Discipline That Works, Part Two 129

LESSON 8
Motivating Children To Do What They Don't Want To Do 149

LESSON 9
Preventing and Dealing with Rebellion 167

LESSON 10
Teaching Precept Upon Precept 197

LESSON 11
Your Child's Future: Disaster or Delight? 215

LESSON 12
Resolving Children's Problems 235

APPENDIX
Lesson Answers & Memory Verse Cards 259

About the Author

Debi and her husband Tom have been active in local church ministries for over thirty years. For the past twenty-five years, Debi has taught and led various women's ministries including seminar speaking, college-level teaching, Sunday school classes, soul-winning and visitation classes, counseling, and Bible studies. Debi is a certified Biblical counselor through Institute of Biblical Counseling in San Diego, California.

Debi and Tom reside in San Dimas, California, and continue to be active in their local church through teaching and counseling. They have two married children who are also involved in local church ministries.

How To Use Titus 2 Series Bible Study Books

The Titus 2 series of Bible study books was originally written for a ladies' Bible study group that met once a week. At that time, there were no question and answer sections, side margins for note taking, or Bible memory verses in the back. What the ladies received was a "bare bones" outline of the lesson being taught. In time, several women began asking for copies of the notes to use with their own Bible studies and expressed their desire for material that would save them time in preparation, but would allow them the freedom to use the material in their own way and with their own illustrations. What they wanted was a "skeleton" they could hang some meat on that would reflect their own teaching style and personality. One particularly enthusiastic pastor's wife suggested the format that became the first published version of the books. As the Bible study books became more widely available to others, it became obvious that the book was useful, not only for group study but for personal Bible study, one-on-one discipleship, and Biblical counseling material as well. Soon we were receiving feedback from women in various ministries who were telling us how they were using the books and how various study formats were working out for them. Following is a description of some of the more common ways people have utilized the material as well as an explanation of how the books "evolved" and why they are presented in the present format.

The original ladies' Bible group spent two or three weeks going through the material in each chapter. The material has always been very condensed which allows teachers to expand on topics within the chapter as they feel led. The major emphasis and presupposition that formed the foundation of each class session was the sufficiency of the Scriptures to provide practical guidance for women seeking to know and serve God on His terms. With time, we discovered the greatest need was not for personal illustrations, stories, or examples to be included in the notes; the greatest need was for references to Scripture that would give direction to women who were in various stages of Christian growth and who were facing a variety of challenges unique to their own age group and life circumstances. Finding life-guiding principles became very important to the ladies and led to more time being spent on explanations of Scripture passages and a greater emphasis on definitions to concepts found in the Bible.

As the studies progressed, it also became evident that some ladies were depending on "spoon feeding" rather than on learning how to study and search the Scriptures for themselves. To offset this tendency, each chapter was opened with a discussion that was developed around one related phrase of Scripture. Unlike many other passages that are explained in the notes, no hints or explanations were provided. The purpose was to provoke thought and encourage the ladies to engage in personal Bible searching, comparing Scripture with Scripture. Eventually, this one verse and phrase was given as an assignment for the following week. This worked well, but it seemed to become even more enjoyable when we grew enough to divide in little groups of three or four ladies who discussed and studied the phrase with the help of a Nave's Topical Bible, Strong's Concordance, International Standard Bible Encyclopedia, and other study aids provided for each group.

The ladies kept their own personal notes in a notebook where the three-hole punched Bible study notes were kept. They were instructed to write three things in their notes—what encouraged them in the study, what they wanted more information or help with, and what points they wanted to remember. They were also encouraged to write personal thoughts and ways they would apply the concepts to their own individual lives as a review at home. Later the notes were arranged in a workbook format with a margin on each side of the page to write these things. Once the notes were put into workbooks, the ladies adopted a system for Scripture. Eventually, this one verse and phrase was given as an assignment for the following week. This worked well, but it seemed to become even more enjoyable when we grew enough to divide in little groups of three or four ladies who discussed and studied the phrase with the help of a Nave's Topical Bible, Strong's Concordance, International Standard Bible Encyclopedia, and other study aids provided for each group.

The ladies kept their own personal notes in a notebook where the three-hole punched Bible study notes were kept. They were instructed to write three things in their notes—what encouraged them in the study, what they wanted more information or help with, and what points they wanted to remember. They were also encouraged to write personal thoughts and ways they would apply the concepts to their own individual lives as a review at home. Later the notes were arranged in a workbook format with a margin on each side of the page to write these things. Once the notes were put into workbooks, the ladies adopted a system for marking, which has become standard instruction to groups as well as counselees—put an exclamation point after comments that encourage you, put a question mark next to concepts you do not understand or want more information on, and underline points you want to remember. Personal notes and applications were written in the wide margins.

When using the books as a discipleship tool or one-on-one counseling, these marks and notes provide the springboard for discussion at each meeting and help the counselor gain understanding into the needs and thoughts of the counselee. It allows counselors to personalize the material to fit the particulars of the person with whom they are working. Many ladies have written years later commenting how precious their notes became when they reviewed their study or used it to teach others. Many leaders use the margins to write speaking notes or comments they want to include in their lessons. Counselors have said they write questions in the margins that have proven to be helpful when using the book in counseling.

You will notice that there are memory verse cards in the back of each workbook that coordinate with each chapter. Before these memory cards were included with the book, instruction was given to write the verse on a 3 x 5 card and simply read it each night before going to bed. Many of the ladies decorated little recipe boxes that were used to store the verse cards next to their bed. Each week the ladies memorized one verse, which the group practiced together. The Bible memory cards worked so well that we eventually added the "already done" cards that are now in the back of each book ready to be cut out. One group of ladies hole punches the corner of the verse cards and adds a card a week to a metal ring designed for keys. Other groups have made little pouches for the cards so the ladies can store them safely in a purse.

We are often asked if the ladies should read the lesson before or after a leader teaches it. Our group was instructed to read the lesson and do the worksheets before the meeting. The first part of the class was devoted to discussion, but we limited the discussion to those who had read the material beforehand. We found that the ladies retained more and enjoyed the lessons more when they had read ahead of time. Because the lessons will naturally vary and emphasize different concepts found in the chapter, it was not repetitious in a way that made the lesson boring. Rather, we discovered that the women who had some familiarity with the concepts because they read their homework actually enjoyed the time the most and retained the most information. The review from a different personality seems to produce better results and more significant life changes. Most groups who give us feedback agree that reading the lesson beforehand works best for them. When we use the book for one-on-one discipleship, we ask the disciplee to let us know when the material has been read and completed, and then we schedule the next meeting.

Many group leaders have written to ask how fast the material is to be taught. There is really no set timetable for teaching the material. Some teachers expand the topics and spend a month on each chapter; others like to go through a chapter a week. Our group settled into a two week per chapter schedule that worked well for them. Some leaders spend one week going through the Bible study on the first page of each chapter and the next the body of the material. Others broke the study up by breaking into small groups for the study questions and discussion and then immediately followed this with the general lesson taught to the entire group by one teacher. This system seems to be the most commonly practiced format.

One of the most interesting ways the books have been used is as an outreach to unsaved neighbors. One church spent several weeks advertising and enlisting young mothers in a neighborhood to attend a 12-week study of Biblical parenting using Parenting With Wisdom. To everyone's surprise and delight, the study interested several unsaved women, some who thought they were believers and others who readily admitted they were not, but were curious how Christians raised children. By the end of the series, many of the unsaved women were beginning to understand salvation and over sixteen ladies professed faith in the Lord Jesus Christ after the last lesson was taught on the subject of teaching children about salvation.

I have personally used the books as curriculum that satisfies many judges who assign court-ordered counseling to mothers involved in domestic violence or child abuse. When the books are used with supplemental material that addresses individual needs, they provide a structured course that can be used in a variety of ways to educate and correct problems. Twelve lessons seem to be the optimum number of lessons on one given topic, providing a start and a finish to give a sense of accomplishment and completion. One church uses the books in a discipleship program that is open to any woman wanting to participate and gives certificates of completion to those who complete all twelve lessons. I have often taken women to lunch to celebrate the completion of their book. The completion was something we both looked forward to with special anticipation and delight.

As you can see, there is not one particular way to use these books. We have one God, one way of salvation, and one Bible; yet God is also the master of variety Who delights to create snowflakes so diverse not one of them is like another. It is His pleasure to give His church many gifts, methods, and personalities to communicate the unchangeable principles of His Word. Perhaps you have ideas and suggestions unique to your group or ministry that would provide creative spark to others seeking the best approach for them. Please let us hear from you so your successes (and failures) can be a source of inspiration and direction to others! May the Lord bless your efforts to feed His sheep and may He give you special wisdom and direction as you prepare your heart to teach and encourage women.

Debi Pryde

Before You Begin

There's no such thing as a perfect mother, one who makes no mistakes. (What a relief!) The fact is, about the time you've finally gotten motherhood nailed down, your children will be grown. There were two thoughts that helped me through a lot of the bumpy stages of parenting—"Love covers a multitude of sins" and "This too shall pass."

For many years I have been burdened to write down the things I've learned about mothering that have helped me survive and live to tell about it. Some things I learned from experience, some from Bible study, and some from older mothers who have passed along things they learned to others. Most of what I have learned, however, came from my mother, who learned much from her mother.

Mom taught her four children the two most important things in life—to love God and to love others. She had the wonderful privilege of leading each of us to the Lord and saw all of us grow up to become active Christians before she unexpectedly went home to be with the Lord.

My mom has been my best friend, my confidante, my encourager, and my inspiration to be a loving mother. We spent countless hours over the years talking about children and children's problems. I could always depend on her to have uncanny wisdom when it came to understanding a child's special quirks and ways. I will miss her greatly.

The evening before Mom passed away, we were laughing and joking together. Suddenly she grew very serious and said, "You know, our life is but a vapor that appears for a moment and vanishes away." I don't remember what I said in return, but I do remember thinking it was an odd thing to say at that particular moment. She had no idea her doctor would accidentally puncture her heart during a routine procedure and she would wake up in heaven in a few short hours. As I pondered her comment I couldn't help smiling, because it was so much like my mother, and sums up her success as a mom. As she had so many times in our growing up years, she was viewing life from heaven's perspective and sharing her confidence and love for the Lord. That day, I kissed my mother good-bye, said I love you, and for the last time, saw her loving smile.

I would like to say, "Thank you, Lord, for giving me a Christian mom and a Christian dad who truly love You and their children. That is what has made all the difference in the world in our lives. Thank you, Mom and Dad, for all you invested in us. I pray I can be an encouragement to other young mothers, as you have been so often to me."

Finally, let me say thank you to my sister-in-law, Robin Milby; my dear friend, Barbara Needham; and my daughter Michelle who helped with editing and advising; my son Thomas who gave much input and advice; my husband Tom for doing all the tedious computer work; and to my Dad, who finished the editing my mother was doing, and who sacrificially gave his time to assemble the first printing of books. Precept Upon Precept was truly a family project!

With Love to All of You,

Debi

Lesson 1

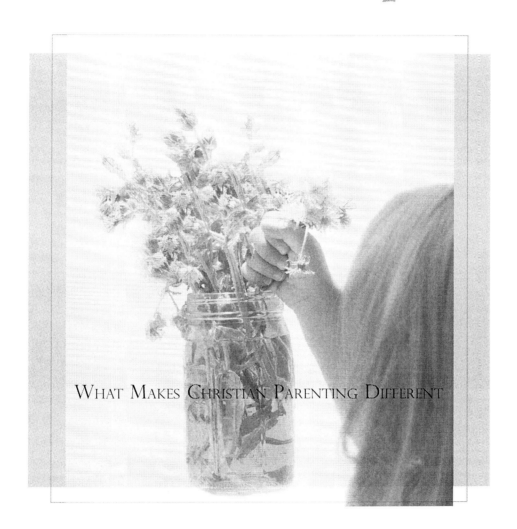

What Makes Christian Parenting Different

The father of the righteous shall greatly rejoice: and he that begetteth a wise child shall have joy of him. Thy father and thy mother shall be glad, and she that bare thee shall rejoice.
Proverbs 23:24-25

Whatsoever ye do, do all to the glory of God.
1 Corinthians 10:31b

Key THOUGHTS

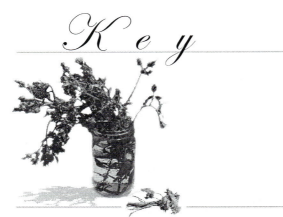

Christian parenting is built on the foundation of God's love and the authority of God's Word. The primary focus is on raising children for the glory of God, by God's strength and grace. A non-Christian philosophy of parenting has as its focus raising children for the glory of the parent through the parent's skill and ability to provide an ideal environment.

Discussion Problem

Tony, a fifteen year old, has recently announced that he doesn't want to go to church anymore. Over the past few years Tony has gradually become more lethargic at home, has taken to watching television every chance he can, and spends more and more time with a cousin who is not a Christian.

Tony's parents don't understand why Tony isn't interested in spiritual things since they have taken him to church all his life, have kept him in Christian school, and warn him constantly about bad things they do not want him to do. They spend very little time with him since they are so busy with church activities. However, they do take time to read the Bible with the family each day, emphasizing God's judgment, and using the time to preach to and correct their children.

Tony's parents openly criticize people who do not conform to their opinions, and regularly express their anger over wickedness they see in the world. They take pride in the fact that they are strict disciplinarians.

Use the principles outlined in chapter one to find possible reasons Tony could be rebelling. How could Mom and Dad be contributing to the problem? What could they do to change the situation? Do you believe their motives have been Biblical?

Bible Study

1. According to Deuteronomy 6:5-7, what is the first thing a parent must do before she can successfully teach her children about the Lord? _Love the Lord w/ all their ♥, Soul + Mind. + Teach these thing DILIGENTLY · Talk about them all ways._

2. Deuteronomy 31:12-13 explains that God wants even children to hear the Word of God so they will __hear__, __learn__, __fear__, and __observe__.

3. According to Deuteronomy 12:28, what two things does God say we must do before He will bless our home? _That which is Good + right in the sight of God._

"You can do everything else right as a parent, but if you don't begin with loving God, you're going to fail."
Alvin Griend

The Difference

Suppose an unbelieving neighbor asked you how Christian parenting differs from any other approach to raising children. What would you say? Would you begin by telling your friend how Christians discipline their children? Or would you mention differing household rules or differences in what is considered acceptable activity? Suppose your unbelieving neighbor told you she didn't believe any parent could be assured her child wouldn't one day rebel and become a wicked adult. Would you agree with her?

Many people believe the basic difference between the way Christians and unbelievers raise children is that Christians spank their children, impose strict rules, and frequently attend church services; whereas, others do not. Sadly, some folks who mistakenly believe this are professing Christians, not just unbelievers who disdain the Bible. Oftentimes Christians do not know what makes Christian parenting truly Christian, or what makes some Christian parents successful, while others are not.

The difference certainly is not spankings, rules, or church attendance. Genuine Christian parenting begins with the foundation of God's love and rests wholly on the principles of God's Word. The Bible has much to say about parenting and children—and surprisingly, it even addresses specific reasons for success and failure. The Bible tells us how crucial love is in determining the course of a child's life. The Bible tells us what precepts protect a child from error, and what concepts a child must know about God's character in order to prevent rebellion. The Bible provides parents with all the knowledge, wisdom, comfort, and encouragement they will need to successfully train their children. Most of all, the Bible provides the understanding that is so necessary to guide children toward spiritual maturity.

The goal of Christian parenting is the goal of our Lord Jesus Christ—to train our children in such ways that they will delight to know the Lord who conforms us to be like Christ and gives us His own character. The hopes and dreams of parents who love the Lord and know the joys of walking in His Spirit are for their children to likewise experience the wonders of Christ's love, joy, peace, longsuffering, gentleness, goodness, faith, meekness, and temperance. Such parents desire that their children grow to be mature believers, filled with God's Spirit, ready to be useful members of society, "perfect [mature] thoroughly furnished unto all good works" *(1 Timothy 3:17)*.

Foundation of Biblical Principles

It is not uncommon to hear unreasonable Christian parents defend their harsh actions by angrily quoting Scriptures such as, "Foolishness is bound in the heart of a child; but the rod of correction shall drive it far from him" *(Proverbs 22:15)*. It is interesting to note that such parents rarely quote with the same enthusiasm verses like, "And, ye fathers, provoke not your children to wrath: but bring them up in the nurture and admonition of the Lord" *(Ephesians 6:4)*. The tendency in a vast number of Christians is to isolate one passage of Scripture and build a philosophy or approach to parenting

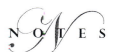

on that one passage, rather than learning the basic themes and principles of the entire Bible in order to understand the context and spirit behind each Scripture passage that deals with parenting and Christian growth.

When we dissect a single passage of Scripture in this way, we risk misinterpreting God's commands and instructions and risk misrepresenting God Himself. Scripture must always be interpreted in its context, comparing Scripture with Scripture and defining Bible words by Bible meanings. The practice of ignoring basic rules of interpretation such as these unnecessarily exposes us as well as our children to possible error and destruction. It leads us to become as the Pharisees—proud people who love to preach the letter of the law while ignoring its intent, or worse, people who add to what God said and construct their own rules of conduct.

> *The strength and wisdom of any parent rests in being a student of the Word who seeks to understand and apply basic Bible truth and precepts to everyday family life.*

Christian parenting, to be Biblical and blessed, not only rests on God's Word, but also rests in the careful handling of God's Word. The strength and wisdom of any parent rests in being a student of the Word who seeks to understand and apply basic Bible truth and precepts to everyday family life. This will require much more than finding all the verses in the Bible that mention children or parents. It requires one to recognize basic principles that have more than one application. While some passages in the Bible do indeed relate directly to parenting, there are many more passages that relate to parenting *indirectly*.

For example, Biblical principles that address our relationships with one another apply to our relationships inside our homes as well as outside. The Bible tells us "Love worketh no ill to his neighbor" *(Romans 13:10a)*. Clearly, our closest neighbors are those in our own family, including our children. This very basic principle of love applies as much to the relationship between a parent and child as it does to a husband and wife, two friends, or a co-worker and boss. This verse teaches us that genuine, godly love never hurts and destroys another person, no matter who it is. Certainly a parent who loves his child will not want to do anything that would hurt or destroy his child.

When we understand basic life principles such as these, Biblical parenting makes much more sense. In fact, if we look at Biblical parenting in the context of the entire Bible, we see that God's commands were not given to make life miserable for His people. Rather, they were given to bless and help us. Likewise, God's ways are designed to bless and help our children, not to be a source of grief and dread to them.

Good and Right, Not Cruel and Harsh

Perhaps you are wondering what part such things as spankings, rules, or church attendance have in Christian parenting. These are not what make Christian parenting Christian, yet they certainly have a place of importance *when* they are used responsibly and righteously. If they are practiced apart from a Biblical motive or outside a godly context, however, they can actually be devastating to the spiritual well being of a child. Sadly, right things done in a wrong way or for a wrong reason have the potential of tearing down the very thing a parent wishes to build.

For example, although discipline is good and right, it is possible to distort the Biblical concept of discipline to such a degree that it is actually destructive to a child and sinful on the part of the adult. Most Christians are deeply grieved when they hear about parents who cruelly beat their children and excuse it as discipline. It causes us to cringe when we hear of those who use the Bible as a weapon, who hurl distorted interpretations of Scripture at their children as a means of justifying their own selfish demands and anger. Tears come to our eyes when we encounter misguided parents who invent rules and restrictions even the Pharisees couldn't have thought up. This is not Christian parenting. In fact, it bears no resemblance to parenting that is, indeed, Biblical.

Such parenting practices ought to sadden every Christian who loves the Lord and loves His Word. It is sad because God's ways are misrepresented, God's plan for families is distorted, and we who are believers give unbelievers cause to blaspheme the goodness and wisdom of the God we serve. It is also tragic because children are severely wounded and confused by such treatment. Rather than learning how God's ways are good and right, mistreated children assume God is cruel and harsh. Proper correction may indeed involve spanking a child, but there is far more to Biblical discipline than spanking. Biblical principles of love, self-control, responsibility, and patience also play a part in correcting a child.

In the same way discipline can be distorted, so rules and restrictions can be twisted with disastrous results. Christian parenting does include enforcing reasonable limitations and healthy guidelines for a child. Yet again, the Biblical principle of love, mercy, and wisdom must also bear on the restrictions imposed on children. Likewise, Christians believe church attendance should be an important part of every child's life. However, the Lord Jesus Christ instituted the local church to be a place of loving fellowship, care, instruction, and joy. It should never be a place where children are forgotten or treated with contempt.

In the chapters that follow, we will discuss many parenting concepts that differ from a secular, non-Christian view as well as many that differ from a traditionally Christian, but unBiblical view of parenting. In doing this, our goal is to help you construct a parenting philosophy that is able to withstand Biblical scrutiny and at the same time, produce methods that will correctly and successfully implement godly principles.

No sincere believing parent wishes to fail in his or her responsibility to raise children in the nurture and admonition of the Lord, and certainly, no loving parent wishes to raise a foolish or wicked adult. Yet oftentimes, sincere and loving parents do fail to understand God's ways and implement His instructions, relying instead upon their own reasoning rather than the Bible. As in so many areas of life, "there is a way which seemeth right unto a man, but the end thereof are the ways of death" *(Proverbs 14:12)*. For this reason, it is crucial for Christian parents to resist the tendency to trust their own heart and determine instead to learn God's truth, as He defines truth, and seek His way in the matter of raising children.

Successful Christian Parenting Centers on Christ

Christian parenting is different because it has as its foundation and focus the wonderful love and mercy of a gracious God. There are moms and dads, believers and unbelievers alike, who incorporate many Christian principles into their parenting. Yet, if their motivation and focus is only their own desires, they are not practicing Biblical parenting at all. The Lord Jesus Christ is always the primary focus and motivation behind successful parenting.

	PARENTAL SELF FOCUS	**PARENTAL GOD-FOCUS**
PURPOSE OF LOVE	To bring glory to parents for raising such a successful, smart, good child.	To bring glory to God for His unmerited grace and wisdom that enables imperfect parents to raise godly children.
PURPOSE OF DISCIPLINE	To punish wrong behavior. To prevent parents from being embarrassed or disappointed. To make child easier to live with. To vent anger and intolerance for child's immaturity.	To correct wrong behavior. To instill in child a love for God's commandments that will enable him to avoid the consequences of foolish choices and help him live a life that is pleasing to God.
PURPOSE OF MOTIVATION	To instill a desire to fulfill a child's dreams and desires and win the applause of men.	To instill a desire to fulfill God's special plan for child's life and win the applause of God.
PURPOSE OF TRAINING	To develop talents and personality in such a way as to achieve success and status.	To develop God-given talents, gifts, and character in such a way as to prosper and to achieve goals through godly principles and hard work.
PURPOSE OF EXAMPLE	To instill a desire to be like parents.	To instill a desire to be like Christ.
PURPOSE OF CHRISTIAN TRAINING	To enforce rules that will prevent your child from developing undesirable habits and choices. To influence child's actions.	To prepare child to receive salvation and develop a growing, loving relationship with Christ. To influence child's heart.

Why Do Some Parents Fail?

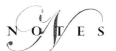

Failure often occurs when parents focus *primarily* on rules, correction, punishment, and children's mistakes rather than giving primary importance to teaching children about God's love for them, His mercy when they do make mistakes, and His great commandments and available help. So often, parents choose what is easiest and what seems to be right rather than carefully choosing what is Biblical and consequently, most effective. In this case, pointing out what is wrong and zeroing in on what is wicked is preferred over patiently taking the time to teach a child to love what is right or engaging a child in thought-provoking conversation and reasoning that will lead him to love God and love what is right. The assumption is that severe warnings will instill a fear of consequences that will cause a child to avoid sinful and destructive conduct.

First, such a conclusion ignores the fact that God says, "By the fear of the Lord men depart from evil" *(Proverbs 16:6b)*, not simply by the fear of consequences. Second, emphasizing what is wicked instead of leading a child to God's love ignores the fact that God puts major emphasis on learning what is right than learning all about evil. It is far better to encourage children to learn what is right before wrong ever becomes an issue, than to be forced to correct what is wrong later. No parent has ever succeeded in teaching a child to hate sin without first teaching the child to love righteousness. *Psalm 78* illustrates this principle very well. Read it carefully, noting the three things God instructs parents to teach their children so they will keep His commandments and not become stubborn and rebellious.

> *Psalm 78:4-8*
>
> "We will not hide *them* [God's words and commandments] from their children, showing to the generation to come the praises of the LORD, and his strength, and his wonderful works that he hath done. For he established a testimony in Jacob, and appointed a law in Israel, which he commanded our fathers, that they should make them known to their children: that the generation to come might know *them*, even the children *which* should be born; *who* should arise and declare *them* to their children: that they might set their hope in God, and not forget the works of God, but keep his commandments: and might not be as their fathers, a stubborn and rebellious generation; a generation *that* set not their heart aright, and whose spirit was not steadfast with God."

Truths To Teach Children

1. To praise the Lord.
2. To marvel at God's strength.

3. To remember the wonderful works God has done.

Reasons We Teach These Truths

1. So the children will know about them.
2. So the children will set their hope in God.
3. So the children will not forget the works of God.
4. So the children will keep God's good and gracious commandments.
5. So the children will not become stubborn and rebellious against God.

Of course children need correction and reproof. The Bible says in *Proverbs 6:23* th[at] "reproof of instruction is a way of life." *Proverbs 19:18* says, "Chasten thy son whi[le] there is hope, and let not thy soul spare for his crying." Teaching children about th[e] painful consequences of sin is absolutely necessary if they are to learn to fear it in [a] healthy way. The Bible says, "By mercy and truth iniquity is purged: and by the fe[ar] of the LORD men depart from evil" *(Proverbs 16:6)*. While the *fear of the Lord* do[es] include fearing God's consequences, it envelopes a much broader understanding [of] *fear*.

One cannot fear God without some measure of understanding with regard to God['s] character and holiness. The consequences of sin are feared *because* sin is first hated and the character and righteousness of God loved. It is this awareness of *who* Go[d] is that causes a mortal being to reverence, love, and respect Him. This is the fea[r] of God that changes who we *are*. The fear of consequences may temporarily curta[il] sinful behavior, but it will never change a child's heart or character. God want[s] parents to address the heart of the child and teach them much more than a fear [of] consequences. They are to teach them to love and respect God with the whole hear[t.] The goal is to help children mature in such a way that they learn to be motivated b[y] their love of God and desire to please Him rather than by the self-focused desire t[o] avoid pain.

According to *Galatians 5:16*, the way we overcome temptations to sin is to pou[r] our energy into walking in the Spirit, or living an obedient life by the power tha[t] indwells every believer (children included). To the degree we depend on God['s] power to work in us as we deliberately learn to obey and love doing what is right[,] is the degree we will not have a desire to do what is wrong. If we are constantl[y] focusing on the wrong we are not to do, and fail to fill our mind and time doing wha[t] is right, the wrong we desire will eventually be the very thing we will be drawn t[o] do. Parents who concentrate on filling their children's lives with good activities[,] wholesome conversation, godly goals, and God-loving people don't spend muc[h] time talking or worrying about the bad things they don't want their children to do.

Children who are brought up in this kind of happy, godly environment, and wh[o] learn to *love* godly living, do not develop a compelling desire for wicked endeavors[.] Thoughts of rebelling and desires for sinful vices are not aroused in a child's hear[t] at the same time he is enjoying the love and happiness of a truly joyful Christia[n] home. On the other hand, children brought up in an atmosphere of constant rebuke, hostility, and constant focusing on the evil they are to avoid, sometimes develop a curiosity about the very sins the parents are trying to urge them to reject. Very often, when children begin to sense that their life is oppressive, they begin to desire the very things they are being warned to avoid.

God exhorts parents not only to teach God's commands, but also to teach the benefits of keeping God's commands. He tells them not to neglect to teach their children the happy praises of the Lord. He tells them to describe His strength and wisdom to the children and teach them all about the wonderful works God does on behalf of the people He loves. We are instructed to dwell on God's infinite goodness and grace toward us. It is the first duty of parents to make the Bible precious and the Lord delightful to their children. We are to "adorn the doctrine of God our Savior in all things" (Titus 2:10b). And this, the Bible says, is what keeps children from disregarding God's commandments and becoming rebellious and stubborn.

Parents fail when they do not evangelize and spiritually nurture children.

Parents often underestimate the importance of properly evangelizing and spiritually training their children. They fail to recognize the fact that a parent can force a child to obey and conform for only so long. Eventually, if a child hasn't developed a desire to obey, he will choose his own ways and disregard God's ways. A parent's responsibility is only half done if a child is only *made* to obey. Godly parents must make every reasonable effort to instill in them a *desire* to obey as well. Sound impossible? It is, unless the child's heart is changed through salvation and taught to respond to God's gracious and loving will. Keep in mind that we are not raising puppies that have no soul or responsibility to God, or who only learn by cause and affect alone. We are involved in raising heirs to immortal life who will one day give an account of their life to their Creator. We are given the awesome responsibility of engaging a child's heart, not just his mind.

Unlike Pavlov's dogs, a child's behavior originates in his heart, and is far more than a function of his brain or operant conditioning. The heart, according to the Bible, speaks of the place where a child reasons and decides what he believes, where he weighs choices and harbors his passions and desires. What a child does, says, or thinks will ultimately be consistent with what he desires and believes at any given moment. Although parents are able to direct their attention toward affecting what a child desires and believes, only God can transform a heart, even a child's heart. Our efforts to teach our children properly are vital, yet we must have God's power and strength in order for them to be effective. Apart from God, truly we can do nothing (John 15:5).

The child whose heart is filled with resentment towards God will not conform to godly standards of living when he is finally out from under the control of his parents. External controls will cease to be an effective deterrent if a child is not governed internally by the law of God written on his heart. For this reason, every believing parent should pray and strive toward helping his child develop a sincere love for God, as well as a love for God's Word and God's ways. The place to begin is by making sure our own life reflects our sincere love for God and love for God's Word and God's ways. How often we hear reminders to diligently teach God's Word to our children as instructed in *Deuteronomy 6:6-7*. Yet how seldom we hear the command in its full context, which is preceded by the command to parents to "love the Lord thy God with all thine heart, and with all thy soul, and with all thy might." God wants his love and His Word to be in a parent's heart first—then the parent is able to spontaneously and joyfully teach children with genuine passion and conviction. Parents who ignore the first half of the command cannot presume to expect God to honor their efforts to fulfill the last half.

Parents fail when they do not have right motives.

Christian parents often fail when their motivation for parenting falls under selfish reasons rather than godly reasons. Many good parents do the right things for the wrong reasons.

For example, on the surface it would appear that a parent who sends his child to a Christian school has only the noblest motivations in mind. Yet such a choice may be futile if a parent's underlying motive is to protect his child from evil merely to avoid embarrassment for himself. A Christian school is good if a parent's motive is to give the child the best training and environment possible in order to equip his child to live a life pleasing to God.

James 1:27 says, "Pure religion and undefiled before God and the Father is this, to visit the fatherless and widows in their affliction, and to keep himself unspotted from the world." When we, or our children, keep away from the evil influences of the world, it pleases God and protects us from acquiring bad habits and destructive ways of thinking that are contrary to the truth God wants us to know. So obviously, a Christian education is a good choice for a parent to make. Nevertheless, even a good choice such as this can turn out wrong if the parent's underlying motives are wrong.

A good Christian school should be regarded as a ministry to Christian parents, not to relieve parents of their responsibility to educate and train their children, but for the purpose of helping Christian families and churches fulfill their God given responsibility to properly protect, prepare, and train children. Because a godly parent's greatest desire should be to see a child grow to be Christ-like, it is noble to want a high quality, yet truly Christian education for ones children in an environment that will help, not hinder, the development of Christian character and Christ-likeness. Nevertheless, such a parent must understand that a Christian education begins first in the home, for it is to parents that God gives the ultimate responsibility of training and educating children *(Deuteronomy 6:7, Ephesians 6:4)*.

Christian school should never be considered a substitute for the parental responsibility to train children to live the Christian life. We are never to send them in an effort to ease our conscience, to provide discipline we ourselves are responsible to give, or to protect ourselves from future embarrassment. Countless numbers of parents have sent their children to a Christian school at great personal sacrifice to keep them off drugs, out of bars, and away from sexual immorality only to wind up brokenhearted in the end. No matter how good the school, these are not godly reasons to send your children.

The issue of education is only one of many decisions that must be rooted in truly Biblical motivations. This truth applies to disciplining your children, taking them to church, imposing rules, and other similar areas. These things are good and right, but God does not bless them if our underlying motivation is for our own glory and not God's.

Parents fail when they do not receive godly instruction.

Christian parents may fail if they assume there is nothing special they need to learn about Christian parenting, or they are never given the opportunity to hear godly instruction through the ministries of a good local church. *Hosea 4:6* says, "My people are destroyed for lack of knowledge: because thou hast rejected knowledge, I will also reject thee, that thou shalt be no priest to me: seeing thou hast forgotten the law of thy God, I will also forget thy children."

Many parents learn what it means to raise children in the nurture and admonition of the Lord only after their children have grown and left home. This is a tragedy, and certainly not God's plan. All of God's children have gifts and talents that enable them to have a part in helping others grow into mature believers. God gives churches gifted people who are needed to provide good administrators, teachers, pastors, deacons, and helpers. In God's plan, He intends the mature believers to teach the younger. Specifically, God commands the older women to teach the younger mothers how to love their children.

Often older women fail to assume this responsibility and have no burden to teach and encourage the younger women. In other cases pastors fail to encourage or use qualified women to fulfill this need. Lack of knowledge often leads to failure, whether the lack of knowledge is a result of a parent's prideful refusal to believe he needs instruction, or the mature women's failure to assume their responsibility to impart knowledge, or a church's failure to give qualified parents an opportunity to fulfill this important ministry.

The Ultimate Parental Failure

Has the parent failed when a child chooses to sin? If a child makes an immature or foolish choice that results in sorrow, have his parents failed? What if a child becomes cold spiritually, and in this condition, he makes wrong decisions? Is that a direct consequence of parental failure? When we ask these questions in reference to "little" sins and little mistakes we tend to say, "Of course not. It's the nature of sinners to sin,

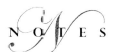

whether it involves an adult or a child." However, when we ask the same questions in reference to sins that cause major trials or devastation in a child's life, we tend to believe the parents are at fault in some way.

Perhaps in heaven we will learn that the greatest failure of parents is the failure to pray for their children's salvation, and failure to live their lives in such a way that their children are drawn to Christ.

It is true that children sometimes do make mistakes and errors in judgment because their parents failed to instruct or correct them in the way God commanded. However, it is also true that even children who were disciplined and instructed *do* sin, grievously at times.

King David knew God's law intimately, yet he sinned. Can we say his parents were at fault? When Adam sinned, was it because of some flaw in God's instruction to him or some flaw in the environment God had provided? A child's choice to sin is not always a result of poor parenting. Children, like adults, have sinful hearts that are prone to fulfilling their selfish desires and prone to resisting God's authority. They, like us, are growing and maturing spiritually. God uses the "all things" in their lives as well as in ours, to work all things together for good *(Romans 8:28)*. If our children know the Lord as their Savior, God will be faithful to correct them when sin and get off track. God uses parents in this diciplining process, but when the child is grown, He does not cease to discipline. Rather, He uses other means. It might grieve us as parents to see grown children suffering the consequences of their poor choices, but even this is part of God's plan to bring them up to spiritual maturity.

The believer can be confident that God will work in the lives of her children, if they have truly been converted. Our children's development isn't done when they leave home. The work is only done when God takes them home to heaven. God promises, "Being confident of this very thing, that he which hath begun a good work in you will perform it until the day of Jesus Christ" *(Philippians 1:6)*.

The Way He Should Go

Perhaps you have pondered the passage of Scripture that says, "Train up a child in the way he should go: and when he is old, he will not depart from it"*(Proverbs 22:6)*. Let's first determine what this verse does *not* say. This verse does not promise that your child will not sin, or suffer consequences as a result of his sin. This verse also does not promise that your child will not backslide. This verse *does* say that if you bring up your child in the way he should go, he will not depart from it when he is grown. This promise refers to bringing up a child in such a way that he would trust the Lord as his Savior and that he, as a child brought up to trust the Lord, would never grow up and reject Christ or salvation.

Many Bible scholars firmly believe that a child who grows up in a Christian home where he is lovingly taught the way he should go will never die a rebellious unbeliever. The child who is disciplined properly, loved, and trained is not going to reject salvation. However, many a godly mother has had to wait and pray fervently

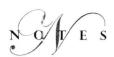

for a child's repentance and salvation. Many *negligent* parents raise moral children who do *not* grow up to be drug addicts, adulterers, or social misfits. However, the child may also never receive the Lord as his Savior. The *good* child, raised in a Christian home, who does not repent and receive salvation, was not brought up "in the way he should go." A socially acceptable, moral child who is never saved is the ultimate parental failure *(Mark 8:36)*. Remember, success as the world defines success is not how any of us will define the word in eternity.

No parent is capable of being perfect enough to raise a sinless child. No parent can impose enough rules and discipline to raise a sinless child. No parent will provide such an ideal environment that his child loses his propensity to sin. The fact is that *every* parent can make a personal list of parental failures. Every one of us is wholly dependent on God's grace and work on our children's behalf and none can take credit for what God so graciously does in the hearts of our children. What affects a child's behavior and attitude is the miraculous change of heart that takes place when the child understands repentance towards God and a loving relationship with Jesus Christ. Never forget that the salvation of our children is the result of God's grace. Parents who seek God's grace to win their children to Christ and bring them up to love God reap the blessings of a Christian home. This is successful parenting!

Do not be quick to assume a parent whose child sins is at fault. Sometimes the cause is faulty parenting, but sometimes it is not. If the child is so rebellious and worldly that he displays absolutely no evidence of salvation in his life, we do well to assume he was never really saved in the first place. In this case, the failure of the parent isn't necessarily the manner in which he raised his child, but a failure to live his own life fully surrendered to Christ, or failure to take seriously the salvation of the child and recognize the fact that it is a miracle brought by God's Spirit.

Perhaps in heaven we will learn that the greatest failure of parents is the failure to pray for their children's salvation, and failure to live their lives in such a way that their children are drawn to Christ. God promises those who live wholly surrendered to Him that they might ask what they will and it shall be done for them *(John 15:7)*. What good thing could a godly parent desire more than the salvation of his children? God cannot lie. He will save the children of parents who are saved and living godly lives.

Six Foundational Parental Responsibilities

As preparation for the remainder of this study, prayerfully consider the following six foundational responsibilities of Christian parents. Read the Bible passages with each heading, noting the direct and indirect principles that apply to parenting children. If you are doing this study with a group, discuss the passages, adding others that come to mind. Then, use the statements at the close of this chapter to self-evaluate your Biblical parenting skills, noting where you most need improvement. Fill in the blank with numbers from ten as the highest degree of master, to zero as the lowest level of practice.

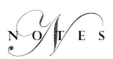

1. **Love your children.**

Love requires sacrificially investing the time, discipline, and attention children require. It means a parent will accept and love each child's unique personality, talents, physical characteristics, capabilities, and limitations as God made them. *Philippians 2:3-5; Titus 2:4*

2. **Discipline your children.**

Parents must establish reasonable limitations and consistently enforce them without going to the extremes of harsh oppression or indulgent permissiveness. The purpose of discipline, according to the Bible, is to instill a sense of personal responsibility for the consequences of actions, to help a child understand his accountability to God and others, and to lead a child to respect authority. *Proverbs 3:3-4; 1:8-9; 6:20-22*

3. **Motivate, build up, and encourage your children.**

A parent's encouragement ought to instill a desire to act upon what is right. Children who are encouraged in the way the Bible teaches develop a healthy understanding of themselves and their limitations as well as a confidence in God and God's willingness to help and guide them. *Proverbs 15:15-17; Isaiah 66:12-13; Exodus 4:11-12; Jeremiah 1:5-8*

4. **Diligently train your children.**

Parents need to daily teach principles and skills that will prepare their children to live godly, productive lives. Christian parents are to give their children the tools and knowledge they need to achieve and succeed. *2 Timothy 1:5; Proverbs 22:6*

5. **Provide a living example of all you teach for your child.**

Have God's Word and a love for God in your own heart so you are able to effectively teach your children. Lead your children by living right before them and by letting them see the difference God makes in your lives. *2 Thessalonians 3:7-9; Psalm 78:4*

6. **Have the utmost concern for the eternal soul of your child.**

Your child's relationship to the Lord Jesus Christ is the most important relationship he will ever develop. Understand the nature of a human heart. Realize only God's Spirit can change the heart of a child or adult. Be far more concerned with what your child is going to be like when he grows up instead of merely what you want your child to do. *2 Timothy 3:14-15*

Evaluate Your Parenting Skills

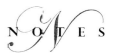

_____ I am building a genuine bond of friendship with my child that will enable him to turn to me for help and support when he fails.

_____ I take time to listen to my child with undivided attention and establish eye contact with him daily.

_____ I reinforce good behavior and praise my child twice as much as I correct him.

_____ I build up (edify) my child by finding, understanding, and encouraging his individual strengths and potential talents.

_____ I consider childhood a time when lifelong memories are created, and take seriously my role in building memories and creating impressions that will have an indelible effect on my child's future life.

_____ I understand the general characteristics and limitations of my child's age group and deal with him accordingly.

_____ I use corporal punishment for deliberate defiance (disobedience) or disrespect, but not for childish infractions.

_____ I never provoke or discourage my child by threatening him, berating him, or humiliating him.

_____ I always define the boundaries to my child before I enforce them.

_____ If I make a request to my child and he disregards me, I follow up every time with firm, deliberate action rather than with screaming.

_____ I consistently and confidently insist my child respects and obeys me.

_____ I never challenge my husband's authority, discipline, or decisions in the presence of my children, knowing disunity would breed insecurity and disrespect.

_____ I go out of my way to provide good activities, playmates, and companions, family friends, and role models for my child.

_____ I do not hesitate to restrict or remove any activity or person from my child's life that threatens to influence him in a negative way.

_____ I understand my child has an eternal soul and understand his ultimate emotional and spiritual well-being depends on the spiritual training I provide for him.

Lesson 2

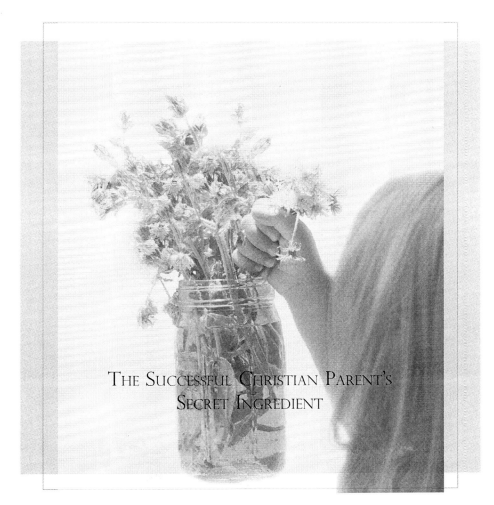

The Successful Christian Parent's Secret Ingredient

And when they shall say unto you, Seek unto them that have familiar spirits, and unto wizards that peep, and that mutter: should not a people seek unto their God? For the living to the dead? To the law and to the testimony: if they speak not according to this word, it is because there is no light in them

Isaiah 8:19-20

Wisdom is the principal thing; therefore get wisdom; and with all thy getting get understanding. Exalt her, and she shall promote thee; she shall bring thee to honor, when thou dost embrace her.

Proverbs 4:7-8

Key THOUGHTS

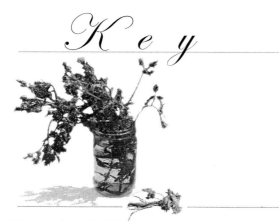

Christian parents are not to rely on their own ideas, experiences, intuition, or any worldly source for advice and direction in raising their children. Rather, they are to seek to know and understand God's Word and rely on God's precepts and wisdom to give guidance in raising children.

Discussion Problem

Judy is an intelligent, active mother who takes a great deal of interest in her children. She is a faithful church member and active in Awanas. She is an avid reader, loves to keep up with popular talk shows, and loves to listen to Christian radio discussions concerning family issues. She is pleased that she has accumulated so much information and describes herself as being very open and broad-minded about current issues.

When anyone in the church nursery brings up a problem with children, Judy is quick to offer advice, and carefully cites expert opinions and statistics along with it. Many of the young mothers are intimidated by Judy's confidence and knowledge and do not question the validity of her suggestions. In fact, many come to her for help with their problems.

None of Judy's children are active in church. In fact, two have left home and want nothing to do with living for the Lord. Julie's husband displays no enthusiasm for serving the Lord and pretty much lets his headstrong wife run the show.

After you read lesson two use the principles you learn to discuss reasons Judy's advice may not be wise. Also consider what errors she is making in the way she collects and applies her knowledge.

Bible Study

1. According to Proverbs 1, what is the beginning of knowledge? *vs 7* __To fear the Lord__

2. What are four results of wisdom listed in Proverbs 2? *vs 5+9* __understand the fear of the Lord, find knowledge of God, understand righteousness, judgment, equity + every good path.__

3. What two questions does Job ask in Job 28:12-28? Where does he say it can be found? __vs 12 Where shall wisdom be found? Where is the place of understanding? vs 20 vs 28 God knew were. The fear of God is wisdom to depart from evil is understanding.__

4. What two things prevented the people in 1 Corinthians 3:1-3 and Hebrews 5:11-14 from being able to discern spiritual things? __They were carnal + babies in Christ.__

"When home is ruled according to God's Word, angels might be asked to stay with us, and they would not find themselves out of their element."
Charles Spurgeon

Secret Ingredient

When was the last time you ever read or heard someone tell you that the one thing absolutely necessary to raising godly children is <u>wisdom</u>? The topic of wisdom is conspicuously absent in the most popular child-rearing books by some of the most distinguished and respected Christian authors. One would not expect wisdom, as God defines it, to be discussed in a secular, non-Christian book for parents. Wisdom's absence from Christian books, however, is most troubling. Of all the Christian graces needed for the guidance of children, none is more crucial than wisdom. Without wisdom, knowledge is useless, for wisdom is the ability to apply truth and knowledge in a practical way.

Wisdom, according to the Bible, is what enables believers to implement truth. It is the means by which believers judge what course of action is just, proper, or useful. God's wisdom empowers us in such a way that we are able to recognize and avoid evil as well as to accomplish good. It makes possible the ability to discern what is right or wrong, true or false, good or bad. We read that the "law of the wise is a fountain of life, to depart from the snares of death" *(Proverbs 13:14)*. And again God reminds us that, "strong meat belongeth to them that are of full age, even those who by reason of used have their senses exercised [trained] to discern both good and evil" *(Hebrews 5:14)*. Repeatedly, the Scriptures warn that apart from wisdom, we do not have the ability to correctly interpret God's Word nor apply it to our life and we certainly do not have the ability to foresee evil and avoid it *(Ecclesiastes 8:5; Proverbs 2:10-12; Proverbs 22:3)*.

Ask a young mother with several children what she spends most her time doing and she will likely tell you she is a constant "referee" for her children. Some mothers describe their role as judge, jury, and executioner, as well as cheerleader, guide, teacher, counselor and physician. One thing is certain—mothers and fathers judge, discern, and decide on courses of action that affect their children's lives on an hourly basis. Or in other words, parents *govern* the lives of their children and play an extremely crucial role in the development of their character. Notice the statement God makes in *Proverbs 8:14-16* as He describes the attributes of godly wisdom and its relationship to those who govern others. "Counsel is mine, and sound wisdom; I am understanding; I have strength. By me kings reign, and princes rule, and nobles, even all the judges of the earth." Wisdom is necessary for any ruler to govern successfully or judge people fairly. How much more is wisdom necessary to mothers who desire to govern their children successfully and correctly judge daily decisions involving them?

Wisdom is the most important element in successful parenting, the secret ingredient rarely mentioned in the many "recipes" for well adjusted, happy children.

The Experts and the Bible

Christian parents may now choose from a virtual smorgasbord of child-rearing books. The amount of information and advice available to parents is staggering. In fact, the

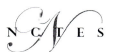

mega-information is enough to discourage a young mother into believing she is not able to raise happy, productive, well-adjusted Christian children without the help of professional experts. Child-rearing books and magazine articles seem to emphasize "new" ideas that presume to be the *key* to successful parenting. Some put the major emphasis on discipline, scheduling, "quality" time, an early education, self-esteem, or parental dominance, among others. We have how-to books, child development books, books about children's problems, and books that tell us it's okay if we're not super moms. But are these books always accurate, and more importantly, do they really make the difference between success and failure?

I once listened to a gentleman give child-rearing advice who had probably never spent an entire twenty-four hour day alone with three small children in his life. His descriptions were charming, accurate, and easy for a mother to identify with. His book was well written, humorous, and sure to make money for its publisher. Never mind that his advice was, for the most part, vague and downright unrealistic—he had an earned Ph.D. so he commanded our attention and respect. Another "expert" gives advice that violates sound medical reasoning and ignores reputable doctor's warnings of error. Never mind that he has no medical expertise that would enable him to understand the dangers of what he proposes to young mothers—he *sounds* competent and sincere, gives powerful testimonies, and writes books…so he *must* be good, right? Wrong.

Have you ever wondered how godly mothers managed to raise children for so many centuries without the advice and expert opinions of child psychologists? How is it so many succeeded in raising mighty men and women who made an enormous impact on the world for the cause of Christ? If one believes the comments and claims of many modern child-rearing experts, one might wonder if it is possible to raise well-adjusted children unless parents provide an ideal environment and somehow accumulate a massive amount of child-rearing know-how. Young mothers are sometimes so intimidated by strong leaders who forcefully promote their own theories and philosophies that they cease exercising godly discernment and capitulate to whatever they are taught, even when it violates clear Biblical principles and commands.

Homes become strong and happy through God-given wisdom, through understanding God's ways, and through an intimate knowledge of God's Word.

Christians who would otherwise immediately reject human reasoning as a basis for making life decisions tend to lose their wariness if someone they hold in high esteem is doing the reasoning. Because an author holds academic credentials, is regarded highly by respected Christians, or is accomplished in some area of life does not eliminate his propensity to error or eradicate sin's effects on the human heart and mind. *All* human beings, no matter how sincere and knowledgeable, have a heart described by Jeremiah as "deceitful above all things, and desperately wicked" *(Jeremiah 17:9a)*. This truth is precisely why God warns us not to put our trust in *any* man *(Jeremiah 17:5)* and not to trust in our own heart. The alternative to living foolishly is to live wisely by humbly putting one's trust in the

Lord rather than self or others. "He that trusteth in his own heart is a fool," the Lord warns, "but whoso walketh [lives] wisely, he shall be delivered" *(Proverbs 28:26)*. To live wisely is to live in dependence on the Word of God, and the God of the Word.

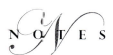

Once mothers begin to lean on human reasoning as their main source of direction in raising children, the Bible ceases to have the preeminence as the basis for all conduct and decisions. Consequently, such mothers do not have the confidence to believe they are able, with God's help, to discern what's best for their children *against the advice of an expert*. The Bible is no longer the plumb line for discerning right and wrong. At some imperceptible point, the expert has quietly pushed God into a corner and taken center stage. What a tragedy, for God did not abandon young mothers or leave them without adequate help and encouragement these thousands of years until the real experts could show up on the scene and save the day.

Parents do not build strong homes that are able to withstand the storms of life through the advice of "experts." God plainly tells us "Through wisdom is an house builded; and by understanding it is established; and by knowledge shall the chambers be filled with all precious and pleasant riches" *(Proverbs 24:3)*. Homes become strong and happy through God-given wisdom, through understanding God's ways, and through an intimate knowledge of God's Word. To lose sight of this important truth is to ignore the treasures of God's plentiful provisions and search the garbage cans of human efforts for our sustenance and strength.

Any author, speaker, teacher, or pastor who exalts himself, a book, a school, or any other human instrument of learning or authority as the basis of success is deceiving you as well as himself. If you never read a book about children and never attend a seminar or class on child development, you can be successful in raising children *if* you build your home God's way by establishing your home in His wisdom and Word. Books *can* be helpful, but just as often, they can be harmful. In this day of increased knowledge, we are easily "spoiled through philosophy and vain deceit, after the tradition of men, after the rudiments of the world, and not after Christ. For in Him dwelleth all the fullness of the Godhead bodily. And ye are complete in him, which is the head of all principality and power" *(Colossians 2:8-10)*. Beware, as Paul said, and stay rooted and built up in Christ. Judge your books by the criteria provided in the Bible and never put more confidence in them than God does.

God Wrote Only One Manual

Job asked a question many moms and dads ask today, "But where shall wisdom be found? And where is the place of understanding?" *(Job 28:12)*. Do we find wisdom by listening to the words of genuinely godly people who love the Word of God and are gifted teachers? Can wisdom be obtained in training seminars conducted by successful parents or through the counseling of wise and compassionate mentors? None of these resources are in themselves sinful, and all may be genuinely helpful, but none are listed in the Bible as *the* source of wisdom, and none are able to replace wisdom. People may be able to inspire us to seek God's wisdom, they may be able to point us in the right direction so we might find God's wisdom, and they may be the means God uses to motivate us to open our Bibles and cry out to God for wisdom. Yet never one time does God direct us to people as the source of wisdom. People may direct us to God, but God does not point us toward people. Job came to the right conclusion, "And unto man he said, Behold, the fear of the Lord, that is wisdom; and to depart from evil is understanding."

If God has blessed our lives with the godly influence of wise people, may they always point us to the *source* of their wisdom, not the by-product of their relationship with God. To God we must go for such a precious treasure. James tell us "If any of you lack wisdom, let him ask of God, that giveth to all men liberally, and upbraideth not; and it shall be given him" *(James 1:5)*. Solomon, the wisest man in the world, does not direct his sons to look to him for wisdom. Rather, he exhorts them to listen to him as he points them to God and His Word. Notice his passionate exhortation in *Proverbs 2*. "Yea, if thou criest after knowledge, and liftest up thy voice for understanding; if thou seekest her as silver, and searchest for her as for hid treasures; then shalt thou understand the fear of the Lord, and find the knowledge of God. For the Lord giveth wisdom; out of his mouth [Word of God] cometh knowledge and understanding." Note the condition for receiving wisdom and the source of wisdom. It must be asked for, it must be searched for diligently, and it must be found in the Word of God.

Our priorities will always reflect our life focus, and they will change when our life focus changes.

Mothers and fathers who are hungry for advice first need wisdom in order to critically evaluate what's accurate, what's unrealistic, what's Biblical, and what's merely someone's interesting opinion. God does use godly people, imperfect as they are, to teach and guide us, yet these people are never to supercede God's Word or the Holy Spirit who indwells us. Paul instructed us to be followers of him, even as he was of Christ *(1 Corinthians 11:1)*. He did not ask us to follow him blindly and believe what he said on the basis of his education or upbringing. Paul told us to follow him even as He followed Christ. How do we know Paul is following Christ? We can only discern Paul's actions by knowing Christ and knowing the Word. This is why Paul commended the Bereans. They were willing to diligently search the Scripture to see if what Paul was saying was true. This searching did not offend Paul—it delighted him. They didn't throw out the words of Paul because they were human words. Rather, they wisely used the Bible to evaluate the merit and authenticity of Paul's message.

Unless a Christian develops good judgment and acquires wisdom that comes only from learning godly principles, all the books and advice in the world will not make up for the lack of it. Mothers who attempt to do what others think is right invite confusion and error into their lives in the long run. Instead, women need to learn how to wisely evaluate and implement whatever God would have them do in any circumstance unique to their family's life. We do need wise people in our lives—

wise people who will teach us to think Biblically and challenge us to recognize and reject the vain philosophies of this world.

If our major life focus is to learn and apply God's Word, we will have precious little time to pursue things that will not matter in eternity, nor will we desire any such pursuit. Our life focus is defined by our priorities and the importance we give to God's Word. Our priorities will always reflect our life focus, and they will change when our life focus changes. Be sure, therefore, that your focus is firmly fixed on Christ and your affections on things above, not on the things of this earth. This focus is the essence of wise and effective parenting. The home that is blessed by God is the home where the Lord Jesus Christ reigns supreme and rules in the hearts of parents. "For whoso findeth me findeth life, and shall obtain favor of the Lord. The curse of the Lord is in the house of the wicked; but he blesseth the habitation of the just. Surely he scorneth the scorners; but he giveth grace unto the lowly. The wise shall inherit glory; but shame shall be the promotion of fools" *(Proverbs 8:35-36)*.

Raising Children by Principle Isn't So Difficult

Have you noticed that parenting is not a black-and-white undertaking that can be readily charted out in a book? We might learn how to raise a puppy in ten easy steps, but children definitely are not puppies. They are complex, living souls. The variables in their personality, experiences, and individual decisions are innumerable. Consequently, no mother has the ability to orchestrate all the events that will occur in her child's life, nor does she have the wisdom in herself to solve all her children's problems. To provide mothering instructions for every possible variation, experience, or circumstance that could come up in a child's life would require more books than could be contained in any library. Most mothers get a headache just trying to remember the instructions given in one book, let alone trying to implement the ideas and advice given in many books. Add to that the advice of mothers and friends, and it's no wonder many women decide daycare is a better alternative to staying home to raise children. No book or books can prepare a mother for every situation she will face.

Our God, who is a master of variety, does not make two snowflakes alike. Should it surprise us, then, that no two lives are alike and no two children are exactly alike? As much as we can find common denominators and similarities, we cannot find any two people in God's creation that are exactly alike in every single way. Neither will we find two people whose experiences are exact duplicates. This presents a challenge to those who must find an exact duplication of experience in order to accurately obtain instruction. Typically this challenge leads to a search for someone who we believe shares our experience in such a way that we can compare ourselves to that person. When we believe we have found a person who is successfully managing an experience like ours, we commonly attempt to duplicate his or her solution hoping for duplicate results.

Such a method of finding help and instruction invariably leads to disappointment after the initial euphoria of discovering common ground subsides. God tells us we are not wise if we compare ourselves to others. We are certainly not wise to compare our children to other children. Paul warns, "But they measuring themselves by themselves, and comparing themselves among themselves are not wise" *(2 Corinthians 10:12b)*. This truth is not saying that common experiences do not have any merit whatsoever as a means to better understand or guide one another. Paul stated in the same epistle that we learn how to comfort others with the same comfort that God uses to comfort us in any trouble *(2 Corinthians 1:3)*. It does mean that we are not to make judgments on the basis of experience alone—ours or any other person's.

Our experience, to be profitable to another, must have its substance in Biblical precepts. If I were to offer comfort to you in a trial, it would be right to base that comfort on my experience of finding God faithful and His Word true in times of difficulty. I would not be righteous or wise to provide you comfort by telling you your trial will end the same way mine did because it is so similar. Hope, to be genuinely Biblical hope, must be based in God's truth and God's character, not in probabilities or common experiences. Instruction, likewise, to be Biblical instruction, must have its basis in precepts that can be validated in God's Word, not simply in experiences that look exactly like ours.

The Bible does not attempt to instruct us with exact instructions as to how to deal with every single circumstance that could possibly come up in life. Can you find a specific command in the Bible not to smoke marijuana? Where would one find explicit instructions not to sing in the church choir wearing a bikini? Or where would one find a direct reference to Christians being required to obey a speed limit? We chuckle because we intuitively know these are obviously ungodly behaviors. But can you support your conclusion with a Biblical principle? Remember, a principle, or precept, is a basic truth or assumption that provides a rule or standard for behavior.

In the case of smoking marijuana we could list numerable Bible principles that such an action would violate. One would be the principle of being controlled by the Holy Spirit rather than a substance such as alcohol or drugs. The desired effect of the drug, a sense of well being, joy, peace, confidence etc., is to be found in Christ, not a drug. Wearing a bikini in the church choir would likely violate the principle of church unity, not to mention Biblical principles of modesty. Driving a car without regard to speed limits violates principles of governing authority, love for others, and the responsibility to protect rather than jeopardize life. The very same principles that govern our behavior in each of these three situations also govern our behavior in numerous other ways. One principle has many applications. Wisdom enables us to apply basic principles to complex situations and determine a particular course of action.

God provides us with basic principles (or truths) found in His Word so they can serve as foundational rules of action. We use them as a guide even as we weigh the tremendous number of variables that might occur in any one situation. The

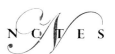

Wisdom enables us to apply basic principles to complex situations and determine a particular course of action.

major purpose of this workbook isn't to provide a lot of miscellaneous information or specific advice about children. This book's major purpose is to help you learn basic Biblical principles, or precepts, that will enable you to make truly wise and specific decisions on behalf of your children no matter what circumstances present themselves in your particular experiences. Information can be good and helpful, but information alone is not enough to give you success in raising your children. Information must always be coupled with God's wisdom if it is to benefit your family.

Three Ways Parents Rear Children

Parents tend to make decisions with regard to raising children in one of three ways. They are most influenced by advice from other people, they make decisions by impulse, or they seek to apply godly principles through wisdom. The first set of parents leans on the understanding of others and trusts in them. The second set of parents is leaning on their own understanding and trusting their own heart to guide them. Only the third set is approaching the responsibilities of parenting with a humble and godly perspective. To presume we, or anyone else has within our own heart or mind the ability to make wise, godly choices as parents, is the epitome of arrogance. We are wholly dependent on God to give the necessary wisdom and ability to discern His Word and apply it to life's circumstances in practical ways.

Of all the many wonders of God that we could teach our children, one of the most precious is the concept that apart from Christ neither our children nor we can do anything. Jesus said, "I am the vine, ye are the branches; He that abideth in me, and I in him, the same bringeth forth much fruit; for without me ye can do nothing" *(John 15:5)*. What a tragedy it would be to teach our children to depend on Christ while we ourselves demonstrate our unbelief by depending on others or ourselves. We as parents desperately need to become aware of our dependence on Christ before we can successfully train our children to "trust in the Lord with all thine heart; and lean not unto thine own understanding. In all thy ways acknowledge him, and he shall direct thy paths" *(Proverbs 3:5-6)*.

Perhaps we need to pay special attention to the two verses following the more familiar ones we just mentioned. "Be not wise in thine own eyes; fear the Lord, and depart from evil. It shall be health to thy navel, and marrow to thy bones" *(Proverbs 3:7-8)*. To be wise in our own eyes is to believe we can understand and choose what is best apart from God or His Word. It is also a reference to the kind of pride and self-sufficiency that results in a life full of heartache and devastation. When Jeremiah warns us not to put our trust in man's abilities or power of reasoning, he prefaces his warning with a strong pronouncement that such dependence brings a curse. "Cursed be the man that trusteth in man, and maketh flesh his arm, and whose heart departeth from the Lord" *(Jeremiah 17:5)*.

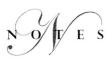

Jeremiah then goes on to describe in vivid word pictures the life of those who put their trust in human ability in contrast with those who put their trust in God. One picture features a lifeless tumbleweed blowing aimlessly in the dry, barren desert sand. The other features a beautiful thriving tree planted by a river, consistently bearing fruit no matter what weather prevails around it. We all make a choice to either be a lifeless tumbleweed blowing unproductively in the wind, or a strong mature tree that produces fruit that is a blessing and source of life to others. We make that choice when we choose to either put our trust in what God says, or put our trust in what we or anyone else says or thinks. You may be one lone person making choices on the basis of what God says rather than what even the godly crowd says. But you may also end up being one lone tree thriving in an oasis in the desert with tumbleweeds blowing all around you. Take your pick.

No tenderhearted Christian parent would ever want to be cursed by God in any way. You, like others, no doubt desire God's blessings, and you may have them. All that it will cost you is your pride. "Wherefore He saith, God resisteth the proud, but giveth grace unto the humble. Submit yourselves therefore to God" *(James 4:6-7a)*. God gives His grace, meaning the desire and ability to do His will, to those who are humble and dependent on Him. But He resists, or is opposed to, those who maintain their pride and their own self-sufficiency. As you study the following chart, consider how you may be unwittingly following an unBiblical approach to parenting children. Then take some time to pray and seek the Lord's wisdom and direction as you commit yourself to learning Biblical precepts that will enable you to raise your children for God's glory.

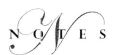

Impulse	I do what comes naturally and trust my own instincts. I believe women who need teachers and books are silly. I don't need anyone telling me how to raise my children. **Conflicts with:** *Proverbs 28:26*—He that trusteth in his own heart is a fool: but whoso walketh wisely, he shall be delivered.
Advice	I prefer doing what the experts tell me to do. I believe they are smarter than I and must know better than I how to raise children. I trust the expert's advice more than anyone else's. I question the sufficiency of God and His Word in making decisions on behalf of my children. **Conflicts with:** *Proverbs 19:21*—There are many devices in a man's heart; nevertheless the counsel of the LORD, that shall stand. *Psalm 118:8*—It is better to trust in the LORD than to put confidence in man. See also *Isaiah 30:1*
Principle	I do what conforms to Biblical principles and trust God to guide me as I weigh information and advice given by godly teachers. I know I need encouragement and instruction, but I also know God is able to give me wisdom to discern what is useful to my particular situations. I don't hesitate to disregard the advice of any experienced mother or child psychologist if it conflicts with Biblical principles. **Agrees with:** *Proverbs 3:5-6*—Trust in the LORD with all thine heart; and lean not unto thine own understanding. In all thy ways acknowledge him, and he shall direct thy paths.

More Wisdom—Not More Books

How important is wisdom to a mother raising children? Wisdom is more important than a comfortable income or a sprawling home with a yard. Wisdom is more important than years of experience with children or a degree from a prestigious university.

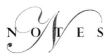

A woman can be a good mother without any of these earthly things, but no woman can be a good mother without God's wisdom. Wisdom is the one thing a mother absolutely *cannot* do without!

A wise mother is a happy pleasant mother to be around.

Proverbs 3:13-35—Happy *is* the man *that* findeth wisdom, and the man *that* getteth understanding. For the merchandise of it *is* better than the merchandise of silver, and the gain thereof than fine gold. She *is* more precious than rubies: and all the things thou canst desire are not to be compared unto her… My son, let not them depart from thine eyes: keep sound wisdom and discretion: so shall they be life unto thy soul, and grace to thy neck. Then shalt thou walk in thy way safely, and thy foot shall not stumble. When thou liest down, thou shalt not be afraid: yea, thou shalt lie down, and thy sleep shall be sweet….

A wise mother is blessed of God.

Proverbs 8:35-36—For whoso findeth me findeth life, and shall obtain favor of the LORD. The curse of the LORD *is* in the house of the wicked: but he blesseth the habitation of the just. Surely he scorneth the scorners: but he giveth grace unto the lowly. The wise shall inherit glory: but shame shall be the promotion of fools.

A wise mother is able to understand the Word of God.

Proverbs 14:6—A scorner seeketh wisdom, and findeth it not: but knowledge is easy unto him that understandeth. *Psalm 25:12*—What man is he that feareth the LORD? him shall he teach in the way that he shall choose.

She is sensitive to the guiding of the Holy Spirit and is able to apply scriptural principles to life's everyday circumstances and trials. The foolish mother, on the other hand, finds the Word of God impossible to understand or enjoy and does not know how to apply it to her life. She does not recognize God's quiet promptings that would help her guide and instruct her children.

A wise mother knows how to influence her family and others for good.

Proverbs 14:1—Every wise woman buildeth her house: but the foolish plucketh it down with her hands. *Proverbs 16:20-22*—He that handleth a matter wisely shall find good: and whoso trusteth in the LORD, happy is he. The wise in heart shall be called prudent: and the sweetness of the lips increaseth learning. Understanding is a wellspring of life unto him that hath it: but the instruction of fools is folly.

A foolish mother, on the other hand, will end up wasting her resources and time on herself.

A wise mother is able to discern good from evil.

Hebrews 5:14—But strong meat belongeth to them that are of full age, even those who by reason of use have their senses exercised to discern both good and evil.

Ecclesiastes 8:1, 5b—Who is as the wise man? And who knoweth the interpretation of a thing? A man's wisdom maketh his face to shine, and the boldness of his face shall be changed . . . a wise man's heart discerneth both time and judgment.

A wise woman is able to sense danger and error and therefore steer her children out of harm's way. A foolish mother, however, is ruled by her emotions and lacks discernment. She does not foresee the consequences of selfish or evil influences on her children until they have irrevocably affected her children.

A wise mother understands the love of God and can communicate it to her children.

Psalm 107:43—Whoso is wise, and will observe these *things*, even they shall understand the lovingkindness of the LORD.

A wise mother reaps the future blessings of wisdom.

Proverbs 31:28-31—Her children arise up, and call her blessed; her husband *also*, and he praiseth her. Many daughters have done virtuously, but thou excellest them all. Favor *is* deceitful, and beauty *is* vain: *but* a woman *that* feareth the LORD, she shall be praised. Give her of the fruit of her hands; and let her own works praise her in the gates.

Furthermore, wisdom is the only thing that has the power to ultimately make a woman a joyful, fulfilled mother of children.

Lesson 3

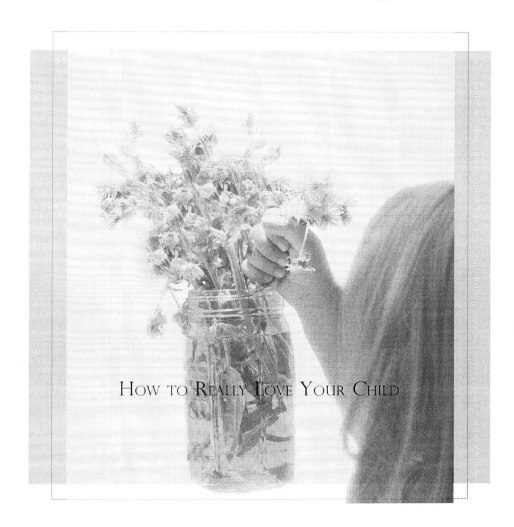

How to Really Love Your Child

This is my commandment, That ye love one another, as I have loved you. Greater love hath no man than this, that a man lay down his life for his friends.
John 15:12-13

With all lowliness and meekness, with longsuffering, forbearing one another in love; Be ye kind one to another, tenderhearted, forgiving one another, even as God for Christ's sake hath forgiven you.
Ephesians 4:2, 32

Key THOUGHTS

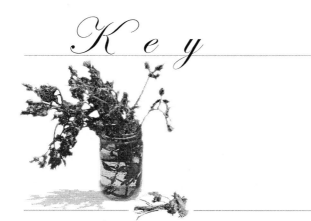

The way in which we sacrificially give of ourselves to train, discipline, and nurture our children is an expression of our love for them. Love is the cornerstone of a mother's influence on her children. It is an art, not a feeling, and is learned by emulating the love of God.

Discussion Problem

Cheryl has three small children under the age of five. She has a challenging career in desktop publishing and leaves her children in a day care center while she is at work. Cheryl loves her job and sometimes even brings work home so she can get ahead and win more promotions. When the children cry and want Cheryl's attention, she explains that she needs to work so she can buy them a nicer house and lots of toys. She does not discipline the children because she insists she loves them too much to spank them.

Besides, since she doesn't see them all day she doesn't want to spend her time with them fussing about problems. She explains that she wants her little time with them to be "quality" time. Cheryl depends on the day care center to discipline and train her children and believes they are doing a good job.

However, two of the children are having trouble forming friendships and seem increasingly more distant and detached from Mom and Dad. The third is displaying very aggressive behavior and is whining constantly. Cheryl insists she deeply loves her children and is doing what is best for them.

After reading chapter three, use the principles you have learned to discuss the possible ways Cheryl has misplaced her priorities at this time in her children's lives. Explain how she has misinterpreted the Biblical concept of love.

Bible Study

1. What does Proverbs 23:24-25 say a wise child produces? _____

2. According to Proverbs 19:18, when may we infer is it easiest to effectively discipline a child? _____

3. What two things are needed in order to produce wisdom in a child according to Proverbs 29:15? What produces the opposite and ultimately causes the parent to be ashamed? _____

"Too much love never spoils children. Children become spoiled when we substitute presents for presence."
Dr. A. Witham

Do You Know God Loves You?

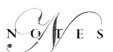

If Jesus were physically present on the earth today, it would doubtless melt our hearts to hear Him tenderly call us by name. To see Him direct His warm and accepting smile toward us personally, or feel His loving embrace would thrill our hearts and bring the strongest among us to tears, for nothing has the power to touch our lives more profoundly than knowing God loves us. The apostle John marveled that we who have trusted Christ would be so loved by God that He would call us His children. John said, "Behold what manner of love the Father hath bestowed upon us, that we should be called the sons of God" *(1 John 3:1)*. David marveled as he pondered the reality that God knew him intimately and understood him so completely. The thought of such a loving and personal God moved David to exclaim, "How precious also are thy thoughts unto me, O God! How great is the sum of them! If I should count them, they are more in number than the sand; when I awake, I am still with thee" *(Psalm 139:1-18)*. All believers who know the realities of God's personal love for them and are assured of His forgiveness want to express their joy and adoration for Him. Indeed, we do love Him because He first loved us, just as John said *(1 John 4:19)*.

Our hearts are touched, but not satisfied to know God loves the world—we want to know He loves us *personally*. It is not enough to know God loves His children—we long to know "Jesus loves *me*," even me. Perhaps that is why Jesus' comment that our Heavenly Father knows how many hairs are on our heads delights and fascinates young Christians. As new believers we are naturally timid and unsure of God's interest in our lives. However, once we begin to grow in our knowledge of Christ and begin to see the many scriptural evidences of God's loving character, fear is replaced with confidence. John has provided us with a wonderful description of this transformation. "And we have known and believed the love that God hath to us. God is love; and he that dwelleth in love dwelleth in God, and God in him. Herein is our love made perfect [mature], that we may have boldness in the day of judgment; because as he is, so are we in this world. There is no fear in love; but perfect [mature] love casteth out fear; because fear hath torment. He that feareth is not made perfect in love" *(1 John 4:16-18)*.

We begin to experience God's love as we daily draw close to Him in prayer, hear Him speak through His Word, and see His love manifested in so many ways. To the degree we grow in our knowledge of the Lord Jesus Christ and believe the testimony of His Word, we become assured He loves us *personally*. As we learn to trust His love more and more, we learn to submit our will to His and imitate His character. Once we understand the nature of God's grace and mercy and the significance of our imputed righteousness in Christ, we begin to understand the joy of God's acceptance. We become intimately acquainted with the peace that follows repentance toward God, and the assurance of His forgiveness. Our delight and our consuming passion is to please the God Who loves us so deeply and provides so freely everything we need. Such a child of God knows he is the apple of God's eye and consequently, becomes happy and secure in his Heavenly Father's love. In a similar way, the little child whose heart is assured of his parent's love and commitment becomes happy and secure, no matter how imperfect or childish he may be.

Children respond to parental love and personal involvement in their lives in much the same way adults respond to assurances of God's love and personal involvement in their lives. Nothing is more powerful or motivating in the life of a child than the assurance his parents love him. The concept of God's existence and involvement in our lives is not easily understood by a child who is not yet able to reason in abstract terms or accept the reality of something he cannot see, hear, or touch. Therefore, children tend to understand the reality of God's love as they experience the realities of a parent's love in concrete ways. To a child, parents are the tender voice of God calling them by name. They are the warm and accepting smile and the comforting and loving embrace of the Lord Jesus Christ. Just as these things have the power to melt our adult heart, so they have the power to melt a child's heart and elicit love, adoration, and obedience toward a parent. Children blessed with loving parents quite naturally embrace the Lord Jesus Himself as they come to understand who He is.

Is it any wonder, then, that God would instruct the older women to teach the younger to love their children *(Titus 2:4)*? In this simple command, there is a world of meaning that is so all encompassing that it summarizes everything a mother needs to raise her child successfully. The word love, as it is used in Titus, implies far more than a mother's natural instinct to nourish and care for her own children. It is more than the *act* of loving. In the Biblical sense, it is the *art* of loving one's child selflessly. More specifically, this love is the learned ability to emulate God's love in her relationship with her children. Paul presumes that older and mature Christian women know the love of God and understand the way He works in our lives. To these mature women, God gives the responsibility of training young mothers to love as He loves us. Such love is a learned response, yet it is also a Christian grace that originates in God and is given by Him. This love is not an emotion or passion of the heart, but a skill that is taught in such a way that mothers learn how to apply it to the every day, nitty-gritty work of raising children in the nurture and admonition of the Lord.

Nothing is more powerful or motivating in the life of a child than the assurance his parents love him.

God Is Love

Far more important than learning "what to do when" is learning "how God responds when." The more a young mother understands God's nature and how His love functions in His children's lives, the more she is able to emulate God's character in her decisions and responses to her own children. No matter what decision a mother makes with regard to her children, it must first follow the principle of love. Therefore, when a mother questions which course of action she should take, she ought first to determine which course follows the law of God's love. "What would Jesus do?" isn't a bad question to have at the forefront of one's mind when contemplating decisions. Nevertheless, this popular question doesn't do much good if one does not know what Jesus *would* do in such a situation.

To know what Jesus would do, one must first know something about Jesus' character and how His love operates in the lives of His children. What does God's love look like in practical everyday life? How does God's love determine the way He deals in our lives? To understand these questions is to understand how our love is to manifest itself in our parenting relationship to our children. The topic of God's love has never been exhausted; and all the books in the world could not convey its depth, let alone adequately exalt its wonder and power. The following is a description of how we can readily see God's love working in our lives, but the descriptions hardly scratch the surface and only vaguely convey God's loving character. They are given with the hope that the descriptions of God's love will inspire and excite you to become better acquainted with the Him who delights to love His children. As you do, it is my prayer that you will want to love your own children in the same way.

Love Gives

One of the most beloved passages in the entire Bible begins with the words, "For God so loved that He gave" *(John 3:16a)*. Love that originates with God always gives. It gives freely, without regard for itself, and without expectation of reciprocation. Love gives self-sacrificially, not grudgingly, with a willing and joyful heart. A mother who chooses to love her children does not hesitate to sacrificially give of herself to fulfill the responsibilities of training and nurturing them. Her love will be reflected in her willingness to give her child a place of priority in her life. She will do what is best for her child, even at great cost to herself, because love will always consider the child more important than self.

Mothers who abuse their authority over their children, who expect their children to cater to their desires and conform to what pleases them, do not love their children in the Biblical sense of the word. Such mothers make decisions for their children based solely on what is most convenient to them, what will cost them the least, or what will bring most pleasure to them. They steer their children away from interests that do not interest them or choices that would be best for the child but costly to the parent. It is not uncommon for such a parent to discourage or forbid a child from serving as a missionary in another country, attending a Bible college far from home, or pursuing hobbies that will inconvenience the parent though it would greatly benefit the child. When a mother truly loves her child, she is willing to accept the hardships in order to do whatever is necessary for her child's benefit and future welfare. To the best of her ability and to the extent it is possible, she gladly gives of herself to meet her children's needs.

Would you be able to give up your personal aspirations, your friends and family, or a comfortable lifestyle if doing so would be in the best interests of your child? Parents are often faced with problems that require them to do just that. Some will refuse to sacrifice their own desires for the cause of their children, choosing to rationalize or justify choices in order to follow their own wishes instead. Others will not hesitate to give up everything they hold dear in order to provide what is needful to their children. Consider the father who sold his beloved business in the city and moved to a rural mountain town in order to build a relationship with his rebelling son and remove him from the influence of bad friends. Or consider the single mother who gave up her desire to have her only son live close to home so he could attend a Christian college far away.

A young woman at the peak of her career baffled her co-workers when she resigned in order to tutor her child with learning disabilities so he could have a fighting chance at academic success. A couple turned down an all-expense paid vacation to Hawaii in order to attend their son's debut in the high school play. A Christian father declined a promotion and job offer in another state in order to keep his children in a Christian school and active youth group. These parents sacrificed something they wanted for something far more precious. What they gained will matter for eternity. What they lost will mean nothing in the end.

When the Bible tells us "God so loved the world that He gave," it emphasizes that He gave what was most precious to Him for the benefit of those who were helpless without His sacrifice. God gave His *only begotten Son*, not for His own pleasure, but for the benefit of others. It was more than a gift; it was the most precious gift God could give—the gift of *Himself*. When parents sacrifice their own desires for their children, they are giving more than an object—they are giving themselves for the just cause of another. Most importantly, they are emulating the love of the Lord Jesus Christ. "We then that are strong ought to bear the infirmities of the weak, and not to please ourselves. Let every one of us please his neighbor for his good to edification. For even Christ pleased not himself; but, as it is written, The reproaches of them that reproached thee fell on me" *(Romans 15:1-3)*. Notice we are instructed to give of ourselves for a specific reason, not to cater to the selfish whims of another, but for our neighbor's good to edification—to build him up and benefit him.

To withhold what is good and needful is to neglect a child, and this neglect represents a form of child abuse of the most subtle and destructive kind.

Love motivates parents to give what is needful to their children, whether it is their time, their resources, their attention, their approval, their participation, or any other thing that a child needs. To withhold what is good and needful is to neglect a child, and this neglect represents a form of child abuse of the most subtle and destructive kind. A lazy parent who does not count the cost of neglecting his child's education thwarts his academic progress and brings untold hardship into his child's future. Another parent neglects to provide spiritual encouragement and training and unwittingly communicates a disregard for spiritual priorities. At the time it may not seem important, but years later, when the child has no interest in the things of the Lord and lives an ungodly adult life, both parent and child reap the heartache of a parent's selfish refusal to give. There are countless ways parents might neglect their children and bring sorrow to the Lord as well as to themselves. It is a sobering thought to remember that the Bible says a parent who neglects to provide for his child denies the faith and is worse than an infidel *(1 Timothy 5:8)*. An infidel, or one who rejects Christ, is one who does not know the love of God or practice Biblical love.

Love Is a Choice

There was a time when believers sang "Amazing grace, how sweet the sound that saved a wretch like me" and believed God's grace truly *was* amazing that He would save a wretched soul. Christians once marveled at God's love for them when they sang, "Alas and did my Savior bleed and did my Savior die, would He forsake that sacred throne for such a worm as I." In today's culture, describing one's self as "wretched" or calling one's self a "worm" makes even Christians cringe. Some have gone so far as to remove such "offensive" words from the hymnal and replace them with descriptions more pleasant to hear. We are living in a time when believers who ought to know better are rejecting sound doctrine and forgetting that the cross is not only foolish to a lost world, but offensive as well. Attempts to make the message of salvation inviting by denying what God says about man's depravity and God's grace is heresy. God did not send Christ to die for lovely sinners that had merit or value. He sent His Son to die for wretched sinners who were enemies, unworthy of His love and mercy. Christ loved us in spite of our wretched condition; and while we were yet sinners, He died for us *(Romans 5:8-10)*.

To understand God's love for the unlovely is to understand His grace. We are saved by grace—something we do not merit (or deserve) in any way for any reason. Salvation is a gift that is based completely on what Christ has done for undeserving sinners, not on what a lost sinner is, or has, done for Christ. We are valuable only because we are God's children, not because we merit His love of ourselves. This is the Christian's greatest joy and triumph—to be so forgiven, so thoroughly cleansed by the blood of Christ that God's love and acceptance does not depend on anything except the immutable promises of God. God forgives us and loves us for Christ's sake, according to *Ephesians 4:32*, not for ours. This means there is nothing we can do that will make Him love us more than He already does, and there is nothing we can do that will make Him love us any less.

After God led Israel out of Egypt and established them as a nation, He did not tell them they were a special people because they had value or attractive qualities. Rather, God reminded the people that He did not set His love upon them, or choose them, because there were great in number or merited His love in any way. Instead, He loved them because he would keep the oath that He had sworn unto their fathers *(Deuteronomy 7:7-8)*. God's love was given because of God's faithful and merciful character, not because of Israel's.

Parents, who love their children as God loves His, love their children simply because they are their own. Love is not based on performance or preference, for such a love would not really be love at all. To be like God's love, it must be given out of a parent's unselfish character and commitment, not on the basis of a child's goodness or attractiveness. Love is not earned or elicited because a child deserves it or because a child possesses special intelligence or beauty. Rather, a loving parent chooses to love and care for the child God gives because it is a life made in the image of God and belongs to God. Parents are to be stewards of the living soul that God gives to them, and parents are accountable to God for the way they care for and nurture their children. In this sense, we love our children, no matter what they look like or act like, for Christ's sake, not our own. We do not reject them because they have flaws or unchangeable imperfections or because they are difficult to care for. We love them in spite of them because they are given by God and are our own.

Loving a child with godly devotion requires, first of all, a commitment to accept one's child as a unique individual with his own peculiar characteristics and potential. No matter what a child's strengths or weaknesses, peculiarities or talents, he has exactly what he needs to do exactly what God wants him to do in this world. At the very moment of conception, each child has his own unique genetic blueprint. The baby is irrevocably male or female. Eye and hair color have already been determined, as well as blood type, physical features, intelligence, and personality. Before the child is even formed or recognizable as a baby, God has equipped him for a specific destiny. In *Exodus 4:11b* God asks Moses, "Who hath made man's mouth? Or who maketh the dumb, or deaf, or the seeing, or the blind? Have not I the LORD?" You can be sure God has allowed whatever our babies are and loves each one, exactly how he is.

No baby is a mistake. Even in the most difficult of circumstances, children are able to thrive and grow when they are loved in spite of themselves and are accepted on the basis of a parent's devotion and commitment, not on their own merit. Every parent can praise the Lord that his child is fearfully and wonderfully made and known by God. David said "…marvellous *are* thy works; and *that* my soul knoweth right well. My substance was not hid from thee, when I was made in secret [quietly hidden], *and* curiously wrought [developed] in the lowest parts of the earth [mother's womb]. Thine eyes did see my substance, yet being unperfect [not yet formed]; and in thy book all *my members* were written, *which* in continuance were fashioned, when *as yet there was* none of them" *(Psalm 139:14-16)*. Mothers too often lament the very characteristics God designed for a purpose. How much better to be thankful for a child's differences and help him refine and use his unique abilities to be all God wants him to be.

Love Motivates

Even the most ungodly researcher recognizes the fact that the quality of a mother's love and acceptance forms indelible impressions on the minds of our tiniest infants. The heart of a baby is educated by the impressions he receives; and the memories of love, gentleness, and patience that are stored in his memory produce lasting effects on his developing personality. Babies thrive when they are cuddled and cherished by a mother who responds to them and speaks gently to them. They are healthier and happier than babies whose mothers are irritable, distant, or cold. As a baby begins to grow, the mere atmosphere of love in his home gives him a sense of security and joy. A mother's smiles, hugs, kisses, and playful attentions all soothe and comfort little children. In fact, nothing will encourage or strengthen a child to do what is right as much as seeing his mother's earnest expressions of love and joy when he attempts to please her.

Love induces children to listen and receive the understanding that they need to become useful and happy throughout life. The kindness of a mother, demonstrated by loving acts of mercy and tenderness, draws children to respond to her and follow her. Children who are disagreeable, immature, or rebellious tend to soften under the firm but gentle hand of adults who genuinely care about them. Many school administrators and teachers know that unless they win the heart of a child, they are powerless to influence him for righteousness. Harsh words, tough gestures of contempt, strict rules, and condemning lectures harden the hearts of children. Yet they often submit to the most difficult corrective measures when they are disciplined with kindness, mercy, and love.

Recognizing the power of love and kindness helps us better understand why God said to Israel, "Yea, I have loved thee with an everlasting love; therefore with lovingkindness have I drawn thee" *(Jeremiah 31:3)*. God uses love and kindness to draw Israel closer to Himself in a relationship of obedience. In Romans we read a fascinating passage addressed to a rebelling soul, "Or despisest thou the riches of his goodness and forbearance and longsuffering; not knowing that the goodness of God leadeth thee to repentance?" *(Romans 2:4)*.

You might think God would immediately judge the wickedness of offenders and exact justice upon them, as they deserve. But God is forbearing and patient, and in love gives sinners space to repent and turn to Him before they experience the righteous judgment of God. As parents, we sometimes become too quick to come down harshly on an erring child and fail to discipline in love with understanding and patience. We often fail to understand the importance of drawing children close to ourselves with love and kindness so that our discipline and instruction is received with a willing heart.

Love Disciplines

On one hand, we are to patiently guide, nurture, and protect our children. We are to love them as Christ loves us, with a willingness to exercise mercy and understanding, as well as a willingness to give ourselves sacrificially for their care. These are obviously pleasant and enjoyable aspects of loving. The other side of love is just as needful for the future welfare of our children, though it is not a pleasant or enjoyable part of parental love. God tells us that we must love our children enough to correct and discipline them, just as He corrects and disciplines us for our own good and future benefit. Parents who indulge their children's every whim, or who do not enforce restraints or discipline in their children's lives, produce children who

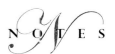

are insecure, self-centered, and rebellious. Far from being merciful, this is actually a cruel form of parental neglect. "He that spareth his rod," God tells us, "hateth his son; but he that loveth him chasteneth him betimes" *(Proverbs 13:24)*.

God instructs parents to use the pain of corporal punishment, properly applied, as a means of dealing with willful disobedience. Reasoning alone does not curtail willful disobedience or change rebellious behavior in a small child. Reasoning might be easier at the moment; but in the end, reasoning without enforcing discipline causes more pain for both the parent and the child. The Bible reminds us that *both* the rod and reproof give wisdom to a child. God tells us to chasten our children while they are young, for it is easier to mold the will and behavior of a small child through the proper use of discipline than to alter the will and behavior of a teenager who has developed a rebellious attitude and can no longer be disciplined in the same way a small child can.

According to the Bible, discipline properly carried out is an act of love and care. In fact, when children are disciplined in a godly, controlled way, they themselves see discipline as a means of helping them overcome what is wrong and harmful to them, not as a sign of anger or rejection. The key is in learning to discipline the right way out of proper motivation. The parent who punishes his child in anger acts out of selfish motives. The angry parent reacts to a child's misbehavior more because it inconveniences and disrupts the parent's wishes than because the parent wishes to train his child for the child's benefit. In contrast, the parent who disciplines his child in a controlled, loving way views discipline as necessary for the future happiness and good of his child, not as retaliation for wrongs committed against him.

Biblical discipline always incorporates a combination of gentleness and firmness. It is never to be carried out with hatefulness or a lack of self-control. This requires a parent to forget about the pain caused to himself and focus instead on what is good for the child. From a godly perspective, love and discipline are a perfectly consistent duo. We see this same combination in the way God disciplines his own children, for He always corrects us without any anger, rejection, or condemnation whatsoever. The Scripture tells us, "Whom the LORD loveth he correcteth; even as a father the son in whom he delighteth" *(Proverbs 3:12)*. And in *Romans 8:1a* we read that, "There is therefore now no condemnation to them which are in Christ Jesus." Jesus took the condemnation for our sin, both our children's and ours. Furthermore, God does not permit us to condemn our Christian brothers and sisters, or our children in any way. We are to love them the same way Jesus does, on the basis of what Christ did at Calvary, not on the basis of whether or not they deserve love. Therefore, we correct our children, but we do not do so with condemnation or malice of any kind.

Learning to administer firm and consistent discipline, together with gentleness and patience, is not something that comes naturally to our human nature. Rather, it requires us to seek God's strength, power, and wisdom as we learn how to master disciplining our children in love. The ability to love, as God would have us love, is not possible apart from a relationship with Christ. We must realize that we cannot do it apart from His strength and grace. The source of love, God's love, is not in our own human heart. The source of Biblical love is God Himself.

Love Looks Ahead

Love sees what a child might become, not necessarily what he is at the moment. Today the child is immature and silly, but tomorrow he may very well be the pastor of a church or the mayor of your city. Love sees past today's childishness and foresees the impact of what is done today on the future of a child. In truth, much of what a parent does is really "time-released teaching" that won't come to fruition until a child reaches adulthood. Much of what God does in the lives of His children is not understood immediately and often times it is not understood until we reach our home in heaven. What God does for us is done for our future benefit as well as our present welfare. He prepares us and disciplines us now so that we might enjoy the benefits of obedience later. Yet God already sees us as we will be when we stand in His presence in the courts of glory, for God who is not bound by time already sees us as holy and without blame before Him in love *(Ephesians 1:3)*.

David praised God for redeeming his life from destruction and crowning it with lovingkindness *(Psalm 103:4)*. Hezekiah likewise praised God when he said, "Behold, for peace I had great bitterness; but thou hast in love to my soul delivered it from the pit of corruption; for thou hast cast all my sins behind thy back" *(Isaiah 38:17)*. Our loving Heavenly Father sees the bitter results of future destruction and acts on our behalf to steer us away from evil and toward the safety of a godly life. Many parents make choices for small children that will have an impact much later and are intended to prevent them from going in a direction away from God. Other parents seem to have no wisdom to see the potential effects careless choices today might have on the future. Love always looks ahead and paves the way in order to protect and spare others from the devastations of sin.

Love Protects

> *A plainly dressed woman was noticed to be picking up something in the street—a poor slum street, where ragged, barefooted little children were accustomed to play. A police officer patrolling nearby noticed the woman's action, and watched her very suspiciously. Several times he saw her stoop and pick up something and hide it in her large coat pocket. Finally he went up to her, and with a gruff voice and threatening manner demanded, "What are you carrying off in your pockets?" The timid woman did not answer at first, whereupon the policeman, thinking she must have found something valuable, threatened her with arrest if she did not show him what she had in her coat. The woman reached into her pocket and revealed a handful of broken glass. "What do you want with that stuff?" asked the officer. The woman replied, "I just thought I'd like to take it out of the way of the children's feet."* [1]

This woman's love caused her to do what she could to protect little children's feet. Hers is the kind of love that motivates parents to remove those things that would cause their child to stumble or bring the pain of sin's devastation into their child's life. While children are young, they are tender and vulnerable to things that would harm them. They do not comprehend life's dangers or have the ability to foresee its pain. Like a fragile plant just beginning to sprout, children need protection from the storms of life until they are grown and become strong enough to withstand them. This is why parents withdraw their children from the public school environment and so often at great sacrifice to themselves, pay a private Christian school to educate them in an atmosphere where they will not be taught the philosophies of the world. It is why parents guard the computer and television and choose more wholesome activities for their children to pursue. Protecting children in this way is like picking up pieces of glass so they will not cut themselves while playing.

Love sees past today's childishness and foresees the impact of what is done today on the future of a child

Loving parents seek an environment for their children that will help, not hinder, the development of Christian character and Christ-likeness. Their purpose is not to shield children from all unpleasantness or to isolate them from the world. Rather their purpose is, or should be, to train and prepare children to live in the world without becoming a part of the world, or loving the world. God provides protection for His children and assures them, "The beloved of the Lord shall dwell in safety by him; and the Lord shall cover him all the day long and he shall dwell between his shoulders" *(Deuteronomy 33:12)*. The place of protection is always close to God and far from the evils of the world. God gives us His good and gracious commands, not to keep us from enjoying the good of the world, but to protect us from the evils in the world and of our own sinful nature. God's love guides us away from evil and into the safety of His presence. David understood this when he sang to the Lord about such lovingkindness and exclaimed, "For this God is our God for ever and ever; he will be our guide even unto death" *(Psalm 48:9,14)*.

Love Forgives

Sometimes it would seem that parents believe they must find and punish every childish action, every flaw, and every sin their child commits. These parents often forget that God Himself does not do this to His own children. David became sad and overwhelmed when he thought of all his sins and confessed they were more than the hairs of his head. He found encouragement and comfort in knowing God was merciful; meaning God in mercy does not give us what we often deserve. David prayed, "Withhold not thou thy tender mercies from me, O Lord; let thy lovingkindness and thy truth continually preserve me" *(Psalm 40:11-13)*. Again David prayed, "If thou, Lord, shouldest mark iniquities, O Lord, who shall stand? But there is forgiveness with thee, that thou mayest be feared" *(Psalm 130:3-4)*.

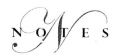

God, in love to our souls, pities we who are His children and remembers that we are but dust and frail. He is quick to show mercy to those who fear Him and love Him. David tells us, "He hath not dealt with us after our sins; nor rewarded us according to our iniquities" *(Psalm 103:10-14)*. As we become aware of God's love and mercy, we respond with devotion, gratitude, and praise to Him. It is because of His mercy that we are not consumed, because His compassions fail not *(Jeremiah 3:22-23)*. God forgives childish infractions and overlooks immaturity. He weighs our actions, considers our weaknesses, and adjusts His response in proportion to our abilities, attitude, and understanding. If He were to mark every sin we committed in a day, we would not be able to function. We would be overwhelmed with sorrow and discouragement. Rather, God deals with His children individually according to His plan and causes us to grow in grace while He progressively moves us toward maturity. He forgives us, David declares, rather than marking every failure.

Parents would do well to consider how merciful and patient God is with them. Before pointing out a child's failure, it would be wise to remember the way we would like to be treated when we fail. We tend to accept correction from those who temper it with love and mercy, who do not correct out of anger or disgust, but deal with us gently for our benefit. Children are no different. They are little people with emotions as tender as our own, and have a spirit that can be easily wounded by harshness. They cannot withstand an onslaught of demands and corrections. They become easily agitated and discouraged when parents do not use wisdom in choosing what really needs to be dealt with and what needs to be overlooked.

Children also become discouraged when parents do not forgive offenses, but bring up past failures repeatedly, and constantly remind children of failures. Parents who love their children are ready and eager to forgive, just as God our Father is good and ready to forgive *(Psalm 86:5)*. Once a sin is dealt with, it is forgotten in the sense that it will not be brought up or used against the child again. The seriousness of a child's sin does not diminish the loving parent's willingness to forgive; rather, it moves the parent to wait patiently, if necessary, until the child comes to repentance. The prodigal son's father did not disown his son when he left home and spent his inheritance living in sin. He was waiting, ready to forgive the moment his son repented and came home. He did not impose more consequences upon the repentant son as his older brother wanted to do, but gladly took him in his arms and forgave, restoring him immediately in full fellowship. A forgiving heart will keep parents from reacting in anger and keep children from becoming discouraged.

Many who have observed well-adjusted children note that they invariably have parents who manifest two specific qualities. First, the parents are empathic and loving towards their children. To *empathize* means we are able to identify with and understand another's situation, feelings, and motives. Empathetic parents will love their children with the kind of love described in *1 Corinthians 13:4-7*. "Charity suffereth long, and is kind; charity envieth not; charity vaunteth not itself, is not puffed up, doth not behave itself unseemly, seeketh not her own, is not easily provoked, thinketh no evil; rejoiceth not in iniquity, but rejoiceth in the truth;

beareth all things, believeth all things, hopeth all things, endureth all things. Charity never faileth." The Bible teaches us that this kind of tenderhearted, sacrificial love is the greatest motivating force known to mankind.

Second, it has been observed that successful parents are firm in setting limitations and are non-indulgent towards their children. It is simply the other side of the same coin. Firm parents love their children with the kind of love described in *Proverbs 13:24*. "He that spareth his rod hateth his son: but he that loveth him chasteneth him betimes." The Bible teaches us that setting definite limits for our children's benefit, and caring enough to take the pains required to enforce those limits, is the outcome of our choice to love them.

Children Spell Love: T-I-M-E

The Bible warns, "And, ye fathers, provoke not your children to wrath: but bring them up in the nurture and admonition of the Lord" *(Ephesians 6:4)*. When parents do not practice Biblical love, they provoke their children to act in anger or become discouraged. Children often act up, or display frustration or anger, when they feel misunderstood or hurt, when they sense their parents are acting out of selfish motives, or when they sense their parents are not interested in investing time into their lives.

Children very quickly discern whether those in authority over them are governed by a genuine interest in their good or by selfish motives. Very often, problems arise when parents love themselves too much, and fail to love their children enough to adequately invest the time required to train them and guide them properly.

Parents communicate a lack of love when they fail to

- Take the time to respond to disciplinary needs consistently, justly, and mercifully.
- Take the time to provide for the legitimate emotional, physical, and spiritual needs of their children.
- Take the time to listen, understand, and attend to a child's individual fears, problems, and concerns.
- Take the time to teach their child how to complete tasks, how to succeed, and how to live.

There is no such thing as quality time without quantity. While it's true that we often spend time with our children in unproductive, or less than enjoyable ways, it is not true that quality time miraculously erases the need for a quantity of it. It requires time to help children learn to tie their shoes or help them with their homework, (especially if a parent has to re-learn algebra to do it). It requires time to read bedtime stories (over and over again), to play games, or help a child learn a new skill. It takes time to listen to a child tell about his daily thoughts and fears, hopes and dreams, disappointments and achievements (and money if they go away to college

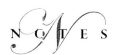

and need to talk on the phone often). You can be sure that good communication with family members doesn't just happen. Good communication requires time to develop.

It takes a lot of time to patiently referee a dispute between children, and teach them how to resolve their problems. It takes an enormous amount of time (and repetition) to daily discipline and train a toddler to become an obedient and self-controlled child. It takes an investment of time to organize and discipline a child's life, to follow up on requests, to see that schedules and responsibilities are met. It requires time to teach children godly principles of living, and time to have leisurely discussions (usually at night when you'd rather be sleeping) about living happily and successfully in a world that is hostile towards Christians. It requires time to explain Scripture passages and how they can be applied to specific situations.

It requires time to prepare balanced meals for a family and favorite home baked goodies that warm a child's heart (not to mention time to clean up the mess). It requires time to care for a sick child, to bandage scrapes (or sit in an emergency room), and to get to the dentist before a toothache interrupts everyone's life. It takes time to keep children bathed (especially boys), and their hair cut and fixed neatly. It takes time to teach children how to select clothes that reflect good Christian taste and keep them washed, ironed, and mended. It requires time to take children to soccer practice, baseball practice, piano practice, swimming lessons, and youth activities. It takes time to fix broken bike chains, to play catch, and to go on hikes. It takes even more time and energy to cheer at their games and participate or help in their activities. It takes time to teach children how to work, how to manage money, how to develop interests and skills necessary to live happily and responsibly in years to come.

It takes time to sponsor a slumber party (and recover the following day), to plan a birthday party, or make special days truly special. It takes time to pray for your children, to take them to church faithfully, and to involve them in projects of Christian service. It takes time to teach a little girl to be a lady and a little boy to be a man.

It takes more than quality, my friend. It takes a great deal of *quantity* to raise good children and be a good mother and good father. In fact, it requires more than an enormous investment of your time and life to raise well-adjusted children. It requires *a sacrifice of your time and life*. And isn't that what love is all about? Love is sacrificing ourselves to meet the true and legitimate needs of another, just as Jesus did for us.

When we see a well-trained dog delighting to respond to his owner's commands, we know that owner invested time in his training. It would be silly to assume such an obedient dog learned obedience without time and effort on the part of its owner. It is just as ludicrous to think obedient children learned obedience without an investment of time and effort on the part of his parents. You cannot possibly expect to reap the benefits of happy, well-behaved and godly children if you are not willing to invest your life in the project.

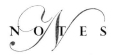

How Much Time Do You Spend Each Week

_____ talking   _____ listening

_____ playing   _____ teaching

_____ praying   _____ helping

What are the special needs of each of your children that require your time?

[1] Banks, Louis Albert. *Anecdotes and Morals*. London: Funk and Wagnalls, 1898. Page 12.

Lesson 4

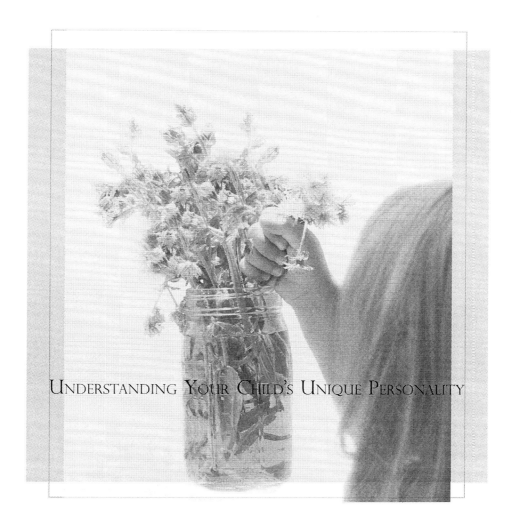

Understanding Your Child's Unique Personality

But now, O LORD, thou *art* our father; we *are* the clay, and thou our potter; and we all *are* the work of thy hand.
Isaiah 64:8

I will praise thee; for I am fearfully *and* wonderfully made: marvelous *are* thy works; and *that* my soul knoweth right well.
Psalm 139:14

Key THOUGHTS

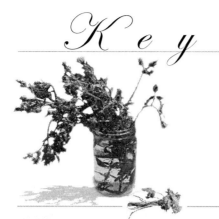

Parents need to recognize how greatly they influence their children's personality development. They must accept the responsibility God has given them by diligently influencing their children in loving, godly ways. They must also learn to understand and recognize that their children possess many God-given, inborn personality traits that can be refined, but not changed. Finally, Christian parents need to remember that spiritual growth produces the greatest impact on personality development, which is not recognized by child development experts who do not understand the power of the gospel to change lives.

Discussion Problem

Brenda has four children. Her oldest seventeen-year-old son is on the honor roll at school, is very athletic and sociable. He is often called the "life of the party" and is full of energy. Brenda's fifteen-year-old daughter is also very bright. She is quiet and sensitive, but well liked and talented in music and art. The youngest is a cute and lovable little girl who is easy going, non-demanding, and adored by friends and family members alike. Brenda's third child is eight-year-old Danny. Danny is not very aggressive or coordinated in sports, lacks social maturity, and struggles in school. Brenda and her husband Pete describe Danny (even in his presence) as their *problem child*. It seems no matter what they do, they cannot get Danny to excel as the two older children have. Pete forces Danny to play baseball even though Danny hates it, and tries to get his son to be more manly and athletic like he and Danny's older brother. Most of the time, Pete ends up scolding Danny in frustration and screaming that Danny just isn't trying.

Lately Danny has been waking up with stomachaches and begs his mother to let him stay home from school. He often cries and says that no one understands him, and that he can't do anything right. Danny likes animals and enjoys building and fixing things, but Pete and Brenda believe his dawdling over animals and broken toys is a waste of time. They want him to be more aggressive, more sociable, and more successful in school so he can win a college scholarship someday as their oldest son has done.

After reading lesson four, use the principles you have learned to discuss what is different about Danny, what could be contributing to his discouragement and lack of confidence, and what his parents could do to change the situation. Also, see if you can identify which personality traits most characterize Danny.

Bible Study

1. According to Psalm 10:14, 17-18, parents who oppress and neglect their children will be _____ when the children cry out to God.

2. From Exodus 22:22-23, Deuteronomy 10:18, and Job 29:12 we learn that God is especially attentive and responds to the _____ of a child who is mistreated, in particular, a child who does not have _____ or someone to help him.

3. In Psalm 127:3 David recognized that children are a _____.

"A mother understands what a child does not say."
Author Unknown

Longing To Be Understood

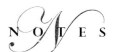

Stan was a quiet, soft spoken college senior of slight build, studious, polite, and determined to work his way through college; certainly not the kind of college student one would expect to see in the back of a police car. As you read about Stan's nightmarish ordeal in the following paragraphs, imagine you are Stan. What would you be experiencing emotionally? How would you respond to the same kind of treatment? What caused the misinterpretations? What good qualities do you see in Stan? Most importantly, note your reactions at being misunderstood as opposed to being treated with understanding.

Wise parents are able to put themselves in their child's place and see events through their child's eyes. They listen carefully (without interrupting), and work at understanding what their child is experiencing and what kind of response would be most appropriate and encouraging. Children and teens tend to listen to those who convey their understanding and compassion in times of distress. What will impact children and teens most isn't agreement or disagreement, but understanding. Evaluate how well you are able to see events through Stan's eyes and how keenly you can empathize with his emotions and reactions based on what you might infer regarding his personality and unique situation.

Stan's day had begun normal enough with a 7:00 mid-term exam that he had studied for late into the night. After two more exams on opposite ends of the campus, Stan rushed off to work to make it on time. Business was heavy and men were out sick making it an exhausting night's work. Stan couldn't wait to climb into his pickup and head home to a nice warm bed—even if home was a college dorm shared with several rambunctious freshmen that hadn't yet found jobs. Stan drove through the local McDonalds and devoured his Big Mac, coke, and fries before he even reached the highway leading home. The only thing on his mind was sleep and pleasant thoughts about Jenny, the girl he planned to propose to, once her overpowering father was convinced he was the kind of person he wanted his daughter to marry.

As Stan turned off the highway onto a winding canyon road, he felt a sense of relief to be minutes away from the comfort of his bed. He was so lost in his thoughts that he almost didn't notice the thump from under his truck; but looking back through his rear view mirror, he could see the form of a dog on the road and feared he had run over him. Stan pulled off to the side of the road and slowly backed up until he reached the lifeless dog, bleeding and obviously dead. Tears came to his eyes as he felt for the dog's collar and turned it until he could read the tags. Sure enough, they included the dog's name and an address just a few blocks away. Stan carefully lifted the animal into the back of his truck, covered him with a blanket and drove to the address printed on the dog tag. As he pulled into the driveway he noticed two men standing to the side talking. The men looked at him suspiciously as he climbed out of his truck and walked toward them. "Do either of you own a dog named Buck?" Stan asked quietly. "Yeah, one gentleman mumbled, what about it?" "I, uh, I…I'm so sorry," Stan whispered, "I'm afraid he ran in front of my truck and…and…I have him in back…"

At that moment the owner became enraged and began yelling obscenities as he ran to the back of the pickup. He tore the blanket off the dog and hugged it close to his chest weeping one moment and screaming hateful threats at Stan the next. Stan stood back, stunned, not quite knowing what he should do next. The man's friend finally convinced the owner to let him take the dog to the side of the yard for him, all the while the man continued threatening and yelling. At that moment, the man's wife ran from the house and reached the truck about the time her husband was pushing Stan and calling him a murderer. Hearing this, the woman turned and ran back to the house and called the police.

Officers arrived moments later with the dog owner still screaming at Stan and hollering to the policeman that Stan had hit him. As the officer ran toward the men with a flashlight he immediately saw the blood on the dog owner's shirt and ordered his partner to get Stan into the police car. Although Stan tried to explain the situation to the officers, they were lost in the confusion and gruffly ordered him to turn around while they handcuffed him and put him into the car. Eventually, they did sort out the situation and realized the blood wasn't the man's but the dog's and Stan hadn't done anything to the man but try to fulfill his obligation to report the accident. Before the problem was resolved, however, fellow students from the college had driven by and recognized Stan's truck. Seeing Stan handcuffed and hearing the man yelling, they wondered what was happening but were ordered to leave by the officers. Of course, they excitedly rushed back to the dorm and found school authorities to report their story.

The report that had been given included details of how Stan had "pulled off the road and beaten up a man after getting into an argument with him." Supposedly, the man's wife called the police who then arrived to pull Stan off the man who was bleeding and angry. Stan, they reported, had been arrested and was probably on his way to the police station. This set in motion all kinds of excitement in the dorm as students discussed what they had heard. By the time Stan arrived back at the school, weary and distressed, the story had snowballed into a major incident that in no way resembled the actual event. Before he could explain what had taken place, the dorm supervisor told him he was expelled, his things were already packed, and his parents on their way to get him. At that point he buried his head in his hands and wept, too exhausted to defend himself further.

Stan went home that night with his parents and returned the next day to talk with the dean of men who had requested an appointment with him. Stan's emotions were intense as he entered the office, and though he certainly tried, he couldn't hide his sense of injustice and the flash of anger in his eyes as he returned the dean's greeting and sat down. Stan began to pour out the details of his story with a less than gracious tone as he anticipated a cold response or lecture from the dean. Instead of answering roughly as Stan had expected, the gray-headed gentleman listened intently as Stan explained the events that had transpired, and nodded with obvious concern and compassion. The dean immediately expressed his understanding and expressed his regrets about the way the incident had been handled. Stan relaxed and sighed with relief. The anger seemed to melt away in the warmth of the dean's kindness and empathy. Stan found himself anxious to put the incident behind him and get back to his studies, and surprised himself that he was leaving the dean's office encouraged and ready to forgive.

Sadly, Jenny's father couldn't be convinced of Stan's innocence, and refused to allow her to continue a relationship with him. He interpreted Stan's quiet response as evidence of guilt and weakness. He was certain, he told his daughter, that Stan's judgment was questionable and that his absentmindedness a detriment to future success. Stan was brokenhearted and his confidence badly shaken after being delivered this news. He found himself longing for an understanding friend and attempted to convey his disappointment to several of his dorm mates. Their "help," however, was more a discouragement than a comfort.

One friend listened politely, then interrupted Stan and said, "You know, it's no big deal. Someday you'll laugh about it. And I wouldn't get mixed up with any girl whose father has to give his permission in order for her to marry someone." Another said, "Hey, dude, why did you hit the dog in the first place? Didn't you see him run in front of you? And why didn't you just turn around and leave when the dog owner started yelling? I'd have been out of there by then. That was kind of stupid to just stand there, don't you think? What were you thinking?" Still another offered his contribution to the debate and said, "I can understand how the dog owner would feel, hearing his dog that he loved was dead. He was probably just in shock and not thinking straight since it was such a traumatic thing. You should be glad he didn't pull a gun out and shoot you. As for Jenny, just be glad you found out what her family was like before you married her." When one of the more spiritually minded in the group piped up and said, "Hey Stan, you know *Romans 8:28* don't you?" Stan decided he'd had enough of the conversation and walked out, slamming the door behind him.

Stan wandered around the campus for several hours, trying to look occupied, but becoming more distressed by the moment as his thoughts churned with the memory of everything that had been said. He toyed with the idea of leaving school even though graduation was just weeks away, or going to Jenny's house and trying to talk with her dad once more. His stomach was in knots as he pondered his choices and sensed the bitterness that was beginning to settle over him like a fog. By chance he found himself in the vicinity of the dean's office, and remembering the dean's kindness decided to see if he had time to talk. The man welcomed Stan into his office and listened as though he had all the time in the world. Stan decided to stay in school, and met with the gracious school dean on several occasions. Though his hopes for a future with Jenny were dashed and the relationship was never regained, Stan did find the understanding and encouragement he was looking for. Stan grew to respect the kind and wise gentleman's manner and as a result, listened and learned from him through the experience.

Stan almost graduated a brokenhearted and bitter young man, but instead, he was able to rejoice with his classmates and look forward to his future with hope and enthusiasm. Several years later, he testified at a men's prayer meeting that one man's love and kindness at a crucial time in his life kept his heart tender toward the Lord and made a difference in his life. Every time he was tempted to be bitter and doubt God's work in his life, he remembered the gentle words of this man, urging him to keep trusting God and commending him for his desire to do what was right to the best of his ability. "I learned so many valuable lessons though this experience," Stan told the men, "but one of the best is the way it has taught me to be sensitive to my own little boy and listen patiently when he is experiencing moments of distress."

It is not uncommon for parents to catch themselves responding to their children's predicaments somewhat like Stan's dorm mates, with impatient declarations of what they should or should not have done, dishing out advice, lecturing, questioning suspiciously, or denying the significance or validity of the child's feelings. Some parents' typical response is to compare their child's situation with something that happened to them as a child or to minimize a child's problems, while others overreact with pity and become angry at whoever or whatever caused their children to suffer. Still other parents become adept at eliciting guilt and treat the child as though he has brought untold suffering upon them. These and other insensitive responses turn conversations with children into arguments, build walls of resentment, and break down any kind of meaningful communication between parent and child. Such parents often report that they just "can't get through" to their kids, or they just can't understand why their kids have a "chip on their shoulder" or don't respect them as they desire.

Misunderstandings, emotional outbursts, anger, and icy stares are only a few of the consequences that occur when parents do not learn how to listen, understand, and appreciate their children's unique qualities and problems from the child's point of view. On the other hand, parents who are able to recognize and value their children's individual abilities and limitations in light of God's sovereign gifts work in their children's lives to build bridges instead of walls between themselves and their children. Such parents are better able to think as the child is thinking and are able to more naturally follow the best course of action. Children and teens do want to talk, and they will, to whomever will listen with a loving and understanding ear. When parents listen with understanding, they will find that children listen better too.

King David went through some distressing times during which he expressed this same human longing to be understood. Note the disappointment permeating his words, "I looked on my right hand, and beheld, but there was no man that would know me; refuge failed me; no man cared for my soul" (Psalm 142:4). David expressed dismay in his search for understanding, and concluded that nobody really cared. When he said, "No man would know me," he was saying that no one understood him. Like many of us have done, he concluded that no one cared for his soul; no one loved him for what he really was inside.

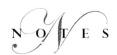

Thankfully, David came to the realization that someone did love him dearly and understood him thoroughly as no one else can. In Psalm 142:5 David acknowledges his complete dependence on the Lord and says, "I cried unto thee, O LORD; I said, Thou art my refuge and my portion in the land of the living." Then David praises his God who perfectly understands every heartache, injustice, and longing of his heart. When David understood this truth, he found peace and comfort just we and our children will find encouragement in realizing our Heavenly Father loves us. Unlike adults, however, children need to be shown this truth by someone who will demonstrate love and understanding. More than anything, children need parents who will invest time and effort into knowing them, and assuring them that they are loved and understood by them, as well as by God.

Different for a Reason

The greatest way to influence our children and help them grow to be well-adjusted, happy people is to love and nurture them within the framework of a loving family; and if we love them, we will take the time to listen to and understand each one individually to the best of our frail human ability. Differences in personality, interests, and ability should not be regarded as good and bad, but as gifts God gives each individual for a specific reason. If everyone were born with the exact same combination of inborn personality traits, people would not be motivated to pursue the diversity of interests, talents, and activities that they do. Nor would they accomplish the variety of purposes that God wants each of us to accomplish within the context of His great plan.

Our differences allow us to fulfill God's will for our lives. They also force us to learn how to harmonize and cooperate together as a team. If everyone were an extroverted social butterfly, we'd have a bumper crop of entertainers, salesmen, and social workers, but few artists, scientists, musicians, or engineers. If everyone were quiet and contemplative, we would have lots of musicians and engineers, but few performers and salespeople. Some people do best as inventors. Others shine as managers. Some have a knack for manufacturing. Others thrive on a zeal for sales. All these personalities are needed to make a company productive, a family enriched, or a church blessed.

It is interesting to see how God equips each local church with many members who have a vast diversity of gifts, talents, and personalities. Some people have been given a special desire and aptitude to teach. Others have a keen sense of organizational and administrative abilities. Some people love to help. Others have a special desire for ministering to those who are sick or discouraged. Still others are gifted in their ability to discern problems and apply practical and Biblical solutions to them. Some have a gift for preaching and evangelizing. Churches have members who are musically talented as well as members who are gifted to work with children's programs. There are some who have exceptional secretarial skills, and others who are able to use their artistic expertise to bless the church ministries in artistic ways.

The important thing to remember is that God brings together many different people, each one having something unique and vital to contribute. The church family is merely a larger picture of the smaller family unit. Each provides a context in which God expects us to grow to learn how to interact with others and how to develop patience and humility, love and forgiveness, cooperation and understanding for others different than ourselves. The experience of childhood is meant to teach us how to interact with others in a godly way in a larger context as adults. The experience of parenting further teaches us to grow in grace, depend on the Lord, seek God's wisdom, develop spiritual discernment, and turn away from selfishness and intolerance. Differences are not always easy to understand or deal with, nor were they intended to be. They do, however, prompt us to grow spiritually; and they do open our eyes to God's ways versus our own.

Differences in personality, interests, and ability should not be regarded as good and bad, but as gifts God gives each individual for a specific reason.

The Bible teaches us that there is one Lord, one salvation, one baptism, and one faith. However, our personalities, experiences, inborn traits, talents, and aspirations are all as numerous and different as the snowflakes that fall from the sky. God, Who is the master of variety, delights to make us different for reasons that are sometimes known to Him, but not to us. It is He who is the architect of our lives and who determines the factors that make us unique. This realization ought to cause us to marvel at God's wisdom and grace, but also ought to humble us to put aside our own aspirations and plans for our children and seek *His* plan for each of them instead.

We can be certain that our children's differences have a purpose; and that they have been given everything they need to do exactly what God would have them to do. Not one of them is deficient in any way when we understand that God has a destiny for every single one to fulfill, and each has the potential to glorify God with his life. We measure success and determine value so differently than God. Accomplishment in our eyes so often means a child achieves a successful career or ministry, fame, money, material possessions, and talent. Yet many children accomplish exactly what God wants them to accomplish and never receive so much as one award or trophy their entire life. When Jesus sought out the twelve men who would be his disciples and hold a place of honor in heaven for eternity, He did not seek out powerful, successful men by the world's standard. He chose common, ordinary, sinful men who were humble and willing to follow Him.

Simple men that no one suspected, such as the man born blind that we read about in the book of John, had a special place in God's plan. Jesus' disciples pitied the man and assumed his parents were given this child as some kind of punishment for sin. They asked Christ, "Master, who did sin, this man, or his parents, that he was born blind? Jesus answered, Neither hath this man sinned, nor his parents; but that the works of God should be made manifest in him" *(John 9:2-3)*. When Jesus allowed Lazarus to die, he told his disciples that, "This sickness is not unto death, but for the glory of God that the Son of God might be glorified thereby" *(John 11:4)*.

Many times difficulties produce eternal accomplishments that we don't readily see any more than the disciples immediately saw the eternal significance of earthly imperfections in these cases. Our children's differences and even their difficulties give us opportunities to learn things we would not learn in any other context, just as their differences cause *them* to learn things they would not learn in any other context. Out of the most unlikely circumstances and imperfections have come some of the greatest stories of God's grace and work ever seen among God's people. Never underestimate the great potential of the most mundane!

God's Evaluation System

Given a choice, we are naturally more drawn to things that are beautiful than things that appear plain or unattractive. Children want the biggest and prettiest Christmas gift under the tree. Parents want the house that has curb appeal and character. Teenagers want the cutest outfit, the coolest car, and the most youthful looking teacher. After we have what we want, however, we often discover that the biggest and prettiest gift under the tree isn't always the most desirable once it is opened. The house with curb appeal and character may have structural problems that make it a money pit. The cutest outfit may not flatter everyone's figure, the coolest car may be the most troublesome, and the most attractive teacher may not be able to teach at all. On the other hand, we are often given gifts that don't look very attractive on the outside or don't seem desirable at first, but later prove to be most valuable. Sometimes we have to peel away the wrappings to discover that the inside is precious, appropriate, and beautiful.

Parents who are given the gift of a child may be disappointed that the child isn't as attractive as they had hoped. The child is not the smartest, the most beautiful, the most talented, or the most socially graceful. In fact, the child may very well come appearing to be broken or defective in some way. Though it may not seem so at first, the parent who trusts the goodness and wise heart of God soon discovers that what's inside is precious and desirable, and what seems defective at first is found to be the perfect gift after all. Every gift that comes from God is to be received with thankfulness and joy, knowing it is given with love and wisdom. But to be genuinely thankful, we will need to reject the human value system that ascribes special significance and virtue to some talents, gifts, and personalities over others. We will have to resist the temptation to go for the prettiest gift, and be content instead with the one we may not have originally picked out for ourselves.

In *1 Corinthians 12*, Paul warns us not to think one person is more important or valuable to God because he has any specific gift or talent. Paul reminds us that everything we have, our intelligence, physical abilities, and special advantages, are given by God. Everything we have the power to achieve or obtain comes from God. This includes our power to have wealth and our parental heritage. All we do or do not have is ordained by God to accomplish something specific for His glory and His purpose. We have nothing to boast about and no cause to feel superior or inferior. In fact, the more gifted and privileged we are, the more God holds us responsible to account for properly using our talents and gifts for His glory. Children cannot be anything they wish to be by sheer willpower and determination. To teach such a thing sets children up for disappointment and failure. They can, however, be everything God wants them to be, by His strength and power. "I can do all things through Christ, which strengtheneth me" *(Philippians 4:13)*.

The most gifted people often have a greater tendency to become proud and critical. The person who knows he is less talented and therefore, less desirable, has a tendency to get bogged down in self-pity and discontentment. The problem isn't that we have too much or not enough. The problem is that we base our evaluations on what *we* want and what *we* believe is valuable, not on what *God* wants and what *God* determines to be valuable. God is honored and pleased when we humbly accept the way He made us and seek to fulfill the unique place He wants us to fulfill, no matter where that place is, or how it is esteemed in the eyes of others. When we as parents truly understand and accept *ourselves* in this way, we are then able to teach our children how to be thankful and content with the way God made *them*. This Biblical view of acceptance prevents children from developing an attitude of either superiority *or* inferiority; both are emotionally and spiritually debilitating.

A Parent's Hopes and Dreams

Imagine the futility of trying to make a cow act like a horse. You might be able to fashion a saddle and bridle for him, but he's never going to win the Kentucky Derby or draw anything but laughter at the hunt club. Parents who are wise will not try to mold their child's personality into a carbon copy of their own, nor will they attempt to make their child fulfill a purpose the child was never made to fulfill. Wise parents do not attempt to call their own children to preach or preordain their children to pursue a specific vocation of their own choosing. Instead, discerning parents seek to discover the particular qualities God has given each of their children and encourage them to develop their own unique interests and talents. They occupy themselves with their responsibility to teach their children to love and serve God, letting God call their children to do what He desires them to.

Children who are encouraged to become something God did not give them the ability to become often develop feelings of failure or frustration. They typically lose their motivation to achieve, and fail to develop the confidence that they need to succeed. Very often such children attempt to please their parents or others who urge them to follow the direction they might like to go only to end up falling miserably short of the dreams the parents tried so hard to instill in them. Many children grow up to be adults who struggle for years in ministries and occupations they did not choose and were not ever well suited for. Some are never able to go back and regain the ability to pursue their own hopes and dreams.

Let me tell you about three fathers. The first believed all boys who enjoyed music or played the piano were effeminate. He declared that he would never allow his son to pursue music. Instead, he said, his boys would all be football players and pursue

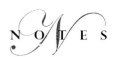

more manly interests. Another father vowed that all his children would go to college and succeed as professionals. Still another proudly announced that every child of his would someday be a preacher or missionary or marry one. These fathers all reaped disastrous consequences as a result of their presumptuous expectations.

The first had several sons who did, indeed, pursue sports and "manly" vocations. However, he had one who hated contact sports but was gifted musically and longed to learn an instrument. This son was a constant source of embarrassment to the father and the son became so discouraged that he one day hung himself in despair. The second father had two children, neither of which went to college, let alone became successful professionals. One child was dyslexic and struggled just to graduate from high school, but happily found work as an auto mechanic. The other had absolutely no interest in a career and chose instead to marry a Christian schoolteacher and raise a family. The third father managed to coerce every child into Bible college and ministry as he had predicted, but none of the children are happy, have any respect for their father, or have any desire to emulate his spiritual walk. One after another the children have confessed their anger toward their father and struggled to overcome bitterness.

What a tragedy it is for any child to be pushed and pulled in directions God did not equip him to go. How much better it is when parents observe the natural inborn traits, special interests, abilities, and talents of each individual child as his personality unfolds throughout his childhood. Then, as a child's differences and strengths are distinguished, the parents seek to guide him in developing and using his personality and talents to the greatest extent for God's glory.

As you assess your child's natural personality style, you will find it easier to understand things that are most likely to motivate, interest, or discourage him. Remember that every child longs to be known and understood. When children believe they are understood, they are more willing to listen and communicate openly with parents. Consequently, understanding your child gives you greater opportunity to influence him for good and guide him in the direction God wants him to go. Take time to observe, understand, and appreciate your child's differences. You will never regret it.

Personality Development

Many complex factors contribute to the development of personality. Some factors are orchestrated by God Himself, such as our parental heritage, the circumstances which exist in our parent's life at the time we are born, our birth order, or other life-changing events such as illness or experiences which alter the way we must live our lives. Our personality is also a reflection of inborn traits that are part of our God-given nature. These aspects of our personality are determined at conception in the same way our eye color is determined the moment we are conceived. Our sin nature influences the way our personalities develop, as well as the individual spiritual choices we make, including our choice to either obey the Gospel or reject it, or to live an obedient or rebellious Christian life. Finally, our environment, individual experiences, and people we associate with all have the potential to affect our personality.

1. Sin changes a personality.

Our personality is influenced by the sin nature we are born with. When we, or our children, do not choose to love God or learn to live for Him, our sinful hearts automatically gravitate toward a sinful, selfish way of life. We develop attitudes and behavior patterns depending on how our sinful inclinations are aroused or brought under control during our young lives. Left undisciplined or unrestrained, children remain self-centered and deceitful into adulthood and become miserable people.

Parents play a tremendous role in the way they influence their children toward sin and self-will or toward love and obedience. The influence for good or evil depends in how parents discipline and curtail their children's naturally sinful urges and desires. If parents do not control and bring into submission their children's sin nature, sinful characteristics will become all the more integrated into the child's developing personality.

The desires of our sinful nature (and our children's sinful natures) are easily identified. In *1 John 2:16* we read, "For all that is in the world, the lust of the flesh, and the lust of the eyes, and the pride of life, is not of the Father, but is of the world." We can describe the lust of the flesh as our unlawful physical desires, the lust of the eyes as our unlawful desires for possessions, and the pride of life as our unlawful desire to govern our own life and be exalted. Even the youngest of our children manifest these three characteristics of man's sinful nature. They do not need to be taught to say, "That's *mine*!"—lust of the flesh; "I *want*"—lust of the eyes; or "You don't pay enough attention to *me* so I don't like you!"—pride of life.

Any mother who has refereed a childhood squabble can attest to the fact that children can be stingy, self-centered, and possessive. If these natural, sinful attitudes are not curbed with loving discipline and control, selfishness, self-indulgence, and arrogance *will* be a molding influence on a child's developing personality. Most importantly, if a child does not grow in spiritual understanding and come to a saving knowledge of the Lord Jesus Christ, his heart will remain unregenerate and unchanged by the power of the Holy Spirit Who conforms all believers to be like Christ. Just as children bear the marks or traits of genetics and human nature, so they also bear the birthmarks of salvation when their hearts are transformed by God's power and brought into conformity with the Word of God by faith in Christ. Nothing has the power to transform a child's personality in the way salvation and loving obedience to Christ does. The fruit of the Spirit is not the result of genetics or environment; the fruit of the Spirit is the result of one's relationship to Christ regardless whether one is a child or an adult.

2. Heart-decisions alter personality.

A child's personality is profoundly affected by the individual choices he makes. Identical twins who have similar temperaments, expressions, inborn personality traits, and talents nevertheless become uniquely different adults as a result of personal choices they each make throughout their lives. One may choose a sinful path and the other a life of obedience to God; each choice produces distinctive differences in personality even while they remain quite remarkably alike.

Choices such as these originate in what the Bible describes as our heart. Our heart is the place where thoughts and actions are weighed and acted upon. It is the place of our most cherished desires and deeply held beliefs. Identical twins with the same genes, chromosomes, and environmental advantages or disadvantages are able to develop into separate people who differ drastically in personality style because every individual is given both the freedom and responsibility to make choices about what he believes and does. Personality is greatly influenced by what we come to believe and desire as well as how we choose to respond to life experiences.

3. Environment and experiences affect personality.

A child's personality is not only influenced by his sin nature, his decisions, and his circumstances, but also by his environment and experiences. Mothers are able to influence the development of their children's character and personality to a large degree because character and personality are, in part, a reflection of the environment and experiences that a parent *can* control.

Because children are particularly susceptible to absorbing both good and bad information, suggestions, and impressions, they do become, to a great extent, whatever they are exposed to and whatever they are allowed to do or believe. Consequently, parents have a tremendous responsibility and opportunity to influence their children's developing personalities in ways that will help them grow up to be happy, well-adjusted adults who love and glorify God. Though we cannot possibly control all the factors that will mold our children's personalities, we *can* play an important part by pleasing God and teaching our children to please Him.

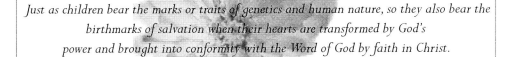

> *Just as children bear the marks or traits of genetics and human nature, so they also bear the birthmarks of salvation when their hearts are transformed by God's power and brought into conformity with the Word of God by faith in Christ.*

A popular and often repeated verse entitled "Children Learn What They Live" reminds us that children *are* influenced, and their personalities affected, by the way parents live and interact with them. Isn't it interesting that many of the qualities listed in this poem reflect qualities God's Word teaches are natural to those who have trusted Christ as their Savior and are obedient to the Word of God? Since our spiritual nature is produced as we walk in faith and obedience, we may conclude that parents who love God will reflect spiritual qualities which will greatly influence their children's personality development and future well being.

> **Children Learn What They Live**
> Copyright © 1972 by Dorothy Law Nolte
>
> If children live with criticism, they learn to condemn.
> If children live with hostility, they learn to fight.
> If children live with fear, they learn to be apprehensive.
> If children live with pity, they learn to feel sorry for themselves.
> If children live with ridicule, they learn to feel shy.
> If children live with jealousy, they learn to feel envy.
> If children live with shame, they learn to feel guilty.
> If children live with encouragement, they learn confidence.
> If children live with tolerance, they learn patience.
> If children live with acceptance, they learn to love.
> If children live with honesty, they learn truthfulness.
> If children live with fairness, they learn justice.
> If children live with kindness and consideration, they learn respect.

4. Personality is partly inherited at conception.

The "nurture or nature" debate continues to be an issue with some who insist it has to be one or the other. If we look at the issue in light of what we learn in the study of Scripture we have no problem admitting personality is both the result of "nature," or inherited God-given personality traits, *and* "nurture" or that which modifies our particular style of thinking and behaving by external influences. Observant mothers have always been able to differentiate between contrasting personalities in babies and children. Mothers who give birth to more than one child or care for several different children don't need a Ph.D. to tell them their children do not begin life as a blank slate. From day one, mothers recognize each baby is distinctively different. One will be easy-going, another more fretful, one more explosive, or one more social. Furthermore, mothers recognize gender differences and know little girls gravitate toward dolls just as naturally as boys gravitate toward dirt and cars without any assistance or encouragement whatsoever from anyone. Mothers may not know the categories some have developed to describe personality traits in modern professional

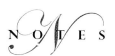

jargon, but they recognize distinct differences even without the labels and will be found enthusiastically discussing such differences with fellow mothers.

It has been observed that similar personalities often gravitate toward similar interests and occupations no matter what pressures are put on them to conform differently. Sometimes intelligence results in personality "quirks" that can be quite predictable and common, and are in no way diminished by outside influence other than to provide understanding and direction that will harness them constructively or unloose them destructively. Many inborn factors provoke individuals to react in similar ways and display similar types of difficulties no matter what environment they live in. Predictable gender differences are apparent in any environment, no matter how hard feminists try to ignore the obvious and convince us otherwise. Outside influences may affect how a person ultimately deals with their characteristics and uses them for good or evil, but quite often, environment seems to have little impact on much personality development that is genetically induced.

Each person's inborn personality is as unique as his fingerprints and is neither sinful nor undesirable. They are merely different qualities that make us unique and equip us for a specific role in life that God desires us to fulfill.

The Four Temperaments Evaluated

In recent years it has become popular to write books extolling the virtues of categorizing people into one of four temperaments. Some authors insist that knowledge of the four temperaments makes the difference between success and failure, stability and instability, happiness and unhappiness. Many authors make a good case for the helpful virtues of understanding human differences that are inherited and recognizing inborn traits that influence behavior patterns. However, their claims cannot go beyond these benefits without drastically contradicting Biblical understanding of what determines a person's success or failure, emotional stability or instability, happiness or unhappiness. Nowhere in the entire Bible will you find Scripture that supports the claim that such an understanding will make the difference in these areas.

When we take the study of personality traits to the extreme and begin seeing others in terms of a label that implies they *are* a certain group of traits, we run the danger of assuming more than we should about ourselves or another person. The Bible teaches us that quick evaluations are never wise *(Proverbs 18:13)*. Rather, after carefully listening and collecting substantiated information, we are to discern a person's actions and character based on scriptural criteria. Categorizing personalities too often leads to hasty conclusions that prove to be misleading and sometimes damaging. Pigeonholing ourselves or other people into a combination of one or two temperament groups is far too broad and generalized to be accurate. It is true that many traits do tend to go together with others, but there are so many variables and exceptions to the rules that any attempt to understand a person by categorizing him is fraught with many pitfalls.

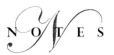

Inborn Traits

The four temperament systems also pose a danger because virtually all its proponents mix traits that are sinful with traits that are not. Outbursts of anger or selfishness, for instance, are never referred to in the Bible as anything other than sins. Assigning a sinful trait as part of one's *temperament* obscures the issue that we have a sinful nature that is capable of turning any good trait into one that has a bad side to it.

The Bible never encourages us to change our behavior by attributing sinful tendencies to our personality style. Rather, we are to recognize the character traits of our sinful nature and walk, instead, by God's righteous nature that indwells every believer. We are instructed to identify, confess, and forsake our sins, but we are never told to identify our "negative inborn temperament traits."

Remember that whatever benefit is derived by studying the man-made four temperament systems falls woefully short of the benefits derived by simply learning to identify God-made spiritual gifts and by learning to recognize character traits of sin and of righteousness. We make mistakes when we describe sinful qualities as temperament or personality traits. Our negative traits are not quirks in our natural personality, but God-given good qualities that have been tainted and changed by our sinful nature.

Behavior Patterns

Observing and identifying differing personality traits, which are neither good nor bad, can be helpful and enlightening. It might also be helpful to observe how inborn traits often go together to form distinctive behavior patterns. However, to avoid the pitfalls of categorizing, you will notice that the following exercise uses no labels. They are grouped only to demonstrate how certain traits are often related to others. Following the first exercise is a second chart, which lists and describes each of the traits in the first exercise and individually shows how each can have both a positive and negative side.

As complex human beings, we might describe our personality, or our children's personality, using any number or any combination of the personality traits listed in the following exercise. I believe it is far better, and far more accurate to say, "My child is outgoing, sociable, and easygoing," than to say, "My child is a *golden retriever* or a *sanguine*." One pinpoints definite characteristics; the other causes us to assume characteristics that may not accurately describe a person.

How to Benefit from Studying Personality Traits

Following are four groups of common personality traits. Notice that none of the traits listed are sinful or undesirable. If you mark all the traits that obviously characterize yourself and each family member, you will probably find that each person in your family has a majority of traits in one group. This is because most people, including children, are characterized by traits that often go together with others and form common patterns of personality styles.

However, you will also discover that each member of your family can be described by traits that are listed in any or all of the groups. There are no absolutes when it comes to personality traits, for we can be made up of any combination and be stronger or weaker in any one of the traits. The patterns and variables are infinite, which is precisely why it is important to understand and observe each trait individually rather than trying to understand them as part of a group of traits.

NOTES

Extrovert	
Talkative	Determined
Happy disposition	Independent spirit
Expressive	Leadership-oriented
Carefree	Tenacious
Social	Decisive
Adaptable to other's moods	Competitive
& situations	Aggressive
Performer	Efficient
Active	Confident
Excitable	Outspoken
Spontaneous	Straightforward
Good at short-term focus	Resolute
Animated	

PERSONALITY TRAITS

Sensitive	
Contemplative	Cooperative
Practical	Careful/cautious
Perceptive	Calm
Analytical	Quiet
Detailed thinker	Diplomatic manner
Emotionally responsive	Logical
Artistic/imaginative	Timid
Innovative	Witty thinker
Serious	Placid
Observant	Slow-paced
Discriminating of slight changes	Unexciteable
Resourceful	

Page 73

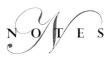

ACTIVE	POSSIBLE PITFALLS
Active people are seldom bored or boring. They have a tremendous capacity for filling their lives with good goals, activities, and achievements. Having a wide variety of interests greatly reduces any tendency towards depressions or deviant behavior. Vivacious individuals tend to have an optimistic outlook on life.	While activity is good, the wrong activity or too much activity can become a major life problem. Overly active people tend to neglect quieter activities and responsibilities. They often try to substitute humanitarian activity for less desirable personal responsibilities. Sometimes personal relationships suffer for lack of quiet care or because the active party has developed a pattern of wanting to be the center of attention.
ADAPTABLE	**POSSIBLE PITFALLS**
Individuals who are easily able to adapt themselves to people and situations take life's changes in stride. They will make the best of just about any situation and aren't resistant to changing their plans or adjusting their expectations when necessary.	Being easily adaptable to situations and people can lead to tolerance for situations that one should not tolerate. Adaptable, enthusiastic people are often easily influenced to buy things they don't really want from persuasive salesmen, or they sympathize with people or causes without taking time to question if they are inappropriate. Adaptable children tend to be followers and can be easily influenced by persuasive friends.
AGGRESSIVE/COMPETITIVE	**POSSIBLE PITFALLS**
Aggressive qualities can be extremely beneficial if aggressiveness is zeal to ardently pursue something good and right. Aggressive people have passion and enthusiasm to eagerly pursue goals and purposes. They can be enterprising, ambitious, energetic, and zealous for the Lord.	Aggressiveness is destructive when it is channeled in such a way that others feelings or rights are not considered and respected. Aggressive individuals sometimes act before they think or zealously pursue endeavors that are not profitable. Their aggressiveness may develop into hostility or belligerence if it is not controlled.
ANALYTICAL/DETAILED THINKER	**POSSIBLE PITFALLS**
People who think analytically have the ability to separate things into parts and break down ideas and actions into smaller principles. This enables such an individual to exercise and discover how things work together. Analytical people are great problem solvers, mathematicians, and teachers. Details are important parts of life to them.	The tendency to want to figure out how things work and systematically organize life into neat columns can cause the analytical great distress when life doesn't work the way it should. Too much attention to detail that isn't significant can cause him to waste time and energy on things that do not matter. He may tend to over-do a project he's working on, whether it is an artistic endeavor or a problem being solved.

ARTISTIC/INNOVATIVE	POSSIBLE PITFALLS
Artistic people add beauty to everything they do. They contribute flair to any hobby or job and excel in music, literature, and art. Artistic people have the ability to see things from differing perspectives, or see how things will look or sound before they're done. They can form mental pictures easily allowing them to construct imaginative solutions while working. They go the extra mile to make something pretty or interesting and add sparkle and inspiration to ideas. They often see problems as puzzles and have a where-there's-a-will-there's-a-way attitude.	Artistic people can become so absorbed in the excitement of creating that they become irritable if distracted. They often lose their train of thought if interrupted. They desire to be sensitive to tension or emotion and are easily affected by it. This earns them the reputation of being rather moody and often self-absorbed. Sometimes imaginative children get into the habit of exaggerating for attention or sliding into self-pity when everything isn't exactly right. Their cleverness can become mischievousness if it's not controlled.

CALM	POSSIBLE PITFALLS
Calm people are usually more patient, optimistic, and flexible. They aren't overly flustered by problems or thrown off course by setbacks and difficulties. They tend to plod along steadily and get things done. They take their own faults in stride and are not easily discouraged.	Calm people can sometimes be inappropriately calm when a serious situation arises. This can make them slow in getting started or in resolving a difficulty before it becomes unmanageable. Calmness can become passivity if it is not controlled. Calm people sometimes have trouble getting motivated and have a more difficult time expressing emotion.

CAREFUL/CAUTIOUS	POSSIBLE PITFALLS
Careful individuals are quick to listen to warnings and learn from the examples of others. They will do whatever they can to avoid making mistakes or getting involved with difficulties. Instead of making quick, impulsive decisions, they collect a large amount of information before proceeding. As a result, they make deliberate, well-thought-out decisions and avoid the mistakes of more impulsive people.	Carefulness can easily become fearfulness, if not balanced. Careful people can become paralyzed with fear and drag their feet when decisions need to be made. Sometimes careful people imagine the worst and develop pessimistic thoughts, which may lead to anxiety and self-inflicted despair.

Notes

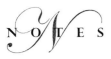

Confident	Possible Pitfalls
Confident individuals approach problems and experiences with courage or boldness. They tend to have a positive mental attitude and trusting approach to life experiences. Confident children will try new things easily, and require little encouragement to attempt an intimidating task. Confident people tend to make friends easily. They pursue goals and achievements zealously.	Confidence can easily turn into a prideful self-reliance; can develop into a false or overrated opinion of one's own ability; may lead to a disregard for the feelings and opinions of others; or may become impatient with others' mistakes, inadequacies, or slower natures. Confidence in self could lesson gratitude to God for abilities, or it could cause difficulty in listening to or submitting to others.
Cooperative	**Possible Pitfalls**
Cooperative people are easy to get along with and tend to tolerate others' imperfections well. They will change for the sake of others and will quietly deny themselves. They tend to take correction well and listen well to instructions. Because cooperative people posses great diplomacy skills, they can become good negotiators and peacemakers.	Sometimes cooperative people can cooperate to a fault in an effort to please or keep peace. They may make compromises that are unwise or unBiblical and give in inappropriately. Their desire for peace may lead them to become wishy-washy or to only express sorrow for wrongs rather than to truly repent.
Contemplative	**Possible Pitfalls**
Contemplative people like to study things and think about them. They watch things closely and muse about what makes them tick. Contemplative people are great problem solvers and inventors. They have a wonderful patience for thoughtfully studying and figuring things out until they come up with improvements or practical solutions.	The tendency to study and think things out can sometimes hinder a contemplative person from accepting God's truth by faith. Their desire to thoroughly understand each point before they act upon it can end up paralyzing or frustrating them spiritually and emotionally. Even though contemplative children want to know why before they obey a command, they should be diligently taught to obey first and then be given explanations when possible.
Decisive	**Possible Pitfalls**
Decisive people sort out information quickly and determine conclusions without undue doubt or deliberation. They tend to be focused and make decisions well.	Decisiveness is a fault when decisions are made too quickly without adequate information. Because decisive people are quick to make judgments, they can be more prone to error or misunderstanding.

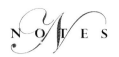

DETERMINED/RESOLUTE	POSSIBLE PITFALLS
Determination is a quality that motivates an individual to complete a desired goal or task. Determined people are not easily distracted from their purpose or resolution, even when problems or discouragement hinder their desired goals. Resolute people tend to be firm and persistent, not easily shaken off course.	Determined people can become so fixed on completing their goals that they refuse to make adjustments in their plans or methods when they cause hardship on others. They tend to believe the end justifies the means, and often bulldoze over people or ignore Biblical character to get what they want or to complete a task. Determination can become stubbornness if not controlled.

DIPLOMATIC	POSSIBLE PITFALLS
Diplomatic people are usually people-oriented and able to make equitable arrangements between others and themselves. They're natural negotiators who keep calm under pressure and think through situations calmly and deliberately. These people find solutions to problems and have a knack for getting people to cooperate with them.	There is a tendency for diplomatic people to compromise in order to make peace between people, even when the situation compromises God's truth. They may find it difficult to take a hard stand when it invites opposition. They may want to soften things God's Word doesn't soften. Their diplomacy may also become manipulation if they do not properly control it.

EFFICIENT	POSSIBLE PITFALLS
Efficient individuals have an organized way of thinking and carrying out tasks without wasting time and effort. Efficient people tend to be productive and practical.	Efficient people often resist changes, new ideas, or new ways of doing things. They can become impatient with anything that gets in their way or disturbs their activity. They may become frustrated when things aren't just right and irritated when they are interrupted or diverted. Efficient children do better in a structured, predictable household, and become easily agitated in one that is undisciplined and unpredictable.

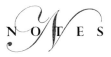

EMOTIONALLY RESPONSIVE	POSSIBLE PITFALLS
People who are emotionally responsive have no problem expressing joy, enthusiasm, sympathy, concern, or compassion. Because they respond to others easily, they are a joy to be around. They have a great capacity to encourage and motivate others and tend to be receptive to the ideas and desires of others.	Emotionally expressive people not only easily express good emotions, but they tend to easily express the more unpleasant emotions as well. They tend to express anger rather than hide it, or express unhappiness rather than conceal it. If they are around sadness, they will be sad. Around negative people they will be negative. They pick up on emotional states very easily and either adapt to them or respond too sympathetically. This can lead emotional people to follow their emotions rather than reason or Biblical admonitions.
EXCITABLE/ANIMATED	**POSSIBLE PITFALLS**
People who are excitable bring enthusiasm to all and greatly motivate others. They are easy to read and tend to be very open and transparent.	Enthusiasm is a wonderful quality so long as it is channeled towards causes and endeavors that merit a Christian's enthusiasm. Unless they are careful, enthusiasm has the capacity to lead people to embrace causes that are destructive or wrong. Excitable people sometimes respond intensely to their inner emotions, and display anger, sadness, happiness, or worry in an outward, dramatic manner. Their emotions change quickly.
EXPRESSIVE	**POSSIBLE PITFALLS**
Expressive individuals communicate emotions and ideas easily and convincingly. They are easy to read and delightful to be around. Speaking and drama come easy to these individuals. If they are musically or artistically inclined, their passion for expression and ability to compel others enhance their work.	Sometimes expressive individuals have a tough time keeping negative or private emotions concealed. Controlling their spirit can often be a difficult challenge. If they are inclined to be angry, they often develop a bad habit of quickly expressing hurtful words towards others. Their mouth is usually their greatest trouble spot.

HAPPY DISPOSITION	POSSIBLE PITFALLS
People who have a naturally happy disposition tend to easily accept discomfort, problems, or wrongs. They often develop a personality that endears them to others. Wherever they are, they help keep morale up.	Happy individuals sometimes fail to take serious matters seriously enough. They might avoid serious conversations or situations, or avoid resolving problems that make them feel uncomfortable. Children with happy natures sometimes learn how to be cute in order to avoid discipline or scolding. |//
INDEPENDENT	**POSSIBLE PITFALLS**
Independent people are able to work, play, and pursue their interests without needing to rely on others for direction, encouragement, or control. They tend to have a greater ability to make decisions without undue bias and without being influenced strongly by the opinions of others. As Christians, they find it easier to stand alone, when necessary, for that which is right.	Independent people have a harder time interacting with others or working together with others cooperatively. They tend to resist authority or subservient roles. As Christians, they may have difficulty submitting to others, as Christ commands each of us to do, or assuming the role of a servant.
LEADERSHIP-ORIENTED	**POSSIBLE PITFALLS**
The ability to lead is a wonderful quality when a leader influences others for good and uses Biblical methods of leadership. Great leaders give others direction and provide motivation, order, and structure to group endeavors. Good leaders have the capacity to make others successful.	Those with leadership qualities often want to lead without first disciplining themselves to do what they want others to do or without having learned to follow others themselves. The tendency to make demands or push others rather than to lead and influence others may be a problem. The ability to lead can easily become a tendency to dominate and control if a leader is not disciplined to practice Biblical leadership and humility. Through wise discipline and training, a parent can teach a child these things.

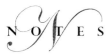

LOGICAL	POSSIBLE PITFALLS
Logical people rarely react out of emotion. They tend to consider the facts and collect data before they make decisions. They have an easier time controlling their spirit and are likely to be slow to wrath. Their dispassionate and careful manner of listening and sorting facts makes them excellent negotiators or mediators who can help adjudicate conflicts.	Logical people can be led astray when logic leads them from the truth. If they do not have a foundation of faith, they may find the Word of God illogical. This makes it hard for them to exercise faith when things don't make sense. Or it can make them very slow to make decisions if the facts aren't clear in their minds. If their logic is based on erroneous assumptions, or assumptions contrary to the Bible, they can stubbornly pursue error.
OBSERVANT	**POSSIBLE PITFALLS**
Observant people notice the little things that can be done to make life easier or more pleasant. They notice things that are wrong and seek to correct them. They tend to understand what makes others tick. Often observant people will develop great patience with others and possess wonderful people skills.	Observant people often become critical and note flaws to a fault. They may concentrate on a speck of dust while the obvious goes undone. Sometimes the observers become the spectators of life rather than participants. They may lack a desire to get involved or try new things.
OUTGOING	**POSSIBLE PITFALLS**
Outgoing people bring an enjoyment to others with their gregarious ways and ability to engage in conversation easily. Because they truly enjoy people, they have a wonderful ability to put people at ease and make them feel welcome and comfortable.	Sometimes outgoing people become so consumed in their socializing and various activities that they fail to develop a disciplined life. People-oriented individuals often prefer social interaction to thinking activity; consequently, they often allow themselves to become easily distracted. They may tend to neglect responsibilities or become disorganized. People-oriented individuals need to be careful they do not fail to please God in an effort to please people.

Outspoken/Straightforward	Possible Pitfalls
People who are both confident and talkative tend to be outspoken communicators. When their thoughts and ideas are godly and pure, they can challenge others to think and do right. They tend to speak up on behalf of those who need help and support, and do not tolerate injustice or abuse without objecting. They are rarely passive but openly speak out when they have a thought or idea. They are often people who *say what they mean and mean what they say*.	Outspoken people have a tendency to think out loud, which can lead to misunderstandings and foot-in-the-mouth trouble. Their greatest problems are in controlling their words and keeping their emotions and thoughts restrained. They tend to believe if they are right, they have a right to say so, and sometimes fail to guard their words. Speaking one's mind is often viewed as a virtue rather than a fault; consequently, this leads outspoken people to say things they later

Performer	Possible Pitfalls
Performance-oriented people are a joy when they use their talents for others to enjoy. They add life to social gatherings and make interesting teachers and communicators.	The tendency to love performing can lead to self-centeredness and a constant desire to be the center of attention. The enjoyment of performing can easily become the motivation for using talents, instead of using talents for the enjoyment of others and the glory of God.

Placid/Slow-paced	Possible Pitfalls
Placid people often submit more readily to authority and are more compliant and yielding in interpersonal relationships than others.	Slower-paced people can become easily apathetic, inactive, or unresponsive to those around them. They have a greater tendency to suppress anger and resentment and may develop a pattern of avoiding conflicts.

Practical	Possible Pitfalls
Practical-thinking people like to reduce knowledge and theories into practical, or useful, applications. They don't like to waste much time with useless details, dreaming, or discussion. Everything they think about tends to gravitate towards usefulness, efficiency, and sensibility. Consequently, practical people help others keep on track and get things done in the most effective way. They also keep others from deviating into thinking and doing things that are destructive.	Sometimes practical people can become so useful-oriented that they fail to learn how to have fun for the sake of having fun. They sometimes view enjoyment as a waste of time, which affects their ability to enjoy life. Practical people often have a hard time trying new activities or being motivated to achieve something desirable. They may become hardheaded and so matter-of-fact that they are unsentimental in good ways or unromantic in marriage.

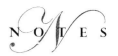

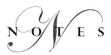

QUIET/UNEXCITEABLE	POSSIBLE PITFALLS
Quiet-natured individuals are easy to get along with and easy to please. They are rarely openly rebellious and do not disrupt others' plans or ideas. Quiet people listen well without interrupting and tend to be contemplative rather than overly excited and impulsive.	While quiet people listen well, they have a difficult time giving feedback or responding to others' efforts to communicate with them. Because give-and-take communication requires an effort for them, as well as for those who try to talk with them, their communication can be inadequate, which may lead to misunderstandings. Quiet individuals can be angry and resentful, or even rebellious, without ever expressing it in an open manner. This can lead to behavior that is difficult to understand, and difficult to resolve.
SENSITIVE/PERCEPTIVE	**POSSIBLE PITFALLS**
Sensitive individuals have a capacity to distinguish and perceive subtle impressions. They are quick to discern slight differences and variations of emotion. Sensitive people have a keen ability to sense others' distress and are often extra compassionate and understanding of others' feelings. They are quick to sense guilt or wrong behavior in their lives, and have a desire to please and keep the peace	People who have a sensitive nature are often excessively emotional to a fault. They tend to govern their lives by feeling rather than by God's commands. They have a hard time ignoring their emotions, even when they know they are unreliable. Sensitive people often read into things too much, and have a hard time tolerating injustice or failure in themselves or others. Children who are sensitive can become depressed, agitated, stubborn, or hyperactive when they live in homes where there is constant screaming, tension, and disorder.
PRACTICAL	**POSSIBLE PITFALLS**
Serious-minded people take on problems no one else will touch. They tend to be realistic and attentive to what's going on around them. They take correction seriously, which makes them conscientious, and are concerned about doing things right. As much as possible, they avoid getting into trouble or making mistakes. They tend to take work and matters of importance seriously and approach life in a purposeful manner.	Sometimes serious individuals can become pessimistic and rigid in their thinking, to the point of being depressing, cynical, or discouraging to others. They might be so serious-minded that it becomes hard for them to see humor or laugh when they make mistakes. Perfectionism can become a problem as they seek to be right in everything. This may lead to self-righteousness and intolerance towards those who do not meet their expectations. They may have a problem understanding God's desire for humility rather than perfection, and God's acceptance of those who trust and believe.

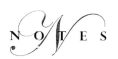

SHORT-TERM FOCUSED	POSSIBLE PITFALLS
People who have a capacity for short-term focus tend to want to complete a task quickly. They seldom drag things out or waste time on unproductive details.	Those who tend to change their focus quickly have trouble sustaining attention on tasks that require longer amounts of time or concentration. Their thinking can become undisciplined, and they're easily distracted. They may have trouble controlling their life and tend to let life happen to them rather than taking charge.

SPONTANEOUS	POSSIBLE PITFALLS
Spontaneous people rarely become upset when problems or changes interrupt their plans. They adjust well to circumstances and find ways to cope or fill their time. Spontaneous people are able to drop what they are doing and move to another activity without feeling upset.	Spontaneous people are often easily distracted and sometimes have problems finishing tasks they begin. They can have trouble realistically assessing their time and priorities.

TALKATIVE	POSSIBLE PITFALLS
Talkative people learn to articulate their thoughts and ideas better than most people. This can be a great asset if they teach or pursue a career that requires good communication skills. Talkers have a wonderful ability in witnessing for Christ and teaching Sunday School classes.	Talkative people are sometimes great talkers but poor listeners. They sometimes develop a tendency to think ahead while other people are talking, instead of listening carefully and patiently to what is being said. This also causes talkers to draw conclusions too quickly, without sufficient data. Talkers can develop the bad habit of quickly expressing hurtful words towards others. Their mouth is usually their greatest trouble spot.

TENACIOUS	POSSIBLE PITFALLS
Tenacious people will hold fast to their goals and beliefs in the face of opposition. They do not often quit or give up on their dreams or goals. They are not easily distracted or discouraged but overcome difficulty and do not sway from their plans.	Tenacity can easily become obstinacy if a goal or desire needs to be changed or abandoned for good reason. Beliefs and opinions that are wrong are not easily given up without a struggle. Children who are tenacious especially need great amounts of input in Christian concepts before they are ever confronted by the world with ungodly concepts. Whichever they learn first will usually sway their direction. They will not change easily.

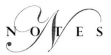

Timid	Possible Pitfalls
Timid people are more naturally modest and sensitive to impropriety. Because they tend to be more reserved, they aren't led into wild escapades very easily, as are the more outgoing personalities. They appreciate good friends and tend to be loyal and loving.	Timidity may cause some to become too self-absorbed, self-aware, or fearful. They may be less willing to interact with or serve others. Because they are more easily embarrassed, they may avoid situations that are uncomfortable and can fail to develop confidence in God. They may be more touchy and withdrawn.
Witty	Possible Pitfalls
Witty people are usually very perceptive, alert, humorous, and enjoyable to be with. They tend to be quick learners, observant, and sensitive to the moods of others.	Sometimes witty people can be tempted to use their wit to manipulate others or avoid responsibility. They may be intimidating to sensitive types if they enjoy using sarcastic humor or are sharp-tongued. They have a tendency to become unthankful, critical, or prideful.

Christians are to be merciful and sensitive to one another's needs and burdens. We are to listen attentively and respect one another's differences, gifts, hopes and dreams. God tells us in *Romans 12:14* that we should, "Rejoice with them that do rejoice, and weep with them that weep." Children are people in transition, who are every bit a whole person as any brother or sister in Christ. Parents do well to regard them with respect and treat them with the same tenderness that the Lord instructs all believers to practice between one another. We often train our little ones to memorize and recite *Ephesians 4:32*, hoping they will learn to be kind to one another. Yet parents too, need the same admonishment when dealing with their children and do well to memorize and recite it too. "And be ye kind one to another, tenderhearted, forgiving one another, even as God for Christ's sake hath forgiven you."

Lesson 5

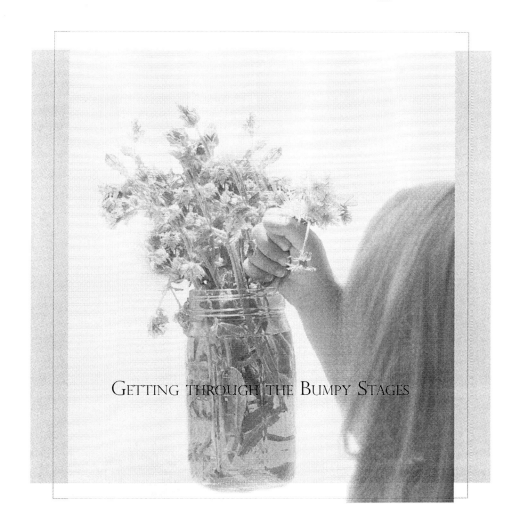

GETTING THROUGH THE BUMPY STAGES

Charity suffereth long, and is kind…beareth all things, believeth all things, hopeth all things, endureth all things.
1 Corinthians 13:4a, 7

Being confident of this very thing, that he which hath begun a good work in you will perform it until the day of Jesus Christ.
Philippians 1:6

Key THOUGHTS

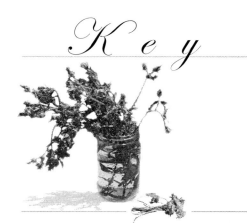

The Bible tells us we can learn much by observing, studying, and discerning behavior in light of Scripture. This means we can also learn how to deal with normal childhood problems by listening to the observations of godly people and by learning to be observant ourselves.

Discussion Problem

Maria has two children. Jennifer is two-months-old, and Jeffrey is thirteen-months-old. Recently, Maria has expressed to her pastor's wife great frustration with mothering. She feels she must be doing something wrong. Neither of her children sleep through the night. The baby cries every evening, and little Jeffrey is into everything. Because she is constantly telling Jeffrey "No," and he is persistently repeating the behavior she is trying to forbid, Maria is beginning to feel like a broken record. Maria was an only child herself and has never been exposed to small children.

After reading lesson five, use the principles you learn to discuss the possible reasons for Maria's frustration. If you were Maria's pastor's wife, how would you encourage her? What could Maria do to build her own confidence? If Maria doesn't receive help, what consequences could take place in years to come as a result?

Bible Study

1. According to Titus 2:3-8, mature Christian women are to display behavior that is holy so they may _____ the young women by their example, so they can be a _____ (role model) for them, and so contrary (rebellious) people will be _____ of their own behavior.

2. In Psalm 107:43 we find that God wants us to be wise and _____ the way He works, and the way people behave. This will cause us to understand the _____ of God.

3. Proverbs 23:26 tells us that the son is encouraged to learn by watching the father's godly _____.

4. From Hebrews 5:13-14 we discover that mature Christians learn to be observant and weigh actions by habitually practicing _____. As they gain this experience they are able to discern _____ and _____.

"A mother fills a place so great that there isn't an angel in heaven who wouldn't be glad to give a bushel of diamonds to come down here and take her place."
Billy Sunday

Bumpy Stages in Your Child's Life

There was a time when parenting children was considered to be the most honorable, important privilege a married couple could embark upon. Fathers were honored to work in order to support their family, and mothers rarely worked outside the home. Families were larger than they are today, and relatives commonly lived in proximity to one another, offering help and support to new mothers. Because mothering children was such a consuming part of most women's lives, young women were exposed to children and children's problems more often than they are today. They had far more opportunities to observe healthy interaction between the mothers and children who lived around them, and consequently they had a good idea what to expect when they had children of their own.

Today, most young mothers and fathers depend more on the advice of friends or books than on direct observation to learn how to handle children's difficulties. If the friends or books they read do not realistically and accurately inform parents what is normal and what is not, mothers and fathers develop a deficient or unrealistic view of normal childhood behavior. When this happens, parents often develop unrealistic expectations, become discouraged, fear being inadequate, worry their children aren't developing normally, or simply lose the joy of parenting. When mothers and fathers lack sensible, practical information, they tend to lack the confidence they need to deal patiently and firmly with their children. Most of all, they lack the necessary information they need to raise well-adjusted, happy Christian children.

It is not uncommon for optimistic young parents to suddenly find themselves older and wiser grandparents who wish they had known years earlier what they now know. Hopefully, this workbook will help prevent such sorrows and produce more grandparents who will be able to say, "I'm glad I did…" rather than, "I wish I had…" Young men and women need to hear about the struggles, mistakes, and solutions that worked for other men and women. They need to know what parents did wrong as much as what they did right. They need to know what problems are common at each stage of a child's life, not just what characteristics and skills children typically achieve at each stage of their development. Young parents benefit from practical, truthful information. They also benefit when they observe the way others have lived before them.

God instructs us to learn not only by receiving instruction, but also by studying and discerning others' behavior. He wants us to develop the skill to weigh actions, compare right and wrong, and choose wise courses of action. The remainder of this chapter lists common problems and characteristics of children in various age groups that might cause them to go through a difficult, or bumpy, stage. Start from the beginning even if your children are older so you can note what things you learned by experience and what things you wish you had known earlier. After you read the observations in this book, write observations of your own, or observations you have gained from other experienced parents.

You will notice there are difficulties that are peculiar to every age. The journey of childhood will be a lot more fun if you recognize that children get through one bumpy stage only to embark on a new one. Knowing the difficulties ahead of time is like reading a roadmap and noting curves and detours before you get to them. Understanding and anticipating bumps in the road give parents more confidence and teaches us to say with a smile, "This too shall pass." For centuries, parents have endured the same fears and problems you will face, and survived. You will too!

Babies In General

Before discussing points typical to specific age groups, I would like to address several "scheduling myths" that seem to be strongly recommended by some mothers.

Myth #1 – "Putting your baby on a schedule is the key to a happy baby."

Scheduling may make a happier mother, but it does not necessarily make a happier baby. As the baby matures, scheduling and predictability do have an impact on his frame of mind, but small infants tend to thrive best with a more flexible and loose schedule. This myth is a close cousin of the "mothers who put their babies on strict schedules are teaching them who is in control" myth.

Myth #2 – "Nursing is merely getting nutrition into the baby and should never be used to comfort a child."

Nursing *is* comforting to babies! God designed mothers in such a way that an infant experiences the warmth of mother's body, the security of mother's arms, and the ability to see mother's smile. Cows and horses do not have this advantage! Then again, baby horses and cows are not human beings who fail to thrive without physical nurturing and comforting. Obviously anything can be taken to an extreme and yes, a mother can become a human pacifier at an age when such a comfort is more a habit than a necessity. However, to say that nursing is *only* for the purpose of feeding is an extreme in the opposite direction! There will be many times when nursing an infant can and should be used to quiet and soothe his fretfulness.

Myth #3 – "Demand-fed babies are always cranky and do not sleep through the night."

The Academy of Pediatrics reports that 70% of babies sleep through the night by six months. Getting a baby to sleep through the night can become a selfish preoccupation of a mother rather than a desire to do what is best for her baby or to obtain sufficient sleep so she can function during the day. Young mothers are often bombarded with people asking if her baby sleeps through the night. Many of them feel the pressure and begin to assume this is an important accomplishment that must be tackled at once. While sleeping through the night is certainly a blessing for a tired new mother, it should not be considered a major milestone to be reached as soon as possible. It also should never be put on the level of a spiritual issue! Different mothers and different babies will approach the sleeping issues with a variety of solutions and approaches.

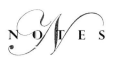

A family's particular routine, the number of other children in the home, how much daddy is available to help, as well as other variables all have an impact on how a mother deals with the sleeping question.

Myth #4 – "A baby should never be allowed to sleep in a parent's bed."

Again, this is more a personal preference issue and is not a spiritual matter. On the realistic side, I believe there will be times when a mother may allow a baby to sleep in bed with her. If a mother chooses to do this for some reason, she should not be made to feel guilty. Certainly, aside from the medical concerns of SIDS and suffocating baby (by rolling over on him), there is not a Biblical reason for or against baby sharing the bed with mom and dad, providing mom and dad *both* are comfortable with the idea. However, parents who do choose to allow this need to be aware of potential consequences that will develop as a result. Keep in mind that you may not always want baby to share the bed with you (particularly when baby is a squirmy toddler), and the habit may be quite hard to break as baby gets older. As well, you may find the practice interferes with your physical relationship as husband and wife, and that does violate a scriptural command. I do think some co-sleeping may be motivated by a mother's laziness: it's a lot easier to leave baby in bed after nursing than risk having him wake up when putting him in a crib. It's also easier to leave him be when you are half asleep and don't feel like getting up in a cold house to put him back in bed. In this case, I believe indulging a lazy desire is sinful.

The Newborn

Perhaps one of the most trying, or "bumpy" aspects of adjusting to a new baby is the need to adjust to a baby's cry. First, it is important to recognize that newborns should have regular intervals of feeding—their tummies are tiny and cannot hold much. The newborn that cries to be fed is often genuinely hungry. Young parents often underestimate how much or how often a baby cries and may become uneasy or agitated when crying is not easily subdued. It helps to remember that crying is a baby's means of communicating his needs and expresses many things other than hunger or discomfort. It will also be helpful for mothers to understand that infants express two basic emotions, fear and anger, by crying. Newborns tend to appear angry when they cry and easily irritated when they are hungry or uncomfortable. They are also easily startled and frightened by loud noises, sudden light, or sudden movements. This sometimes unnerves new mothers who don't understand that this is a normal phase of development that will subside as the infant grows and matures.

Babies cry when they are experiencing pain, when they feel frightened, are cold, bored, lonely, or perplexed. They tend to dislike a cold diaper more than a wet diaper. They are also especially afraid of falling. For this reason, newborns are typically comforted when they are wrapped snuggly in a blanket or placed on their backs between small pillows or a wedge on either side of them. Although they may prefer to be on their tummy, pediatricians do not recommend placing infants on their tummies as it increases the danger of sudden infant death. Until newborns become more comfortable and acquainted with the world around them and eventually learn to express themselves with words, they will communicate their natural fears and discomforts by crying.

With time and understanding, an attentive mother will learn to distinguish between little whimpers that need little or no response and cries that require a mother to comfort and hold her baby. The infant's legitimate needs should be responded to promptly. He will not begin to cry for attention until he is five- to six-months-old, so "spoiling" him does not need to be a concern until that time. Many popular child-rearing books recommend ignoring a crying infant and urge mothers not to indulge "selfishness" by talking to or cuddling a crying infant. Such advice is not only potentially damaging to the emotional development of a newborn child, it violates a mother's natural God-given instinct to protect and comfort her baby. I have found that male authors tend to perpetuate this far more frequently than women. Could this possibly be one reason God commissioned older women, rather than men, to teach the younger women how to love their children?

Two of the most common problems associated with newborns fresh home from the hospital are their tendency to wake at short intervals during the night instead of the day, and the propensity to drift off to sleep while nursing. To encourage him to turn his days and nights around, don't let him sleep longer than three hours at a time during the day. His sleeping intervals at night should lengthen. I would advise young mothers not to make sleeping through the night a major concern. It is wonderful if your baby sleeps longer at night, but it should not be viewed as a major concern if he does not. Babies greatly vary in their sleeping patterns with some infants sleeping 18 to 20 hours a day and others much less. Sleep cycles will gradually lengthen throughout the first year; however, some infants may not sleep through the night until they reach their second or third year.

The emotion of love is taught to a baby; he is not born with it. The newborn has a strong need to establish secure attachment to one or more humans, predominantly mother. The first goal a mother should have for her baby is to establish trust, attachment, love, and acceptance. She accomplishes this by using the sound of her voice to comfort and delight her baby, her body to cuddle and touch, and her self-discipline to feed and care for her child's needs. From infancy to preschool a child is naturally dependent. Don't try to force your baby or toddler to be overly independent too soon. Dependence is a normal part of a baby's make-up, which helps him establish a sense of security, confidence, and trust. Your baby will want his independence soon enough and will gradually begin to see himself separately from his mother. Comforting and soothing a fretful baby provides a child's first experiences of love and acceptance. Give plenty of it.

6-8 Weeks

At this age babies begin smiling, becoming sociable, noticing colors, and responding to seeing a variety of shapes. A tiny baby does not understand words, but he is

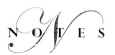

very sensitive to emotions and tones. A mother's gentleness, patience, and loving caresses begin a baby's education. Most babies this age will respond better to a toy that has a happy, smiling face than a toy that is expressionless. Do not display anger or engage in stormy family fights in the presence of any child, but particularly not a baby. A mother's state of mind and the atmosphere she keeps in the home does affect her little children. When your baby is tiny, begin to rely on prayer as a means of governing your emotions and keeping a sweet disposition. Deliberately start your day with happy music, a cheerful attitude, time spent with the Lord, and an outward focus on others. Starting your day well sets a pace for the rest of the day and encourages both you and your family to adopt a sunny disposition. Days that are begun well most often end well.

Establish your baby's routine while he is still young. The secret is to be flexible but predictable. Bad habits established in the early months are hard to change as the baby gets a little older. It's better to get into good routines such as consistent feeding times and bed times, so your baby will already be accustomed to falling into the rhythm of a well-established daily routine as he grows older. You will need to remember, however, that routines need to be adjusted as your baby matures and changes, and need to remain flexible and realistic. Consistency and predictability are crucial elements parents need to master in order to raise secure and happy children. Predictable routines will prevent an enormous number of potential problems and eventually help your child comply with many daily habits such as a bedtime schedule, brushing teeth, picking up toys, making the bed, completing homework, etc.

3-4 Months

A baby this age may begin to sleep through the night and may stay awake half the day. Babies who are breast-fed sometimes take longer to learn to sleep through the night, as breast milk assimilates faster than formula. It's a good idea to let your baby learn to fall asleep on his own so he will fall back to sleep when he wakes during the night. Rather than letting your baby cry until he is exhausted and falls asleep, allow him to cry for three minutes and come back to comfort and pat him. When he is calmed, leave again for three or four minutes and come back again to comfort the baby. Continue doing this, gradually increasing the time away until the baby learns you are near and learns to fall asleep by himself. If you will patiently continue this process, baby will most likely be falling asleep or quieting himself before three minutes.

Three-month-old babies have an easy, congenial mood and begin to love exploring and exercising. They will be extremely responsive to anyone who smiles and tend to want to be in the same room as their mother. A common problem that may disrupt family life is teething pain. Teething babies often become unusually fussy or fretful and may want to be held more than normal or cry more easily. Teething babies also tend to want to chew on something soft or cold and may drool excessively.

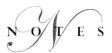

4-5 Months

At this age an infant will intentionally cry for attention. Take care of a baby's needs before he cries for them to be met. For instance, if your baby has been quietly playing on the floor for a while, pick him up *before* he cries and cuddle him. If experience teaches a baby he gets his wants attended to *only* when he screams and cries, do not be surprised if his screaming and crying increase considerably.

If you provide plenty of cuddling and try to anticipate your baby's needs before he has to cry, you do not need to always respond to him immediately if he frets and cries. Don't let his crying unnerve you. Pacifiers will become helpful about this time and often contribute greatly to household peace. Sometimes infants who have previously refused a pacifier want one at this age. Sucking is a means for babies to relieve anxiety and is often most noticeable when the baby is hungry, tired, or stressful. Babies all have a need to suck; so don't be overly concerned about this. It is better for your baby to want a pacifier than his thumb. A pacifier is relatively easy to wean a toddler from later, while thumb sucking can develop into a difficult habit to break. You might be interested to know that mothers throughout the ages have used some rather ingenious methods to provide homemade "pacifiers" for their babies. My grandmother liked to tell how her mother taught her how to fill a rubber glove with gelatin and tie the end so the baby could suck on it. Of course, this horrifies modern mothers who understand the dangers of bacteria and choking on soft objects. Pacifiers made of hard rubber connected to a plastic rim that prevents suffocating are certainly a lot safer and cleaner than methods used in years gone by.

5-6 Months

Because they are limited in moving, babies will often become bored at this age. Walkers and bouncers extend their world and help to keep them occupied and happy. Of course, you will want to be very careful before using a walker, as moveable walkers are a common cause of infant injuries. Boredom, curiosity, and frustration build up just prior to crawling; yet to a large extent, these contribute to motivating a baby to crawl. Babies at this age will begin throwing and banging objects and love to watch others retrieve objects for them.

6-7 Months

Babies older than six months have much more understanding than a four-month-old. About this time, a baby develops a fascination with very small particles such as crumbs, water drops, and fuzz. Because this age baby explores primarily with his mouth, it will require mothers to watch carefully what he puts in his mouth. Toddlers are not yet aware of their limitations and get themselves into all kinds of difficulties as a result. They might crawl off a bed, climb too high up a stairway, touch hot objects, put sharp objects in their mouth, bang on breakable objects, etc. This constant desire to explore and discover how things feel and work will require a mother to be very diligent in watching her baby's activity as well as to be willing to patiently teach limitations. This age group will have abrupt mood changes but will also easily forget what he's crying about when he is distracted. Distraction and ignoring are the first forms of discipline. He won't connect a spank with his behavior just yet. Keep in mind that he won't remember commands for more than twenty-four hours. At this age be sure to refuse to respond to his constant cry for attention.

A common problem may be stranger anxiety. This means he will begin to hesitate going to strangers and needs time to adjust to newcomers. This may last until he is thirteen to fourteen months old. Be sure he is adjusted to being left in the church nursery before this time. You will notice your baby sleeps less than he did in earlier months. Over the next six months, he will sleep less and by one year will likely sleep fourteen to fifteen hours in a twenty-four-hour period.

7-8 Months

By this age, baby will begin to connect the word *no* or a *spank* to his behavior. Words will begin to have more meaning making it possible for a seven-month-old baby to begin learning simple commands such as "be gentle," "come," "no crying," "sit down," etc. His memory greatly improves month by month. He has insatiable curiosity and needs freedom to explore. He will be happier if he has opportunities to see new things and explore environments beyond his own home. A variety of textures, sights, colors, and sounds will help prevent boredom and fussiness and encourage productive mental activity. Babies this age are often fascinated with balls and toys that have moveable features.

A common problem at this age is waking up in the middle of night and wanting to stay awake and play. Check on him. Gently say, "good night," and leave the room. Over-stimulation will often produce as much fussiness as under stimulation and may cause a baby to have difficulty falling asleep.

9-14 Months

This age child explores *everything*! Climbing is a favorite activity. Among other things, he loves to put objects in his mouth, put objects in other objects, play in water, and play with hinged objects such as doors. He will fearfully avoid things that have caused an unpleasant experience for him. Provide for his need to explore new things and practice new skills, but set your limits. Teach him that *no* means *no*. It is important not to let your child have his own way once you have said no.

Do not allow him to infringe on your rights excessively. You will encourage selfishness if you reward his demands by giving in to anything he screams and cries for. Overindulgence will create more problems later though it may appear that giving in is easier. Keep in mind that if he can control you now, he will continue to assert himself and his wants all the more as he grows older.

By this age a baby's memory has improved enough to understand discipline. By twelve months of age he will persistently go back to something he wants, instead of being distracted permanently, as he was earlier. Continue to remove the baby from temptations or the temptations from the baby. However, if he defies your restriction you need to spank to convince him you mean no. Be very certain a spank is administered in a calm but firm manner properly applied to the child's fatty bottom. Anger will only frustrate and confuse your child. While anger may temporarily stop a child's behavior, it will never change the child's behavior and will only lead to increased defiance.

Remember that a small child learns by repetition and will not easily accept no as an answer until mother has declined the wishes or disciplined for the same offense repeatedly and consistently. Calmly and persistently continue enforcing your "no's" with the understanding that this exercise of disciplined training is an important step in your child's development. He will slowly grow in his ability to control himself and accept disappointment or delayed gratification, but it takes lots of time. Self-control is not acquired quickly or instantaneously without much hard work and loving patience. Don't give a baby this age an overload of restrictions since you will be disciplining constantly if you do so and will overwhelm your child. Be willing to be imaginative, available, and *consistent*.

At this age the mother's roll involves three major things:

1. She is the designer of her child's world and experiences.
2. She is consultant, assistant, and encourager all in one.
3. She is the primary authority in her child's life.

14-24 Months

The toddler is beginning to see himself as a separate person. He is able to anticipate consequences and make associations, as well as plan and carry out activities. His most common problems are negativism (rebellion), opposing the will of his parents, and possible hostility towards an older sibling. Often he plays better with older children than those younger. When playmates of the same age are together, they require close, constant supervision.

Your child may begin waking at night afraid because of bad dreams. Toddlers have short attention spans, and short memories. They learn most things by repetition. The first and most important step in disciplining your toddler is to insist that whatever you say must always be done. Do not ever give a command that you cannot or are not willing to enforce. Also do not give a command that is too much for your child to comply with. For example, do not say, "go to sleep." Instead say, "You must stay in the bed."

Every time you give a command and allow your child to ignore it, you increase the likelihood he will disobey you and resist your requests. Do not require too much

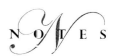

at too young an age. Also do not assume enforcing obedience will get easier if you are inconsistent or lazy about seeing that your toddler obeys. Sometimes you simply need to say no and then quickly physically steer him away from the forbidden object. You may also want to distract him or remove a temptation.

Whenever possible, make your restraints unperceivable to the child. Remember that you are primarily governing the child's life in such a way that he is being directed to do the right thing in order to establish habitual repetition of right activity. Later in your child's development, you will want to focus on reasoning so your child will come to understand the rationale behind right behavior and begin making wise choices apart from the threat of consequences or the promise of rewards. For now, your child does not have the capacity to reason well or understand long term consequences, let alone the ability to reason abstractly. For this reason, the primary focus of your work at this young age is to teach obedience and right behavior by repetitious training until it becomes *habit*. This makes the enforcement of *every* command, and the rewarding of obedience a very crucial part of your training.

Some children are ready to be potty trained as early as fifteen months, but most do not yet have the muscular coordination needed to control bowel or bladder. Most children will urinate or have a bowel movement twenty to thirty minutes after eating or waking from a nap. Many mothers put their toddlers on a potty at these times and "catch" them in the process. However, the child is not truly potty trained as he is not able to actually control or restrain elimination. Most children gain the muscular coordination to control bowel movement between fifteen months and three years. Bladder control usually follows bowel control between the ages of two and three. It's much easier to potty train at the point when children are physically able to learn control and when negativism declines to the place where a toddler has more of a desire to please. Attempting to potty train before a child is ready only frustrates mother and child and produces resistance later.

2 Years

By the time babies approach their second birthday, negativism and contentious behavior diminishes if you have dealt with it well. Some children are more difficult to deal with than others and persist in openly challenging your authority for a longer period. Mothers who understand this behavior do not take it personally or react with fear and anger. They simply continue winning the daily battles with the will until it is under control.

If you have to constantly discipline over trivial things that could be avoided, you may be causing increased defiance.

Typically, your toddler will become more rational as he matures and gains greater control over his emotions and behavior.

Your most challenging problem will likely be consistency in enforcing limitations. It will help if you separate childish infractions that are an inconsequential and normal part of childhood with direct and defiant disobedience that requires a decisive "win" on your part. Encouraging willing obedience should be your major goal. You will accomplish this as much or more by training your child to obey in cheerful ways than by dealing with blatant disobedience. Ask your child to comply with commands that are pleasant and desirable, and then enthusiastically commend him for his obedience. This will help him learn that obedience produces joy and encourages him to obey when given commands that are not so pleasant.

As much as is possible, keep a young child from temptations that are particularly hard for him to resist. This will help minimize the amount of times you will have to tell him no. This will be beneficial since you will probably need to spend a great deal of time teaching obedience. If you have to constantly discipline over trivial things that could be avoided, you may be causing increased defiance. Refusing to "child proof" your house because your toddler needs to learn obedience fails to take into consideration that a multitude of forbidden objects overwhelms such a small child and increases frustration and defiance rather than reduce it. Some mothers go so far as to say they do this on the basis that God put a forbidden tree in the center of the garden. First, such an argument represents a gross misinterpretation of Scripture; and second, it fails to note that God only put one tree in the center of the garden, not multiple forbidden trees! Better to have few forbidden objects at this age and lots of things the baby can explore to aid in stimulation. Remember too, that you will want to encourage, not discourage a toddler's curiosity.

Your commands should be reasonable, not overly restrictive. Once they are given, you must make sure they are obeyed. Hopefully you have enforced limitations and controls, and thus helped to prevent your child from developing into a self-centered, demanding baby. If so, you will undoubtedly enjoy your child at ages two and three immensely more than the mother who has indulged her one-year-old's demands. The indulgent mother needs to expend a much greater effort to bring her child under control. The mother who consistently enforced obedience thus far will most likely enjoy a more cooperative and enjoyable toddler.

The two-year-old can understand about three hundred words. He demonstrates creativity, particularly in coming up with ways to hold his parent's attention. By about age two and a half, he should become less *clingy*. His interest in playing with other children will increase. He usually watches and imitates older children, although he doesn't often interact well with children his same age. Some of the most common problems are hair pulling and biting as defense weapons. These are usually directed toward older siblings. At this age he often will become more aggressive with his older siblings.

If sibling fighting is becoming a problem consider these suggestions:

1. Don't fuss over your toddler in the presence of your older children.
2. Give your older children the opportunity and privilege to participate in activities outside the home.
3. Provide the older children with daily private time.

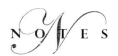

Your greatest challenge will likely be in helping move your child from being *me*-oriented to becoming *others*-oriented, as the two year old finds it very difficult to put himself in another's place. You might also find potty training a challenge if your child is resistant to learning this skill. It will help if you make sitting on the potty a pleasant experience by giving your child a book to read or juice to drink while he sits. Do not attempt to force your child to sit on the potty until he goes. Let him get up when he is "done" but keep trying until he goes and can be rewarded with a small treat kept in a special jar for this purpose. It is not wise to make potty training a discipline issue or to become angry when children do not appear to be making a concentrated effort to use the toilet.

Potty Training in a Day

Your toddler should be between twenty-four and twenty-eight months old and have the physical ability to learn how to control the bladder. Plan a day when you can clear your schedule and concentrate on *nothing* but potty training. Happily talk to your child about "potty training day" that is coming. Let him pick out big girl or boy underpants at the department store and his favorite small treat (M&M's, raisins, peanuts, gummy bears, etc.) to use as rewards. Let him pick out a potty chair or a step stool and toilet insert for the "big" toilet. (Some children dislike potty chairs and prefer to use the big toilet, although most children will prefer the security of their own child-sized potty.) Put these items aside until "potty training day." Continue to build the child's excitement for the coming day by talking about how fun it will be, etc. You might let an older sibling demonstrate the technique or play with dolls, teaching them to "go potty."

On the appointed day, make sure you have lots of salty treats, lots of your child's favorite juices, and lots of time to devote to potty training. Put the child's new underpants on and announce that its potty training day. After breakfast, (which should include lots of liquid) begin trying to "catch" your child's urination on the potty. If he goes, clap enthusiastically and give a treat, but if he doesn't, continue to keep an upbeat positive attitude and let him know maybe next time he will go in the potty. The more your child eats salty things and drinks liquids, the more likely he will need to urinate, so catching him should be fairly easy if you let him sit often and make it a fun thing to do repeatedly throughout the day. The hardest part will be keeping up the excitement and keeping the activity on the fun side. Little boys like to make "bubbles" or aim for a piece of toilet paper, so use your imagination to find ways to make potty time a pleasant experience. Many children will be potty trained by dinnertime using this method.

3 Years

A three-year-old wants social interaction with other children, and he loves to pretend. He is often much happier with one playmate than he is playing with groups of more than two. At this age he begins to share and interact cooperatively with playmates. His thinking is literal, and thus he does not use analogies or view anything as make-believe. Therefore, you must be careful what he sees on television. It is very real to him. He will not understand the concept of play-acting. He will imitate whatever he sees, so guard the content of anything he watches and use this tendency to teach him right behavior.

Help your three-year-old express his emotions verbally by giving them a name. You can do this by deliberately acknowledging his emotions with comments like, "You sound angry." Or, "That must have been very disappointing." Or "That must have hurt." Or, "Sometimes we feel sad when we make mistakes." Such comments not only teach children how to express themselves but convey your understanding and ability to put yourself in the child's situation. This will encourage your child to talk as well as listen when you provide guidance.

Provide social situations in which your child will be able to practice the leading or dominant role, as well as the following or submissive role. You may want to encourage mild competition, but be sure he wins sometimes so he is not discouraged with trying. Three-year-olds hate to lose, but they tend to seek constant approval because they want to please.

You may face two common problems:

1. He readily expresses dislike and dissatisfaction.
2. He refuses to go to bed.

To overcome the second, develop a bedtime routine and stick to it. Avoid strenuous activity before bedtime by choosing quiet and happy activities such as story reading or soft music prior to going to bed. This will help the active preschooler "wind down" and accept sleep. By all means, avoid disciplining children just before they go to sleep or making bedtime a battleground. If necessary, sit in a chair in the child's room to insure he quiets down and stays put. Instituting a quiet bedtime routine will go a long way in settling your children down and easing them into sleep. Once the habit of falling asleep is well established, bedtime battles tend to subside.

Children ages three to five tend to have animal fears or fears of the dark, particularly at night. Nightmares are a common problem that can usually be resolved with reassurance, hugs, and a nightlight or adjustable dimmer switch that the child can control. If your child is taking medication and suddenly experiences nightmares or sleeplessness, consult with your pediatrician, as medications may be responsible.

4 Years

Pretending and role playing are prominent play activities. Your child may invent imaginary friends or delight in constructing stories. His imagination is developing to the point where he loves to be assertive and imaginative and loves to exaggerate. Be careful not to assume your child is deliberately trying to deceive, as this activity is a normal way of learning and exercising imagination. However, you *will* need

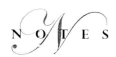

to help him learn to distinguish between fantasy pretending and reality. Enter into your child's fantasizing and pretending when appropriate and become a part of her tea party or his army adventure. He will be delighted with your participation. Never shame or embarrass him in his pretend play, but rather, provide opportunities and "props" for pretending.

Napping will decrease, though he will still benefit from a rest time. Calling naptime "quiet time" will encourage rest. Give children a book to look at during a designated thirty-minute quiet time and quite likely your child will fall asleep if he is tired. Boys tend to nap more than girls at this age.

A few common challenges you will face at this age are selfishness, short attention spans, and whining. You will want your child to know he is very special to you and dearly loved, but at the same time, he is no more special than anyone else in the family. Giving a whining child what he wants is a sure way to ensure whining continues. Try telling your child that mother doesn't hear whining, but hears very well children who ask politely. Ignoring him or her and pretending you do not hear and then responding enthusiastically when the child corrects his tone are usually enough to train a child not to whine.

Short attention spans are a common trial for mothers of more active children. It will be helpful to remember that children vary in their ability to focus on one activity for longer periods of time. Structuring activities and developing daily routines help these children tremendously. Children develop the ability to "sit still" and focus their attention gradually over time, some sooner or later than others. Be patient, work at lengthening the attention span, but don't let a short one bother you.

5 Years

Your five-year-old will most likely enjoy helping, being read to, talking, being silly, doing things himself in his own way, and imitating. He may take special delight in his personal possessions and need a space of his own. Generally five-year-olds prefer to play with children their own age, outdoors if possible.

He may enjoy such activities as listening to favorite music over and over, listening to favorite books read over and over, and watching a favorite cartoon over and over. The love of repetition can be trying for parents, yet is a characteristic that makes learning drills much easier, memorization and language acquisition more successful, and trial and error less discouraging. Boredom is a common problem among five year olds if the child is not involved in schooling. To help, provide learning activities and take advantage of this child's natural desire to read phonetically by teaching simple phonics. Boys tend to be less ready for reading and writing than girls at this age, so don't allow girls to *lord it over* little boys or make them feel stupid.

6-12 Years

A six-year-old loves to be first. He dislikes odd textures in food. He fears bad people, danger, fire, and pain. At this age a child becomes more inquisitive about the opposite sex. Avoid situations where children of the opposite sex are alone at inappropriate times such as potty, bathing, and bedtime. Teach your child to be modest. Many six- year-olds love to ask why, what for, and how come. Elementary school children will identify strongly with the parent of the same sex. Children need heroes so provide them with role models and good patterns for them to follow. About this age, children begin developing the ability to make moral judgments and can be taught Biblical principles and codes of conduct very easily if parents will take the time to talk and explain throughout everyday conversation.

You may find a number of problems occurring during playtime. Often children organize games poorly, dispute rules, and are sensitive to losing and to the cheating of others. The six-year-old child's social immaturity can result in heated arguments with his friends and siblings. This requires tremendous patience from you. Begin to help young children learn how to resolve problems, how to overlook the faults of others, and how to ask forgiveness from others.

Organized and supervised playground activities tend to be most enjoyable and constructive for young children than unorganized play when a group of children are together. This age child likes organized games and responds enthusiastically to children's programs such as AWANA or other organized activity. This is a good age to try little league soccer or baseball since children are generally all at the same level of skill when they are just starting.

Your seven-year-old may tend to be more self-absorbed. About this time his attention span may lengthen. He looks up to older children and teenagers, so be careful who influences him. He may still be very forgetful and distractible. At this time he is more able to put himself in another's place. He now may get embarrassed more easily and may become more perceptive to inconsistencies and changes. You will most likely find he works best when others are working with him.

Seven-year-olds often become more interested in saving money. Encourage him to acquire new skills and interests since as your child gets older, he may not enjoy tackling new interests as much as he does at this age. Remember that every new achievement, no matter how small, is an additional resource that will prevent boredom and depression in years to come.

Eight-year-olds can be very susceptible to jealousy. Their sense of justice and injustice is often more defined. Their feelings can be hurt easily, and they often like to argue. They may be more sympathetic toward others. Generally their bedtime tends to be later, around eight or nine.

At this age girls often have best-friend problems and boys have a problem with clubs. The difficulty may be that they feel excluded or that they are excluding others. Work at teaching your child problem-resolution skills that have a Biblical basis.

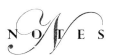

Provide wholesome activities and new experiences. If children are not given useful, constructive things to do, they *will* get into mischief. Do not be tempted to let your children play unsupervised at this age. All children are sinners, and all sinners will sin if they are not engaged in wholesome activity.

You may notice that nine-year-olds are noticeably more self-motivated. They generally organize activities and amuse themselves well. Their conscience is sensitive enabling them to accept blame better than they used to. Children this age often work and play hard. Nine-year-olds can become professional and imaginative at making up excuses. A ten-year-old may be more sensitive to others making fun of him. He may have problems with stomach aches, headaches, or leg cramps. This child will likely be silly, insecure, and self-conscious. He may have a sudden tendency to be withdrawn or lethargic. Ten-year-olds will often begin to use more abstract reasoning.

By the age of twelve, many bodily and personality changes mark the stage of pre-adolescence. On the average this occurs in girls at age twelve and at age thirteen for boys. Commonly, pre-adolescents display more emotional sensitivity than they have previously. They will often become easily fatigued, irritable, negative, or lethargic while they learn to adjust both physically and emotionally to the changes that are quickly taking place in their body. Parents will greatly alleviate anxieties if they understand and prepare their children for this major transition time. Understanding will help reduce the touchy attitudes that commonly arise during this phase. The most common physical symptoms, which signal the onset of puberty, are facial pimples, loss of appetite, increased headaches or stomach aches, and fatigue. Major growth spurts, awkwardness, lack of coordination, body changes, and irritability are all very common.

Beware of your child watching television or playing too many video games at this stage of his development. If you allow it, your pre-teen will spend increasing amounts of time in front of the television or playing video games. Television has the capacity to form perceptions and stimulate desires that will enslave the curious and lethargic. This enslavement will set him on a treacherous course. Remember that what you allow your children to "feed on" mentally is what will come out of them for years to come. Work at teaching your children what is "better" and *more* fun than watching TV. Keep them busy and their minds occupied with good things and you will have less difficulty keeping the television under control.

13-18 Years
Young teens often surprise (and alarm) parents with a sudden interest in friends of the opposite sex; girls generally show interest before boys. Girls tend to form strong attachments that can become a painful problem when their expectations are disappointed. Boys tend to be dangerously curious about sexual issues and often struggle with sexual thoughts and desires making masturbation a temptation. Peer loyalty may create new conflicts with parents. Relationships will tend to be one of

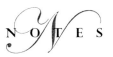

the most difficult areas to navigate in these years, whether they are relationships with friends, relationships with the opposite sex, or relationships with parents.

If you begin early, teenagers can be taught how to have wholesome friendships with the opposite sex. They can be taught how to have fun in groups, how to pace a relationship, how to communicate with other teens in such a way that conversation becomes the center of their friendships rather than sexual exploration. Teens can be taught how to avoid dangerous attachments and deal with the powerful emotions and physical urges that accompany the process of maturing into adulthood. However, they cannot be taught these things without adults who are willing to talk to them or adults who are willing to expend great effort building relationships where the teen is free to discuss and ask questions without fear of rejection. If we do not provide teens with godly and accurate information, they will get it. Quite likely, however, the people and places they get it will be giving them a worldly view of sex instruction rather than an accurate and godly view.

Boys especially need men in their lives who will understand their physical struggles and yet provide guidance and motivation to respect women and keep sexual urges restrained. While masturbation and sexual exploration is very common and should be addressed with compassion, it should not be condoned or allowed to progress into habitual behavior. The habit of self-gratification does not tend to cease with marriage, but brings devastating problems into a future marriage relationship. Sexual tension is not a justifiable reason for masturbation because the flesh is insatiable and does not operate on the principle of tension reduction. Rather than appease desire, the practice of masturbation increases a desire for pornography and self-sex and reduces the potential to enjoy a normal sexual relationship in marriage.

The essence of Biblical sex is the antithesis of self-fulfillment. Sexual intercourse is to be the expression of union and intimate companionship with one's spouse. In contrast, masturbation is the quintessential essence of self-service, self-fulfillment, and self-absorption. It does not require investing one's life in another person or dying to self, which is the nature of companionship in a marriage relationship. Masturbation relies on mental fantasy (primarily a male tendency), which encourages the search for sexually explicit and titillating pictures, movies, or videos. Anything from a Penny's catalog to Internet pornography sites have the potential to elicit arousal and make masturbation desirable. Boys need to learn that the brain is the primary sex organ of the body and must be guarded diligently. They must become aware that it is impossible to be sexually aroused without sexual ideation, making *Matthew 5:27-28* the cornerstone on the issue of mental sexual sin. Avoid giving boys rooms alone or allowing a boy to spend too much time alone in his room. Certainly you will not want to leave your teen unsupervised or allow him to work on a computer without a filter in a private area of the home.

Self-control will be a major issue in the teen years, particularly with regard to attraction to the opposite sex. Teens who are normally self-controlled may be tempted and misled if they are not prepared to deal with their powerful physical and emotional urges. Self-control becomes secondary when the teenage girl's desire for companionship overpowers her desire to restrain herself, or when a teenage boy's desire to satisfy his sexual urges and fantasy overpowers *his* desire to restrain himself. Although boys rarely care in the least about companionship, they quickly key into a girl's desire to hear him pledge his undying love and will take advantage of this more feminine emotional trait. The drive for attachment and companionship is exceedingly strong in the female personality, to the point that young women often believe whatever it is they want most badly to hear. Because teenage girls are too inexperienced to understand the differences in the way boys tend to see relationships or the way they tend to long for a purely physical sexual relationship, they do not comprehend the meaning of the teenage boy's seemingly affectionate touch.

The teen years are an important time for forming goals, ideals, purpose, and meaning. A young teen's mind is very active and susceptible to wrong perceptions of life if the teen's perceptions are not gently countered with truth that is consistent with God's Word. Be sure to provide plenty of wholesome activities and books that provide guidance and understanding of spiritual concepts. Whenever possible, answer questions and deal with problems *before* they arise. Give your teens good role models to emulate. Teens are able to visualize the future more clearly, so take advantage of this by encouraging your child to talk about the future and goals he may want to pursue and the path to getting there.

Avoid lecturing your teen. Rather, engage him in conversation, using questions and brief comments to spark thought. One of the most common problems teens face is the problem of communicating thoughts and ideas. You will help and encourage good communication skills by making special efforts to communicate and reason as you would with a respected young adult. Do not interrupt, ignore, scorn, or treat lightly a teenager's efforts to communicate. Allow your teen to disagree so long as he will disagree respectfully and encourage him to find Biblical principles to support his views. Make talking pleasant and you will find your teen talking about everything with you. If you are not a good and calm listener, you will soon find communication becoming one-sided as the teenager tunes you out and avoids conversations that too often turn into painful personal attacks. Lastly, keep a good sense of humor and have fun talking with your teen. Talking things over with mom and dad ought to be something a teen can look forward to, not something he dreads.

Adolescents begin desiring more independence and showing more individuality in their likes and dislikes. This should not be discouraged, but encouraged. Give your teen choices whenever possible and help him learn *how* to make wise decisions within perimeters that are clearly explained to him. Remember that you are basically working yourself out of a job and preparing your child for responsible adulthood. The ability to resolve problems and make wise decisions is learned gradually through trial and error, much conversation, and spiritual growth that will lead to the ability to apply Biblical principles to real life situations.

Early childhood training and early opportunities to form relationships with spiritually-minded children set the stage for choices that will be made in the teen years with regard to friends.

Provide only enough guidance to ensure your child has the means to make a right decision and then back off so he can exercise sound judgment. Commend him when he makes a wise decision but don't despair when he does not. Help him understand that increasing privileges come with increasing responsibility and growth in character. If you attempt to "micro-manage" his life and decisions rather than expend time and effort teaching him how to govern and manage his own life, you will likely find yourself meeting stiff resistance if not all-out rebellion and resentment at some point in his teen years. Intimidation and force will ensure a teen's compliance up to a point, but the cost to your relationship, not to mention his development, is high and painful.

Early childhood training and early opportunities to form relationships with spiritually minded children set the stage for choices that will be made in the teen years with regard to friends. A teenager invariably chooses friends who have the same values and character level that he does by the time he reaches this stage of his development, not friends that mom and dad want to choose for him. So lay the groundwork early by dealing with heart issues and going to great lengths to provide fellowship for your children with others who love the Lord and find delight in wholesome activities and godly values. Pay special attention to what your child is, not simply what your child does, for he might act one way only to reveal later that his heart was bent toward satisfying sinful desires and delighting in others who share his quest. As children become more independent and begin to function and think with autonomy, their hearts will be revealed with increasing clarity.

Providing opportunities for teens to interact with other Christian young people is an important part of their developing social life. Youth camp, an active church youth group, youth rallies and activities all provide opportunities to reinforce godly values in an atmosphere of uplifting and fun Christian camaraderie that is so important to teens. Teens need a close and warm relationship with parents as well, so they will not be inclined to seek a level of companionship with the opposite sex that the young person is not ready for.

Your daughter may begin having an emotional twenty-eight day cycle even before their menstrual cycle officially begins. You may notice her fluctuating between being more gregarious and loving or to being insecure and needing more affirmation and affection. She will probably be irritable, moody, and unreasonable a few days before her cycle begins. It will alleviate much stress if you are understanding and calm as you teach her how to handle the highs and lows that are a normal part of most women's monthly cycles. Be sure she is getting enough physical activity, nutritious food, and needed sleep; but do not pamper her or excuse unacceptable behavior. She will need to learn that although fluctuating emotions and physical discomfort can be very real, they do not excuse sinful behavior or a lack of self-control. Remind her that God does not have one set of commandments for three weeks out of the month and another set for that special week when it is more difficult to manage or ignore emotions.

Your son's lethargy and fatigue can be a minor problem during growth spurts, but he will nevertheless need a good amount of physical exercise during adolescence. If he does not get enough, you may notice an increase in irritability and moodiness. Mothers will need to avoid dominating teenage boys and encourage them to assume a leadership role when appropriate. This will require wisdom as you must also maintain and insist on complete parental respect.

18 - 21 Years

The young adult poses many challenges while at the same time providing special delight to parents. The enthusiasm and energy of young people is fun and inspiring. They tend to be honest and optimistic about life and are able to interact more as adults than children. At the same time, young adults are sometimes still immature and childlike in many ways, though they live in the body of an energetic adult with all its hormones functioning in full swing. College-age young people still aren't particularly aware of the extent of their parent's sacrifices on their behalf, nor do they always comprehend all the ramifications and importance of personal responsibility. This comprehension usually requires living on their own and experiencing the full weight of family responsibility before they begin to realize how much work goes into meeting day to day living needs and expenses.

The nineteen-year-old wants independence, yet still needs the security of knowing he has a home and understanding parents to give him support and help when needed. Most young adults are not fully independent until the age of twenty six even though they may be college graduates with budding careers or may be embarking on married life. Mom and Dad have a much different role, to be sure, but they are still very much needed and still provide a great deal of security and guidance at times when the young adult needs an understanding and loving pillar to lean upon.

From ages eighteen to twenty one, young people are extremely vulnerable to adopting philosophies of life that they will live by in years to come. For the first time, they are reasoning more as adults and discovering where their values and priorities lie. They will be making some of the most crucial decisions of their lives during this time; decisions that will often be irrevocable or will change the direction of their life forever. Consequently, it is important that young people have as much input from the right sources as possible. Christian friends, good church activities, Christian college, and a close relationship with Mom and Dad will all help give stability and guidance during this transition time.

Young people fresh out of high school are not ready to navigate the treachery of anti-Christian public universities without damage to their moral and spiritual development. The first two years of college are especially crucial years. Young adults who want to pursue a vocation other than full-time Christian service will be strengthened and encouraged by attending a Christian college that will either prepare them for their chosen vocation or provide accreditation that will allow a transfer to another institution once they have completed the typical basic courses required for any major. Parents may need to make financial sacrifices in order to make this possible and young people may need to pull their share of the load by working to contribute to their college expenses as well. The sacrifices are well worth it, however, and seldom regretted.

As exciting as his newfound independence may be, a young adult must realize there is no true independence as a Christian.

Young men are usually less mature than young women, and less likely to know exactly what they want to do with their lives. It is not uncommon for young men to change majors or vocational directions several times before they actually graduate from college. Often the young men are most concerned with vocational decisions regarding their future, while young ladies are most concerned with marriage and family decisions. Both genders tend to be keenly interested in knowing God's will and learning how to make wise decisions. Parents need to provide good materials and instruction in finding God's will long before this point in their child's growth so they will be better able to face this crucial age of decisions with confidence and godly direction.

Remember, a child does not magically become an adult on his eighteenth birthday. Becoming an adult is a gradual process. It is accomplished as parents slowly allow their child freedom to govern himself as an adult without parental interference, and as children gradually gain the confidence and ability to step out on their own. As exciting as his newfound independence may be, a young adult must realize there is no true independence as a Christian. We are to be interdependent with each other and always dependent on God. The young adult is typically so enthralled with his newly acquired adult status in life that it takes some years of maturing before he becomes deeply appreciative and aware of the importance and permanence of family relationships. As difficult as it might be to cease parenting and relinquish all control of your child, you must remember that you will only keep his heart if you give him the complete freedom to fly on his own. To keep him dependent on you will only hinder his growth and cripple him spiritually. The young adult must now be sustained by his own relationship with the Lord and must govern himself by the Word of God as he has been taught.

For personal reflection or discussion:

- What fears did you have when you first learned you were going to be a mother or father?

- What are your hopes and dreams for your child? Do they reflect spiritual values or values that have eternal significance?

- What concerns do you have for your children as they grow toward adulthood?

- What are some of the bumpiest stages you have experienced thus far as a parent?

- How would you most want to encourage parents who have not yet experienced some of the things you have?

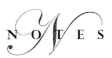

- After reading this chapter, is there anything you wish you had done differently with your child now that he has come through some of these bumpy stages?

- After reading this chapter, is there anything you plan to do differently as a parent?

- Why would wisdom be necessary in dealing with bumpy stages in a child's life?

Lesson 6

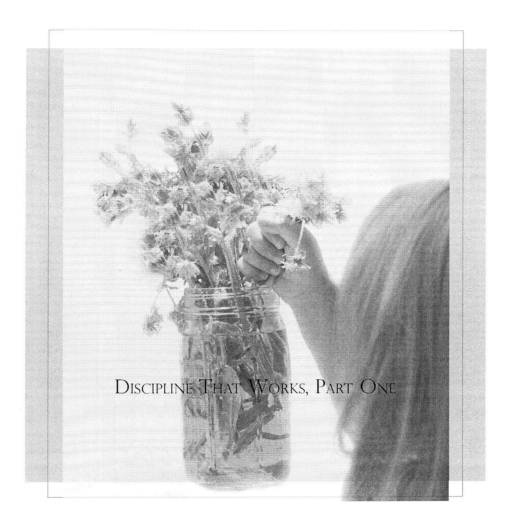

DISCIPLINE THAT WORKS, PART ONE

The rod and reproof give wisdom: but a child left to himself bringeth his mother to shame.
Proverbs 29:15

Correct thy son, and he shall give thee rest; yea, he shall give delight unto thy soul.
Proverbs 29:17

Key Thoughts

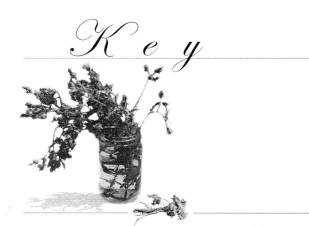

To discipline means to "educate, to prepare by instructing, to correct, to train in principles and habits, to condition by repetition in matters of subordination to authority" (*Webster's 1828 Dictionary*). For the future benefit of their children, God commands Christians to discipline their children. A neglect to discipline constitutes a lack of love for one's child and disobedience to God.

Discussion Problem

Jeff and Bonnie have one child, Katie, who is eighteen-months-old and delights to be into everything. She rarely sits still, creating quite a challenge for her frazzled mother. While Katie eats, she squirms and twists in her chair; and she sometimes runs around in between bites, while Bonnie tries in vain to keep her in one spot while she feeds her.

One evening, Katie's parents decided to take Katie and have dinner at a nearby coffee shop with their good friends Don and Betty. Katie immediately reacted to being confined in the high chair and began squirming and twisting in a successful effort to get down. Bonnie tried to hold her on her lap to keep her happy, but Katie squirmed in protest and began to cry loudly.

Jeff and Bonnie were embarrassed. They did everything possible to appease their daughter and keep her quiet, but Katie promptly threw the spoons on the floor and angrily swept the keys off her tray. Don suggested they just leave because it was late, and Katie was obviously tired. When Betty suggested that Bonnie take Katie to the car to discipline her, Jeff and Bonnie insisted that it wasn't too late for Katie since she won't go to sleep until late. Jeff and Bonnie were horrified to think Don and Betty would spank their children.

Bonnie told them that she and Jeff reasoned with Katie because they believed spanking was cruel and would only lead to violent behavior. Jeff added that Katie would soon grow out of her defiant behavior, and it was best to simply ignore her. He and Bonnie believe they love Katie too much to spank her.

After reading lesson six, use the principles you learn to discuss Katie's behavior and how Jeff and Bonnie are choosing to deal with her. What misconceptions do they have about discipline? Who is in control: Katie or her parents? What do you think of Don and Betty's suggestions? What could be wrong with them?

Bible Study

After reading Hebrews 12:5-11, answer the following questions:

1. For what reasons does God chastise His children? _____
_____
_____
_____

2. How might our children or we misunderstand the purpose of correction? ___
___
___

3. Why would a child feel happy to escape correction as a child, but feel betrayed when he grew to adulthood and remembered he was not corrected? ___
___
___

> *"An infallible way to make your child miserable is to satisfy all his demands."*
> Author Unknown

Discipline That Works

We don't always think of discipline as education, instruction, correction, or repetitious training. More often we think of it in terms of something punitive done to persuade a child not to repeat undesirable behavior. The Bible, however, tells us to train our children, which is synonymous with the word *discipline*. Specifically, parents are to diligently discipline, or train, their children in order to produce Christ-like character. Although correction is a part of discipline, it involves much more than painful consequences that are designed to correct wrong behavior. Painful consequences alone will not transform a child's heart or produce genuine Christ-like character. It may very well stop behavior temporarily, but it will not *change* the will or heart of a child. For this reason many children conform to the will of a parent while the threat of painful consequences is present, but do as they please as soon as the painful consequence is removed. No matter how severe the consequences become, they are powerless to effect real change.

Discipline that works (that produces the kind of change parents desire) involves deliberately guiding and teaching the child in such a way as to change the child's heart, or in other words, change what he believes and what he truly desires. Children, like all people, ultimately behave in ways that are consistent with what they desire and what they believe. When desires and beliefs harmonize with God's desires and God's truth, a child's attitude and behavior naturally reflect God's character. However, when desires and beliefs clash with God's truth and will, the child's attitude and behavior reflect rebellion and self-will. Effective discipline, then, must engage the child's mind and impact the child's heart to the extent that he comes to desire what God Himself desires.

Paul tells us, "to be carnally minded is death; but to be spiritually minded is life and peace" *(Romans 8:6)*. The carnal mind is a mind that is in rebellion against God and results in misery, but the spiritual mind is one that submits to the law of God and results in joy and success. In this passage, Paul is describing the natural bent of two kinds of people. One has not been changed by the Gospel, or has not been saved by believing and putting one's faith in the finished work of Christ for the forgiveness of sin. This person cannot and will not seek to please God on God's terms. The other person has been completely changed as a result of receiving God's grace and is drawn to following or submitting to God. This person pleases God because he has become God's own by faith in Christ, and has God's own Spirit dwelling in him. The difference between the ways these two people respond to what is true and right is like night and day. Basically, one rebels; the other submits.

Because Christian discipline has its basis in the change that takes place when one believes the gospel and puts his trust in the Lord Jesus Christ, discipline cannot be understood apart from salvation. As believers, we both change (at salvation) and are being changed (through sanctification) by the power of God working within us to transform our character as we submit to His Word. We believe that apart from Christ, this heart-level change is impossible. The fruit of the Spirit listed in *Galatians 5* is produced as a result of our union with Christ, when we live in conformity with and dependent upon the Spirit of God and Word of God. This transformation takes place in children who believe as well as in adults who believe. Parents cannot produce the fruit of God's Spirit in their own life by their own power and determination. Neither will they produce it in the lives of their children apart from the power of God. What parent does not want his child to be filled with love, joy, peace, longsuffering, gentleness, goodness, faith, meekness [humility], or temperance [self-control]? Is this not the core goal of *all* our discipline?

A Christian parent restrains and controls his child's behavior in the younger years at the same time that he endeavors to teach his child how to restrain and control his own behavior through a relationship with Christ. A child's natural self-willed nature is brought under loving control as he is deliberately trained to respond to parental authority that is directing the child to obey God's loving commands. Because Christian discipline is carried out in cooperation with the internal work of the Holy Spirit, it must work in harmony with God's Word, not in opposition to it. Parents are the primary means God uses to train children while they are young, but parental control is meant to decrease as the child reaches physical and spiritual maturity and his awareness and understanding of God increases. External motivation to obey a parent must gradually be replaced by internal motivation to obey God. This is how children grow to be strong in the Lord and able to withstand the wiles of the devil at maturity.

Wise parents understand that children can only be *made* to obey and conform for so long. Unless the child's heart is affected to such an extent that he desires to obey and is motivated by internal decisions and beliefs to obey, he will eventually rebel against the restraints and rules that a parent imposes in an effort to control behavior. Discipline that only produces a fear of disobeying rather than a desire to obey will ultimately fail. Therefore, Christian parents must do more than bark out orders and enforce authority. They must be actively disciplining, or *training* children to love God and live a responsible Christian life. The goal is to train children to respond to God, for God goes with him through adulthood; the parents do not.

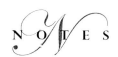

Biblical discipline includes many means of accomplishing this goal, including patient teaching and training, as well as the administration of chastisements when an offense has occurred. Children are to be disciplined, or trained, as they go about the events of daily life, not just when they have committed some kind of offense. Children who are patiently taught how to sweep a floor aren't likely to need correction for sweeping the floor incorrectly. Children who are taught good habits through daily routines aren't as likely to need correction for refusing to go to bed or forgetting to brush their teeth. Children who are taught Biblical reasons for making wise choices aren't likely to need the same kind of correction as children who do or do not do certain things only because mother and dad say it is so. Children who are taught the joys of obeying at times when it is pleasant to do so don't have as much difficulty obeying when it is not pleasant to do so. Try teaching your child to obey by commanding him to get a candy bar from the refrigerator and eat it at the table. Chances are great that your child will obey perfectly, and you will be able to commend him enthusiastically for his quick obedience! Parents who get into the habit of training their children only when they disobey or fail in some way soon find they are meeting resistance and fighting a losing battle. The older the child becomes, the more he tends to resent this kind of intervention.

External motivation to obey a parent must gradually be replaced by internal motivation to obey God.

When offenses occur, as they no doubt will, children need correction as well as instruction. This requires more time than a quick swat or sharp words threatening something more severe. The objective of discipline when an offense has occurred is to correct the child's wrong behavior and attitude and replace it with the correct behavior and attitude. To accomplish this, a parent should seek to understand the child's motives, possible underlying causes of the wrong or sinful behavior, the facts surrounding the incident, and the child's understanding of the offense.

Corrective discipline should include the following:

- **Helping** the child clarify and understand how he specifically chose to behave inappropriately or how he sinned against another individual.
- **Explaining** the violation in Biblical terms.
- **Determining** what corrective measures are appropriate for the offense and explaining the consequences of the child's choice to misbehave.
- **Guiding** the child to understand the purpose of the correction that will be administered and what right behavior must replace the wrong.
- **Instructing** the child how to resolve an offense Biblically or make proper restitution.
- **Assuring** the child of our love, forgiveness, and desire to help him behave appropriately in the future.

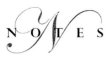

Corrective discipline may require the administration of consequences, or chastisement. When chastisement is warranted, it is always to be administered in love, not anger, for anger never works the righteousness of God and is not profitable to the child. All discipline, including chastisement, is done *for* the child, not *to* the child, and is always for the child's benefit, not the parent's. The aim is not punitive, but corrective. Chastisement is not for the purpose of venting parental anger or expressing parental displeasure. It is not retribution for wrongs committed. It is *not* punishment. Chastisement is a term that refers to God's corrective measures that He uses to discipline His own children. Chastisement is always corrective and restorative, and is done in love for the benefit of the offender. Its purpose is to restore the relationship between God the Father and His child, which was broken by the child's offense.

Punishment is a term God reserves for the heathen, and refers to retributive judgment that will be executed against those who have rejected God. Punishment, as the Bible defines it, is not for the benefit of the offender, but of society, and is the vindication of God's justice. God never *chastises* the unsaved or reprobate, and God never *punishes* those who are His own redeemed children. The Bible makes a clear distinction between punishment and chastisement, or discipline. God punishes the wicked, but He chastises and disciplines His children. Chastisement, even when it is painful, is to be carried out in love, as God's discipline toward His children is carried out in love.

The use of spanking, or the "rod" as it is called in the Bible, is only employed as a means of discipline when direct disobedience, deliberate defiance, or disrespect is involved. Defiant, self-willed, disobedient behavior is referred to as "foolish" behavior in the Bible and requires a deterrent other than verbal reasoning or reproving. The Bible warns us that "The rod and reproof give wisdom: but a child left to himself bringeth his mother to shame" *(Proverbs 29:15)*. Discipline, in the form of a spanking, is to be administered in the proper manner and for the proper reasons. Spanking is never to be used to correct childish behavior that should be dealt with in other ways or overlooked altogether.

Spankings should be limited to specific occasions to train a young child to realize we always suffer painful consequences when we choose to act rebelliously and selfishly. The properly delivered sting of a spanking is designed to alter the behavior of a child so he will not develop habits of behavior that will cause a much greater "sting" and sorrow in his adult life. Proper use of corporal punishment is consistent, limited, controlled, and loving. Pain that is associated with mistakes prevents a child from becoming violent or repeating unacceptable behavior, just as pain experienced in any area of our life usually causes us to avoid whatever we did to bring the pain upon ourselves.

Biblical Discipline Is Balanced

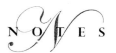

Biblical discipline is accomplished through a balanced attitude of nurturing and teaching, together with parental control that sets definite limits and delivers definite, predictable consequences. This might be referred to as *nurturing dominance*. Nurturing dominance is that wonderful quality of firm control blended with loving, patient teaching. The two together is what arouses a child's respect for those in authority over him, and causes him to respond willingly. Children love a *Mary Poppins*-type mother because she sets definite limits and control, yet also nurtures and teaches the children with love. This is the way God deals with us, and this is the way we are to deal with our children.

Without chastisement, correction, or discipline, the Bible warns that the foolish nature of a child will lead him to rebel against godly authority and to adopt a very self-willed manner of living. Since self-will is at the root of every sin and misery, it is imperative for parents to conquer the will of their children and bring them up to accept godly instruction and discipline. "Poverty and shame shall be to him that refuseth instruction: but he that regardeth reproof shall be honored" *(Proverbs 13:18)*. The right kind of correcting discipline is necessary in order to train a child to *willingly* yield to God's authority. As our children mature, we want them to be governed by convictions in their own heart rather than by external control forced on them against their will by others in authority over them. This does not mean that we do not use external control, but that we couple it with efforts to correct the way the child thinks and believes with regard to the behavior.

Biblical chastisement will

- Drive foolish or rebellious behavior from a child's thinking *(Proverbs 22:15)*.
- Produce godly wisdom and understanding *(Proverbs 15:5)*.
- Lead to a happy home and respect for parent *(Proverbs 29:17)*.
- Produce holy, righteous behavior *(Hebrews 12:10-11)*.
- Cause parents to rejoice in time to come *(Proverbs 29:17)*.

When asked to give specific objectives for disciplining and correcting a child, most Christian parents respond by saying their overall purpose is to enforce obedience. Some add other thoughts, but few have definitively determined ahead of time their objectives for discipline in such a way that they know precisely what they want to accomplish. Following are three major but very specific objectives for disciplining a child:

Parental discipline is designed to produce three major but very specific objectives:

- Appropriate obedience
- Respect for legitimate authority
- Personal responsibility

Obedience - Disobedient children grow up to defy, not only parents and teachers, but government, laws, rules, their boss, or anyone who would attempt to restrict them from doing what they want to do, or compel them to do what they do not want to do—including God. We who know the Lord recognize that God's commands are designed to spare us from the sorrows of sinful choices and lead us to receive the blessings of conforming to God's character. We also recognize that children who refuse to submit to God's limitations and guidance as they grow into adulthood bring into their lives great sorrow. Children greatly benefit by learning to obey legitimate authority. Healthy obedience leads children to become well-adjusted, unselfish, happy people rather than deceitful, selfish, and miserable people.

Israel was a disobedient people primarily because they did not believe God's Word or trust His loving yet just character *(Hebrews 3:16-19)*. Those who obeyed believed. In the New Testament we are told that believing on the Lord Jesus Christ for salvation is synonymous with obedience. Paul said, "But they have not all obeyed the gospel. For Esaias saith, Lord, who hath believed our report? So then faith cometh by hearing, and hearing by the word of God" *(Romans 10:16-17)*. If a proper form of obedience is one goal of discipline, we will want to do more than force our children to obey by chastising them when they do not. We will want to do all in our power to persuade our children to believe obedience is desirable and brings certain blessing just as disobedience brings certain sorrow.

Respect - Respect for God, authority, and other people gives children the skill they need to get along with others and function as a member of society and member of God's family as well. A proper respect for parents and teachers forms a foundational attitude that will later determine a child's attitude towards all other people in his life. Children who are allowed to treat others with contempt, who are not taught to respect the rights and property of others, or who do not regard authority with proper esteem will grow up to be demanding, obnoxious, and arrogant people. They will learn to get what they want at other people's expense, and will use manipulative means to assert their will and satisfy their desire for control and dominance. They will become insensitive to the feelings of others and will lack the humility that is necessary to practice Biblical love and forgiveness between brethren in Christ and others in their community.

Disrespect for parents ought never to be tolerated or excused. Rather, it must be immediately corrected and dealt with decisively. Children need to be taught that they are permitted to disagree and may ask questions of a parent, but may never do so with any kind of disrespect. Others who are in authority over our children must also be given respect, regardless whether the child agrees with them or not. In fact, even in those rare cases when a child is asked by one in authority over him to do something that violates his conscience or is clearly sinful, he is to appeal to that authority in a godly way and ultimately refuse to obey without being disrespectful. We would not want our children to obey all authority without question for to do so would subject them to adults who might exploit their submissiveness and harm them. Rather, we want to teach children how and when authority is limited.

Examples to teach our children include Nathan's appeal to David in *2 Samuel 12*, Daniel's appeal to Melza the prince of the Eunuchs in *Daniel 1*, Esther's appeal to King Ahasuerus in *Esther 4-7*, Jonathan's appeal to Saul in *1 Samuel 19*, and Shadrach, Meshach and Abednego's appeal to Nebuchadnezzar in *Daniel 3*. In each case the one in submission demonstrated careful and appropriate respect.

Furthermore, children who are not taught to reverence or respect God and His Word specifically lack an understanding that would properly lead them to fear God and consequently, depart from evil *(Proverbs 16:6)*. Timothy's mother was commended for her diligence in teaching her young son the Scriptures that were able to make him wise to salvation. Because she placed the fear of God and knowledge of the Scriptures as such a high priority, she chose to give her son a name that means, "one who fears God." It is not surprising that Timothy grew to be a man who not only obeyed and honored his mother, but also obeyed and honored God. It is significant to note that there is no mention of a father in Timothy's life or indication Timothy's father was a believer. Quite possibly Timothy was raised by a single mother and grandmother without the benefit of a believing father. The wisdom of Timothy's mother enabled her to place the proper priority on reverence for God and spiritual understanding, resulting in a godly son even though he did not have a godly father.

Responsibility - Children who learn to be responsible, or accountable, for their own behavior and choices learn to be self-controlled. They develop the satisfaction and security that results when they are able to implement achievements in practical everyday living. Responsible behavior in children prevents many painful consequences, including much of the despair and depression that is always associated with behavior that is irresponsible and undisciplined.

Training children to fulfill obligations and accomplish goals begins with parents learning to do this in their own lives. If parents do not model accepting responsibility for wrongs, fulfilling duties or making responsible decisions, children will not place much importance on responsible behavior either. They will invariably act responsibly only when they are forced to do so. On the other hand, as children see parents fulfilling responsibilities and taking pleasure in it, they tend to follow the example when they are encouraged to do so. Responsibility becomes something desired as children begin to recognize that responsibility brings privileges and is highly valued. Children should be given responsibility and taught how to fulfill their obligations so that they might be given more responsibility and more privileges. This requires parents to train children by *getting in there with* their children and providing the enthusiasm and inspiration that is so vital in helping children *enjoy* fulfilling responsibilities and develop good lifelong habits.

Children learn that they are responsible for their own choices and behavior as they mature. Teaching responsibility begins when children are very young and continues right up to adulthood. Requiring children to take care of their own property by picking up their toys and taking good care of them is only the beginning of teaching responsible behavior. When they are disciplined for disobedience, they need to be asked if they will obey, signaling that it is a choice they make. When they receive consequences for violating limitations placed on them, they need to be reminded that they chose the consequence when they chose to ignore it. When children break or lose things, they need to be taught they are responsible to fix, replace, or restore them. When children make a promise or agreement, they need to learn to keep their word and responsibly fulfill their obligations.

God reminds us that we alone are responsible for our response to Him, that we have obligations to Him that He expects us to fulfill, and that His promises are often dependent on our choice to responsibly fulfill our part. We will all stand before the Lord in the Day of Judgment to give an accounting of how we fulfilled our Christian responsibilities. Children need to understand that they too must give an account to the Lord and cannot blame others for their disobedience any more than parents.

Destructive Misconceptions about Discipline

Misconception #1 - Discipline always means spanking.
Discipline means training. It involves deliberately guiding and teaching a child and uses many means to change a child's attitude and behavior. Spanking is a proper, Biblical form of discipline to use when the child's offense involves direct disobedience, deliberate defiance, or disrespect. However, childish infractions should be dealt with differently, depending on the child's motives and his capacity to understand and learn. Corporal correction must also be tempered with mercy on occasion.

Proverbs 22:6—Train up a child in the way he should go: and when he is old, he will not depart from it.

Misconception #2 - Adequate love makes discipline unnecessary.
Love understands the absolute necessity of both nurturing and disciplining. The two work together in developing responsible, respectful children. Discipline is a direct function of love. Without discipline, training, restraint, and correction, children are left to their own propensity to be rebellious, self-centered, and wicked.

Proverbs 3:12—For whom the LORD loveth he correcteth; even as a father the son *in whom* he delighteth.

Proverbs 13:24—He that spareth his rod hateth his son: but he that loveth him chasteneth him betimes.

Misconception #3 - It's better to wait until a child is older and can understand more before disciplining him.

Children begin developing an understanding and attitude towards parental authority in their first year of life. They are extremely vulnerable to their parent's expectations and training, both good and bad. The most critical period of a child's life is from birth through the age of four or five. After this period, it becomes increasingly more difficult to alter a child's attitudes and personality.

Proverbs 19:18—Chasten thy son while there is hope, and let not thy soul spare for his crying.

Misconception #4 - All confrontations with children can be resolved with love and reasoning.

Reasoning alone is not a deterrent to disobedience. Love demands a response to disobedience that will cause the child realize how unattractive disobedience is. Reasoning, communication, and assurances of love are most effective and constructive after discipline, not before.

Proverbs 29:15—The rod and reproof give wisdom: but a child left *to himself* bringeth his mother to shame.

Misconception #5 - Disrespect for parents is normal and will eventually be outgrown.

A proper respect for parents forms a foundational attitude that will later determine a child's attitude toward all the other people in his life. More importantly, it becomes the framework on which a child begins to build a proper respect (fear) of God.

Proverbs 20:20—Whoso curseth his father or his mother, his lamp shall be put out in obscure darkness.

Ephesians 6:1—Children, obey your parents in the Lord: for this is right.

Colossians 3:20—Children, obey your parents in all things: for this is well pleasing unto the Lord.

Misconception #6 - It's better to ignore a child when he challenges his parent's authority than to make an issue of it.

Ignoring a child's contempt or defiance always encourages repeated episodes of rebellion, disrespect, fighting, or tantrums. Children must know that his parent is in absolute control and will not under any circumstance negotiate his preeminence with regard to parenting. Every challenge to a parent's authority and right to govern the home must be met *confidently* and *calmly* and *won*. *Never* reward defiance by letting a child get away with it. Nor should you indulge a child who makes selfish demands.

Nothing a child cries for ought to be given. No expression of disrespect or resistance ought to go unchallenged.

Proverbs 29:17—Correct thy son, and he shall give thee rest; yea, he shall give delight unto thy soul.

Misconception #7 - Self-discipline and self-control will naturally develop in my child without my help.

Parents must be involved in the instructing and training of their child if they wish him to develop self discipline and self control. Children are naturally undisciplined. Apart from parental intervention or outside motivation, children will generally remain as undisciplined as is possible.

Hebrews 12:11—Now no chastening for the present seemeth to be joyous, but grievous: nevertheless afterward it yieldeth the peaceable fruit of righteousness unto them which are exercised thereby.

Proverbs 16:32—He that is slow to anger is better than the mighty; and he that ruleth his spirit than he that taketh a city.

Misconception #8 - A child is born totally unselfish and good. He only becomes self-centered as he grows older.

A child is born with a totally self-centered nature, which becomes more complex as he grows older. He does not need to be taught to be selfish and disrespectful. This comes all too naturally. As sweet and innocent as children are, they have still inherited a fallen, sinful nature that taints their behavior.

Proverbs 22:15—Foolishness [self will] is bound in the heart of a child; but the rod of correction shall drive it far from him.

Psalm 51:5—Behold, I was shapen in iniquity; and in sin did my mother conceive me.

Romans 3:10—As it is written, there is none righteous, no, not one.

Romans 3:23—For all have sinned, and come short of the glory of God.

Misconception #9 - Yelling and screaming are good forms of discipline. They will make my child respect what I say.

Yelling and screaming may vent your anger, and may stop wrong behavior so long as fear is present, but these methods will *never* accomplish a *change* in behavior, which is the objective of good discipline. Remember that the "the wrath of man worketh not the righteousness of God." *(James 1:20)*

Behavior is changed when parents:

- Define boundaries, rules, and expectations. Avoid harsh or impossible demands.
- Define consequences of misbehavior beforehand. Do not threaten.
- Enforce consequences deliberately, consistently, and confidently. Do not argue.

Immediate action provokes an immediate change of behavior. Screaming provokes a *tune-out* response and results in frustration and anger in both parent and child. This produces *no change* in heart attitude or in behavior.

Colossians 3:21—Fathers, provoke not your children to anger, lest they be discouraged.

Misconception #10 - Spanking and other forms of discipline cause children to become insecure (fearful).

Spanking a child when he has expressed defiance or has willfully disobeyed establishes boundaries in his life that give security much as a railing gives security when standing on the edge of a tall building. Children want limits on their behavior. They will respect adults who lovingly, firmly establish limits for the good of the child. Children with few behavior restraints behavior prove to be prone to insecurity and rebellion.

Proverbs 6:20-23—My son, keep thy father's commandment, and forsake not the law of thy mother: bind them continually upon thine heart, *and* tie them about thy neck. When thou goest, it shall lead thee; when thou sleepest, it shall keep thee; and *when* thou awakest, it shall talk with thee. For the commandment *is* a lamp; and the law *is* light; and reproofs of instruction *are* the way of life.

Misconception #11 - Spanking children causes them to become violent.

Violence and discipline are two totally separate things. It is quite possible for violent and uncontrolled parents to generate hostility, hyperactivity, and aggressiveness in their children. This constitutes abuse and does not in any way represent a Biblical or Christian view of corporal punishment, or more accurately, chastisement. Proper discipline, on the other hand, is consistent, controlled, and loving. It uses pain which is properly delivered to a child's backside as a means to teach that there are always painful consequences when we choose to act rebelliously and selfishly.

Pain which is controlled, limited, and associated with mistakes prevents a child from becoming violent or repeating unacceptable behavior, just as pain experienced in any area of our life causes us to avoid whatever we did to bring the pain upon ourselves.

Proverbs 23:13-14—Withhold not correction from the child: for *if* thou beatest [spank] him with the rod, he shall not die. Thou shalt beat [spank] him with the rod, and shalt deliver his soul from hell.

Misconception #12 - Toddlers should be spanked every time they touch, bite, taste, smell, or break something in their grasp.

Toddlers curiously touch, bite, taste, smell, and handle as a means of learning and investigating their world. They rarely resist the urge to look over an intriguing new object, be it ever so fragile. A toddler should be swatted, or appropriately spanked, when he openly defies a parent's spoken command, but not for merely being childish. The key is distinguishing a child's motive. Is it defiance or childishness?

Ephesians 6:4—And, ye fathers, provoke not your children to wrath: but bring them up in the nurture and admonition of the Lord.

Misconception #13 - It is not good to hug a child after you've spanked or disciplined him.

After discipline has been carried out, children are quite aware that their behavior was not acceptable to the parent. Next they need to be assured with a parent's affection that they themselves are loved. They must understand that it is because we love them that we discipline them and thus will not allow them to behave in a destructive manner. Hugging and reassuring children of our love and forgiveness are important aspects of Biblical discipline.

Psalm 103:13—Like as a father pitieth *his* children, so the LORD pitieth them that fear him.

Isaiah 66:13a—As one whom his mother comforteth, so will I comfort you.

1 Thessalonians 2:11—As ye know how we exhorted and comforted and charged every one of you, as a father *doth* his children.

Misconception #14 - It is not harmful to promise an offense will be disciplined and then decline to carry through with it.

Children must learn that parents can be depended upon to correct rebellious behavior in the exact manner in which they were promised beforehand (not more, nor less). When parents fail to consistently carry out corrective measures, the inconsistency causes a child to believe he might not be corrected. Once he believes there is a remote chance the parent will not carry through, he will tend to risk misbehaving in the hopes this is going to be the case. Every time his risk pays off, he is less inclined to take the parent at his word. The child tends to become bolder and more persistent in his behavior when correction is withheld, changed, or delayed.

Ecclesiastes 8:1—Because sentence against an evil work is not executed speedily, therefore the heart of the sons of men is fully set in them to do evil.

Exodus 8:15—But when Pharaoh saw that there was respite, he hardened his heart, and hearkened not unto them; as the LORD had said.

Isaiah 26:10—Let favor be showed to the wicked, *yet* will he not learn righteousness: in the land of uprightness will he deal unjustly, and will not behold the majesty of the LORD.

Misconception #15 - Children should be disciplined the same, no matter what age they are.

The manner and severity of correction must vary between children of differing ages for several reasons.

- A child's ability to understand varies, depending on his age level. (A four-year-old easily forgets instructions that are too complex or lengthy for him. A fourteen- year-old is able to follow more complex, multiple instructions.)
- A child's capacity to exert self control varies depending on his age level. (A toddler cries easily when he is denied while an older child is able to master accepting denials quietly.)
- A child's motive for certain behaviors differs as he grows older. (A baby may say "no" because it's a new word or because he's imitating his mother. A two-year-old or ten-year-old says "no" because he's rebelling against the will of his parent.)
- A child's maturity level affects his ability to discern right and wrong. (If a three year old taking a bath in Mother's presence touches a sibling's private parts, it is out of curiosity. If a thirteen-year-old in secrecy touches a sibling's private parts, it is for personal pleasure.)
- Certain problems and difficulties are characteristic of a child's age and must be dealt with accordingly. (Babies cry easily because it is their nature to express discomfort in this manner. An adolescent may suddenly cry easily because drastic changes are taking place quickly in his body. An eight-year-old may cry easily because he's learned to get his own way in this manner.)
- A child's age makes a difference in how he will receive various corrective measures. (A toddler can be swatted in the presence of others, while an older child will be embarrassed and resentful if he is swatted in the presence of others.)

Jeremiah 25:14—For many nations and great kings shall serve themselves of them also: and I will recompense them according to their deeds, and according to the works of their own hands.

Ezekiel 36:19—And I scattered them among the heathen, and they were dispersed through the countries: according to their way and according to their doings I judged them.

Ezekiel 39:24—According to their uncleanness and according to their transgressions have I done unto them, and hid my face from them.

Revelation 20:13—And the sea gave up the dead which were in it; and death and hell delivered up the dead which were in them: and they were judged every man according to their works.

Misconception #16 - Embarrassing or shaming a child is a good form of discipline.

Degrading a child is never healthy or constructive to the formation of his character. Shaming him in front of others, forcing him to suffer unnecessary humiliation, or causing him to endure public rebuke will do the following:

- Destroy his sense of confidence
- Engender anger and resentment
- Destroy the loving bond and companionship that is necessary to an effective parent-child relationship
- Cause him to grow up to be overly concerned about the opinion of others

Deuteronomy 12:28—Observe and hear all these words which I command thee, that it may go well with thee, and with thy children after thee for ever, when thou doest that which is good and right in the sight of the LORD thy God.

Misconception #17 - Increasing force is necessary to convince a child to abandon unacceptable behavior.

A spanking needs to sting enough to produce a change in a child's desire to persist in his rebellious behavior. Insufficient force often arouses resentment and anger or indifference rather than a change of heart. However, it is not true that continuing to increase the force and severity of a spanking prevents a child from repeating the behavior. If you believe mere force is the deterrent necessary for prevention, you will tend to spank excessively or uncontrollably.

Excessive discipline may produce compliance for a time, but it also tends to produce anger, nervousness, hyperactivity, a hard heart, or increasingly rebellious desires; and excessive discipline can result in discouraging a child to the point of destroying his confidence, producing depression, or encouraging withdrawal. Calmly, consistently applying the same discipline every time the rebellious offense is repeated is far more effective than increasing the force with which the discipline is applied.

Ephesians 6:4—And, ye fathers, provoke not your children to wrath: but bring them up in the nurture and admonition [chastisement] of the Lord.

Psalm 89:32-33—Then will I visit their transgression with the rod, and their iniquity with stripes. Nevertheless my lovingkindness will I not utterly take from him, nor suffer my faithfulness to fail.

Psalm 118:18—The LORD hath chastened me sore: but he hath not given me over unto death.

Misconception #18- It is important to continue spanking a child until his will is broken.

Usually the idea of breaking a child's will is thought to mean spanking until the child cries sufficiently, displays an acceptable amount of emotion, or appears absolutely compliant. Nowhere in the Scripture will you find a passage to support the idea that a spanking must be continued until a child's will is broken.

Chastisement always has as a goal removing the child's naturally self-willed and rebellious attitude and replacing it with a tender, teachable spirit. However, this cannot always be accomplished in one spanking. It might require repeated spankings, instruction, and encouragement before the larger picture of repentance is truly accomplished.

It is unbiblical, and utter nonsense, to think repentance can be determined by the child's crying, lack of crying, or appearance of sorrow and compliance. Not only do children vary in their emotional responses to spankings, but parents vary in their subjective view of a compliant response. Furthermore, assuming that the force and severity of discipline must be arbitrarily increased in order to produce a certain response can be a dangerous practice. This leads to beating a child into submission, rather than teaching him to respond willingly to correction.

The idea that spanking must *break the child's will but not his spirit* is a vague concept. A child's spirit is damaged when he is beaten into submission by an angry or excessively harsh parent, yet this may look very much like a "broken will" to a well-meaning but misguided parent. The important thing to remember is that true change, or repentance, cannot be determined by how the child reacts to the chastisement, how much he cries, or how much he appears to be sorry. Not until after the correction is administered and the child's subsequent behavior is examined can the measure of repentance be evaluated.

Proverbs 18:14—The spirit of a man will sustain his infirmity; but a wounded spirit who can bear?

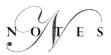

Bible Test for True Repentance—2 Corinthians 7:9-11

Verse 9 — *Now I rejoice, not that ye were made sorry, but that ye sorrowed to repentance; for ye were made sorry after a godly manner, that ye might receive damage by us in nothing.*

Repentance is not just feeling sorry for something, but being sorry enough to turn away from the sin to God. Those who repent want to conquer their problem, even though it may take several failures, corrections, and time before experiencing victory.

Verse 10 — *For godly sorrow worketh repentance to salvation not to be repented of; but the sorrow of the world worketh death.*

There are two kinds of sorrow:

1. Worldly sorrow is painful regret. It focuses on our feelings and is self-condemning and frustrating to us.

2. Sorrow that is godly has primary concern for the good of others and the honor of God. It seeks to right wrongs and to change behavior. Most people will quickly admit that they are a sinner. Few ever admit they are a *helpless* sinner, unable to save or change their own heart.

Worldly sorrow simply admits a wrong. Godly sorrow recognizes the helpless condition sin brings and turns to God to forgive and cleanse. Children who sincerely regret doing what they did or are deeply sorry they got caught are not necessarily repentant. This kind of sorrow doesn't change the heart desires, but merely induces the child to find more sophisticated or deceitful ways to avoid the trauma of getting caught in the future.

Verse 11a — *For behold this selfsame thing, that ye sorrowed after a godly sort,*

Repentant children will have a desire to do what is necessary to right their wrongs and acknowledge their error to those they have wronged and seek forgiveness. They will be eager to pray and seek God's forgiveness, and will sense the need to humbly and honestly confess their sin to God.

Verse 11b   *what carefulness it wrought in you,*

Carefulness means diligence to do right. Children want to do right and will submit to their parent's help to accomplish this.

Verse 11c   *yea, what clearing of yourselves*

The phrase *clearing of yourselves* is referring to the cleared conscious that accompanies repentance. Repentant children who are taught to understand Biblical confession and God's love and forgiveness sense a great emotional relief, and respond with happiness and transparency rather than with sulking and secrecy.

Verse 11d   *yea, what indignation,*

Indignation means moved with displeasure over sin. Repentant children don't like the sin they've confessed, and do not treat sin as though it's an insignificant or unimportant concern of the parents.

Verse 11e   *yea, what fear,*

Fear is referring to a healthy awareness of God. The process of confessing, forsaking, seeking, and accepting forgiveness produces a love and respect for God.

Verse 11f   *yea, what vehement desire, yea, what zeal,*

Zeal refers to an eagerness to serve God. Repentance results in a deep desire to respond to God in ways that are pleasing to Him.

Verse 11g   *yea, what revenge!*

Revenge means a willingness to carry out restitution. A repentant child will accept the consequences of his sin willingly, without making excuses or casting blame. To the best of his ability, he will willingly do whatever is necessary to restore what he has damaged. Parents need to make it possible for their child to carry out restitution and help him in his efforts to do so.

Lesson 7

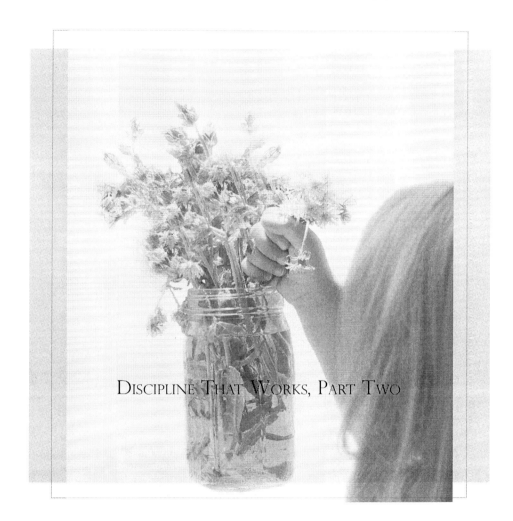

DISCIPLINE THAT WORKS, PART TWO

My son, despise not the chastening of the LORD neither
be weary of his correction: for whom the Lord loveth
he correcteth; even the son in whom he delighteth.
Proverbs 3:11-12

For I have given you an example,
that ye should do as I have done to you.
John 13:15

Key THOUGHTS

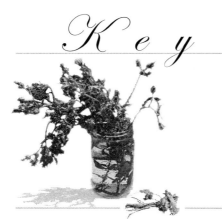

The Bible describes and illustrates God as the perfect father. Thus, God provides parents with the perfect pattern for Christian parenting. Parents are to follow God's example, and observe and learn from others who follow God's example.

Discussion Problem

Jenny is an independent five-year-old who loves to imitate her mother, Pam. One day Jenny quietly studied her mother as she applied her make-up, trimmed the front of her hair, and curled it before going out to dinner. Because Pam was in a hurry, she left the scissors on her dresser and left. Jenny's baby-sitter arrived and quickly sat in front of the television to watch a movie that didn't interest Jenny.

During a commercial an hour later, the babysitter realized she hadn't seen or heard Jenny for quite some time. She went upstairs to find her. She found Jenny with her purse and her lipstick smeared all over her face. The lipstick was ruined because Jenny had pressed it too hard on her lips. The babysitter was angry about losing it. Besides, she was angry Jenny had opened her purse in the first place. It was an established rule that Jenny wasn't to get into anyone's purse.

Jenny also had found her mother's scissors on the dresser and trimmed her own hair, which was quite obviously butchered. When Pam came home she was horrified at the sight of Jenny's hair. The baby-sitter explained about the lipstick and purse, but Pam was very angry about the hair and unconcerned about the lipstick.

After reading lesson seven, apply the principles you learn to decide how Pam should handle this situation. Besides getting a new baby-sitter, what should she should do? Discuss possible reasons she is angry. Why might her reasons be wrong? Pay particular attention to the section entitled "Before You Discipline" (page 151).

Bible Study

After reading Psalm 119:67, 71, and 75, answer the following questions.

1. Why is David glad God corrected (afflicted) him? _____
   _____

2. What does God's correction tell David about God? _____
   _____

3. What causes children to respect their parent's discipline after they have grown? _____
   _____
   _____

After reading Psalm 107:10-13, answer the following questions.

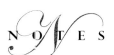

1. Why does God correct (afflict) people? _____
   _____
   _____
   _____

2. When does God cease correction in this instance? _____
   _____
   _____
   _____

3. What means does God use to deliver the people from the errors of their thinking (destructions)? _____
   _____
   _____
   _____

"A torn jacket is soon mended; but hard words bruise the heart of a child."
Henry Longfellow

Operating Instructions

Parents who have no other example to follow other than themselves or other imperfect parents cannot rise above human frailties or become greater than those who are followed. The human heart apart from Christ will always reason incorrectly, deceive itself, and choose paths that lead to dead ends and frightening destinations *(Jeremiah 17:9)*. Furthermore, what seems to be the right route for some does not work for others who are coming from a different place of origin. There is no sure way to find the right course for our children other than seeking directions from the right source. For this reason, we need a roadmap and pattern to follow that exceeds human wisdom and ability, for we cannot hope to lead our children in the right direction if we don't know which way to go ourselves or who is safe to follow. The roadmap God gives parents is His Word, and the example He gives us to follow is none other than Himself.

In *John 13:15* we read, "For I have given you an example, that ye should do as I have done to you." Other Christian parents may provide a good example for us if they themselves follow Christ, but only He is a perfect pattern without fault. The Lord Jesus alone is to be our final authority and perfect pattern by which all others are to be judged. We are able to learn how to respond to our children by learning how to imitate the manner in which God loves, trains, motivates, and corrects *His* children. As we consider how Christ dealt individually with His disciples according to their abilities and personalities and at the same time, consistently led them to the same destination, we begin to grasp the complexity of our task. Christ taught the same principles and same irrevocable truths to all, yet He applied vastly different means to bring people to the same conclusions. No miracle was ever implemented in exactly the same way, yet all brought people to one faith and one God Who never changes.

While we cannot hope to perfectly duplicate Christ's character and wisdom, we certainly have the ability to emulate it if we are His offspring. Learning how to emulate the Lord Jesus, however, will require us to thoughtfully study His example and ponder the ways God works with His own children. He Himself commands us to consider His character and the way He deals with life's situations so that we can know how to respond ourselves. Following are a few examples where we are told to emulate Christ's example.

> *Luke 6:35-36*—But love ye your enemies, and do good, and lend, hoping for nothing again; and your reward shall be great, and ye shall be the children of the Highest: for he is kind unto the unthankful and to the evil. Be ye therefore merciful, **as your Father also is merciful.**
>
> *Romans 15:5*—Now the God of patience and consolation grant you to be **likeminded** one toward another according to Christ Jesus.
>
> *1 Peter 2:21*—For even hereunto were ye called: because Christ also suffered for us, **leaving us an example**, that ye should follow his steps:
>
> *Colossians 3:12*—Put on therefore, **as the elect of God**, holy and beloved, bowels of mercies, kindness, humbleness of mind, meekness, longsuffering.

Just as parents are given an example of parenting that is unsurpassed in its perfection, so children are given an example as well. Christ exemplifies the flawlessly perfect child just as much as the perfect parent. Jesus was one child who really did know more than His earthly parents—yet He obeyed them. He did not always agree with them, but He was able to say so without disrespect or rebellion. Of course this notion excites us as parents, and we are anxious to point it out to our children. May we be just as anxious to see and note how we are to obey *our* Heavenly Father even as we teach our children to obey us. We must remember that we are to exemplify for our children Christ's childlike obedience as much as His compassionate authority as a father. The following comments and passages of Scripture are provided not only as instruction for parenting principles, but to give parents a better understanding of God's fatherhood to them. The more we know and understand our perfect Heavenly Father, the more we will be able to follow His example in the ways we parent our children.

Use the following points as topics of discussion or to prompt personal Bible study. Add Scripture of your own as well as Biblical examples and illustrations. The more examples you can find, the more you will be able to profitably participate in a group discussion or benefit yourself individually. May I also suggest you further your knowledge of God's attributes and character by reading the section under the heading "God" in *Nave's Topical Bible* and by reading such books as Tozer's *Knowledge of the Holy*, where some of God's most notable attributes are discussed. Teachers and counselors may want to utilize such helps when presenting the material in this chapter of *Parenting With Wisdom*.

God Creates in Us a Desire To Obey

God instills a desire to obey just as He warns not to disobey.

Philippians 2:13—For it is God which worketh in you both to will and to do of his good pleasure.

God uses a reward system to provoke His children to be obedient.

John 14:2a—In my Father's house are many mansions: if it were not so, I would have told you.

Hebrews 11:6— But without faith *it is* impossible to please *him*: for he that cometh to God must believe that he is, and *that* he is a rewarder of them that diligently seek him.

Psalm 58:11b—Verily *there is* a reward for the righteous: verily he is a God that judgeth in the earth.

God motivates by openly commending right actions.

Matthew 6:4b—And thy Father which seeth in secret himself shall reward thee openly.

God's lovingkindness is a means to help us trust in His judgment.

Psalm 36:7—How excellent is thy lovingkindness O God! Therefore the children of men put their trust under the shadow of thy wings.

Jeremiah 31:3b—Yea, I have loved thee with an everlasting love: therefore with lovingkindness have I drawn thee.

Romans 2:4—Or despisest thou the riches of his goodness and forbearance and longsuffering; not knowing that the goodness of God leadeth thee to repentance?

Hosea 2:4—And I will not have mercy upon her children; for they *be* the children of whoredoms.

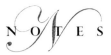

God assures His children of His utmost devotion.

Isaiah 49:15-16—Can a woman forget her sucking child, that she should not have compassion on the son of her womb? Yea, they may forget, yet will I not forget thee. Behold, I have graven thee upon the palms of *my* hands; thy walls *are* continually before me.

God notices the good efforts His children make.

Ephesians 6:8—Knowing that whatsoever good thing any man doeth, the same shall he receive of the Lord, whether he be bond or free.

God is willing to suffer and sacrifice for His children.

Isaiah 63:7-9—I will mention the lovingkindnesses of the LORD, *and* the praises of the LORD, according to all that the LORD hath bestowed on us, and the great goodness toward the house of Israel, which he hath bestowed on them according to his mercies, and according to the multitude of his lovingkindnesses. For he said, Surely they *are* my people, children *that* will not lie: so he was their Saviour. In all their affliction he was afflicted, and the angel of his presence saved them: in his love and in his pity he redeemed them; and he bare them, and carried them all the days of old.

John 10:15—As the Father knoweth me, even so know I the Father: and I lay down my life for the sheep.

God desires and cultivates a close relationship with His children.

Jeremiah 23:23—Am I a God at hand, saith the LORD, and not a God afar off?

2 Corinthians 6:17-18— Wherefore come out from among them, and be ye separate, saith the Lord, and touch not the unclean *thing*; and I will receive you, and will be a Father unto you, and ye shall be my sons and daughters, saith the Lord Almighty.

God both deserves and commands respect because of who He is.

Psalm 89:7—God is greatly to be feared in the assembly of the saints, and to be had in reverence of all them that are about him.

God Listens to and Understands His Children

God is approachable.

Hebrews 4:16—Let us therefore come boldly unto the throne of grace, that we may obtain mercy, and find grace to help in time of need.

Romans 8:15—For ye have not received the spirit of bondage again to fear; but ye have received the Spirit of adoption, whereby we cry, Abba, Father.

God understands His children's individuality and their special needs.

Isaiah 64:8—But now, O LORD, thou art our father; we *are* the clay, and thou our potter; and we all *are* the work of thy hand.

God assures His children of their absolute acceptance and worth, and treats them with respect.

Galatians 4:7—Wherefore thou art no more a servant, but a son; and if a son, then an heir of God through Christ.

1 John 3:1a—Behold, what manner of love the Father hath bestowed upon us, that we should be called the sons of God.

Ephesians 1:6—To the praise of the glory of his grace, wherein he hath made us accepted in the beloved.

God anticipates every approaching need of His children.

Matthew 6:8b—For your Father knoweth what things ye have need of, before ye ask him.

God makes known His desires to give good things to His children.

Matthew 7:11—If ye then, being evil, know how to give good gifts unto your children, how much more shall your Father which is in heaven give good things to them that ask him?

Psalm 84:11b—No good thing will He withhold from them that walk uprightly.

God gives recognition for each of His children's accomplishments.

Hebrews 6:10—For God is not unrighteous to forget your work and labor of love, which ye have shewed toward his name, in that ye have ministered to the saints, and do minister.

When God's children sincerely desire an explanation, God listens; and when it would be in the best interest of His child, He gives explanations.

Jeremiah 12:1—Righteous *art* thou, O LORD, when I plead with thee: yet let me talk with thee of *thy* judgments: Wherefore doth the way of the wicked prosper? Wherefore are all they happy that deal very treacherously?

Psalm 25:4—Show me thy ways, O Lord; teach me thy paths.

God delights to fulfill the good desires of His children.

Psalm 145:16—Thou openest thine hand, and satisfiest the desire of every living thing.

God Trains His Children

God teaches and guides His children.

Psalm 32:8—I will instruct thee and teach thee in the way which thou shalt go: I will guide thee with mine eye.

God's instruction is continual and loving. It is not just something He does before or after correction.

Psalm 139:17—How precious also are thy thoughts unto me, O God! How great is the sum of them!

God instructs with future goals in mind.

1 Thessalonians 3:12-13—And the Lord make you to increase and abound in love one toward another, and toward all *men*, even as we *do* toward you: to the end he may stablish your hearts unblameable in holiness before God, even our Father, at the coming of our Lord Jesus Christ with all his saints.

Deuteronomy 5:29—O that there were such an heart in them, that they would fear me, and keep all my commandments always, that it might be well with them, and with their children for ever!

God uses repetition in His training by His example.

Psalm 78:38-39—But he, *being* full of compassion, forgave *their* iniquity, and destroyed *them* not: yea, many a time turned he his anger away, and did not stir up all his wrath. For he remembered that they *were but* flesh; a wind that passeth away, and cometh not again.

Matthew 18:21-22—Then came Peter to him, and said, Lord, how oft shall my brother sin against me, and I forgive him? Till seven times? Jesus saith unto him, I say not unto thee, until seven times: but, until seventy times seven.

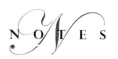

God's expectations are within His children's capabilities when you factor in His grace.

I Corinthians 10:13—There hath no temptation taken you but such as is common to man: but God *is* faithful, who will not suffer you to be tempted above that ye are able; but will with the temptation also make a way to escape, that ye may be able to bear *it*.

God does not make overwhelming demands on His children.

Matthew 11:30—For my yoke is easy, and my burden is light.

God always follows through exactly as He said He would.

Numbers 23:19—God *is* not a man, that he should lie; neither the son of man, that he should repent: hath he said, and shall he not do *it*? Or hath he spoken, and shall he not make it good?

God always keeps His promises.

Joshua 23:14—And, behold, this day I am going the way of all the earth: and ye know in all your hearts and in all your souls, that not one thing hath failed of all the good things which the LORD your God spake concerning you; all are come to pass unto you, and not one thing hath failed thereof.

God never rewards His children with what they want when they try to obtain things sinfully or have a wrong attitude. Their attitude and manner must be adjusted before He grants any request.

1 John 3:22—And whatsoever we ask, we receive of him, because we keep his commandments, and do those things that are pleasing in his sight.

God Exercises Patience in His Discipline

God anticipates failure.

Proverbs 24:16a—For a just man falleth seven times, and riseth up again.

Psalm 37:23-24—The steps of a *good* man are ordered by the LORD: and he delighteth in his way. Though he fall, he shall not be utterly cast down: for the LORD upholdeth *him with* his hand.

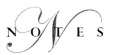

God patiently works toward and waits for maturity.

Isaiah 30:18a—And therefore will the Lord wait, that he may be gracious unto you, and therefore will he be exalted, that he may have mercy upon you.

Philippians 1:6—Being confident of this very thing, that he which hath begun a good work in you will perform it until the day of Jesus Christ.

Philippians 3:12—Not as though I had already attained, either were already perfect: but I follow after, if that I may apprehend that for which also I am apprehended of Christ Jesus.

God recognizes childish weakness and is able to overlook it.

Psalm 103:10—He hath not dealt with us after our sins; nor rewarded us according to our iniquities.

Psalm 103:13-14—Like as a father pitieth *his* children, *so* the LORD pitieth them that fear him. For he knoweth our frame; he remembereth that we *are* dust.

Acts 17:30—And the times of this ignorance God winked at.

God loves and provides for His children though they are immature and sinful.

2 Timothy 2:13,19—If we believe not, *yet* he abideth faithful: he cannot deny himself. Nevertheless the foundation of God standeth sure, having this seal, The Lord knoweth them that are his. And, let every one that nameth the name of Christ depart from iniquity.

Jeremiah 51:5—For Israel *hath* not *been* forsaken, nor Judah of his God, of the LORD of hosts; though their land was filled with sin against the Holy One of Israel.

Nehemiah 9:19-21—Yet thou in thy manifold mercies forsookest them not in the wilderness: the pillar of the cloud departed not from them by day, to lead them in the way; neither the pillar of fire by night, to shew them light, and the way wherein they should go. Thou gavest also thy good spirit to instruct them, and withheldest not thy manna from their mouth, and gavest them water for their thirst. Yea, forty years didst thou sustain them in the wilderness, *so that* they lacked nothing; their clothes waxed not old, and their feet swelled not.

God is longsuffering towards His children.

Colossians 3:12-13—Put on therefore, as the elect of God, holy and beloved, bowels of mercies, kindness, humbleness of mind, meekness, longsuffering; forbearing one another, and forgiving one another, if any man have a quarrel against any: even as Christ forgave you, so also *do* ye.

God never condemns, berates, or uses hateful words on His children though He is grieved by their sinned and must discipline them.

Romans 8:1a—There is therefore now no condemnation to them which are in Christ Jesus.

God encourages His children when they fail. He does not grind them into the ground with continuing lectures.

Psalm 31:7—I will be glad and rejoice in thy mercy: for thou hast considered my trouble.

God Corrects His Children

God's purpose for correction is to change our mind and behavior. Therefore, He withholds correction (not the natural consequences) when we repent.

1 Corinthians 11:31—For if we would judge ourselves, we should not be judged.

God establishes clear limits, behavioral standards, and consequences.

Genesis 2:16-17—And the LORD God commanded the man, saying, Of every tree of the garden thou mayest freely eat: but of the tree of the knowledge of good and evil, thou shalt not eat of it: for in the day that thou eatest thereof thou shalt surely die.

Deuteronomy 11:26-28—Behold, I set before you this day a blessing and a curse; a blessing, if ye obey the commandments of the LORD your God, which I command you this day: and a curse, if ye will not obey the commandments of the LORD your God, but turn aside out of the way which I command you this day, to go after other gods, which ye have not known.

John 14:15—If ye love me, keep my commandments.

Because children have a sin nature, they require correction.

Hebrews 12:5-7—And ye have forgotten the exhortation which speaketh unto you as unto children, My son, despise not thou the chastening of the Lord, nor faint when thou art rebuked of him: for whom the Lord loveth he chasteneth, and scourgeth every son whom he receiveth. If ye endure chastening, God dealeth with you as with sons; for what son is he whom the father chasteneth not?

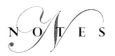

Correction shows God's love and concern for his child.

Proverbs 3:11-12—My son, despise not the chastening of the LORD; neither be weary of his correction: for whom the LORD loveth he correcteth; even as a father the son *in whom* he delighteth.

God's correction is consistent.

2 Peter 3:9—The Lord is not slack concerning his promise, as some men count slackness; but is longsuffering to us-ward, not willing that any should perish, but that all should come to repentance.

God's correction is in proportion to the offense.

2 Samuel 22:25—Therefore the LORD hath recompensed me according to my righteousness; according to my cleanness in his eye sight.

Matthew 12:20a—A bruised reed shall he not break.

1 Samuel 2:3—Talk no more so exceeding proudly; let *not* arrogancy come out of your mouth: for the LORD *is* a God of knowledge, and by him actions are weighed.

God's correction is deliberate and loving, even when He must inflict pain.

Psalm 103:8,10—The LORD *is* merciful and gracious, slow to anger, and plenteous in mercy. He hath not dealt with us after our sins; nor rewarded us according to our iniquities.

God corrects to produce repentance, a genuine change of heart towards the offense. God's discipline is designed to restore.

2 Chronicles 30:9—For if ye turn again unto the LORD, your brethren and your children *shall find* compassion before them that lead them captive, so that they shall come again into this land: for the LORD your God is gracious and merciful, and will not turn away *his* face from you, if ye return unto him.

God corrects willful and deliberate disobedience.

Romans 11:22—Behold therefore the goodness and severity of God: on them which fell, severity; but toward thee, goodness, if thou continue in *his* goodness: otherwise thou also shalt be cut off.

God's correction is for the happiness, well-being, and security of His children.

Psalm 94:12-13—Blessed *is* the man whom thou chastenest, O LORD, and teachest him out of thy law; that thou mayest give him rest from the days of adversity, until the pit be digged for the wicked.

God does not correct to relieve His anger.

Lamentations 3:22-23—It is of the LORD'S mercies that we are not consumed, because his compassions fail not. They are new every morning: great *is* thy faithfulness.

Lamentations 3:32-33—But though he cause grief, yet will he have compassion according to the multitude of his mercies. For he doth not afflict willingly nor grieve the children of men.

Before correction, God establishes responsibility for the offense in an effort to bring about repentance, rather than a defensive response.

Note the way God asks questions of Adam and Eve and Cain in the following verses rather than approaching them with an accusation, even though God knows what they have done.

Genesis 3:9, 11,13a—And the LORD God called unto Adam, and said unto him, Where *art* thou? And he said, Who told thee that thou *wast* naked? Hast thou eaten of the tree, whereof I commanded thee that thou shouldest not eat? And the LORD God said unto the woman, What *is* this *that* thou hast done?

Genesis 4:6-10—And the LORD said unto Cain, Why art thou wroth? And why is thy countenance fallen? If thou doest well, shalt thou not be accepted? And if thou doest not well, sin lieth at the door. And unto thee shall be his desire, and thou shalt rule over him. And Cain talked with Abel his brother: and it came to pass, when they were in the field, that Cain rose up against Abel his brother, and slew him. And the LORD said unto Cain, Where is Abel thy brother? And he said, I know not: Am I my brother's keeper? And he said, What hast thou done? The voice of thy brother's blood crieth unto me from the ground.

God requires restitution after correction. His children are not simply to apologize, but (as much as possible) to make right their wrongs.

Luke 19:8—And Zacchaeus stood, and said unto the Lord, Behold, Lord, the half of my goods I give to the poor; and if I have taken any thing from any man by false accusation, I restore *him* fourfold.

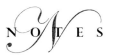

God tempers His correction with mercy and wisely knows when to overlook fault and weakness when the occasion allows it.

Psalm 103:10-14—He hath not dealt with us after our sins; nor rewarded us according to our iniquities. For as the heaven is high above the earth, *so* great is his mercy toward them that fear him. As far as the east is from the west, *so* far hath he removed our transgressions from us. Like as a father pitieth *his* children, *so* the LORD pitieth them that fear him. For he knoweth our frame; he remembereth that we *are* dust.

God loves even His rebellious children. He does not give up on them or shut them out of His life. He is always ready to immediately forgive and restore the most rebellious child the moment he will repent.

Nehemiah 9:17—And refused to obey, neither were mindful of thy wonders that thou didst among them; but hardened their necks, and in their rebellion appointed a captain to return to their bondage: but thou *art* a God ready to pardon, gracious and merciful, slow to anger, and of great kindness, and forsookest them not.

God goes out of His way to restore a wandering, rebellious child.

Luke 15:4-7—What man of you, having an hundred sheep, if he lose one of them, doth not leave the ninety and nine in the wilderness, and go after that which is lost, until he find it? And when he hath found *it*, he layeth *it* on his shoulders, rejoicing. And when he cometh home, he calleth together *his* friends and neighbours, saying unto them, Rejoice with me; for I have found my sheep which was lost. I say unto you, that likewise joy shall be in heaven over one sinner that repenteth, more than over ninety and nine just persons, which need no repentance.

The Discipline Process

The instructions on the following two pages incorporate principles learned in the Scriptures that you have just finished studying. The instructions will naturally feel awkward if you are not already implementing them in your discipline procedure. After you study them, make copies of the pages to post in strategic places where they can be reviewed and learned until the concepts become second nature. Work at keeping your discipline procedure thorough, but as brief as possible. There will be times when it is not necessary or appropriate to engage in a lengthy discipline session and other times when you will need to stop and take a great deal of time to talk through a discipline issue with your child. Generally, small children need brief but frequent discipline and older children require less but more lengthy discipline sessions. Work to make your discipline age appropriate. Note that a good parent-child relationship will make even poor discipline plans work and a poor parent-child relationship will almost always ensure any discipline plan's failure.

Before You Discipline

First, determine the child's motive.

- Have you taken the time to carefully collect information and make certain you know what happened and what the circumstances were at the time of the offense?
- Are you certain the behavior is something the child is able to control? Is the child's age or emotional or physical maturity such that your expectations are reasonable or realistic?
- Is the behavior accidental? Does it represent a childish infraction that will correct itself in time as the child matures?
- Is the child's offense something you are partly responsible for, such as skipping child's nap or neglecting to follow through?
- Is direct disobedience (defiance) or open disrespect involved? Is the behavior something the child has done knowingly and deliberately? (Use a form of discipline other than spanking if this is not the case.)
- Is there possibly an underlying cause to this behavior that you have neglected to see and must correct? Have you considered what might have prompted the behavior other than what is obvious? Have you determined what wrong beliefs or desires might have prompted wrong behavior?

Second, determine your motives for disciplining.

- Are you only reacting out of anger or embarrassment? Is your expectation consistent, no matter what the circumstances, where you are, or whom you are with?
- Is your objective to encourage a change in your child's behavior and aid in the development of his character?
- As much as possible, have you properly defined the limits and consequences beforehand, in anticipation of what your child might be tempted to do wrong?
- Are you able to provide a reasonable and well thought out explanation for your discipline? Are you willing to take the time to teach it?

Third, determine what is needed to correct your child.

- What information does your child need to understand or learn? What cause and effect consequences should he face? What is he capable of learning through this?
- What is needed? Correction? Training and instruction? Motivation?
- If correction is needed, which is appropriate? Spanking? Natural consequences? Restitution? Reconciliation with others? Ignoring? Other?

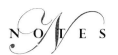

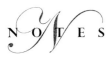

Administering Discipline

1. **Establish** responsibility. Remember, questions produce conviction; condemning accusations produce a defense. Ask the child to tell you in his own words what he did wrong, even if you know exactly what he did wrong. If he's too small to talk, explain in simple words what he did wrong. Avoid asking your child why he did something. "Why" isn't the important issue and tends to only confuse and discourage your child. *What* the child did is important, not why he did what he did. Although there are times when "why?" might be a constructive question in determining what motivated a child to chose the action he did, it is far too often used as an accusation or an expression of incredulous dismay or anger at what the child did. Asking why when it is quite obvious the child simply *wanted* to do what he did because he had a sinful inclination to do so is not constructive. For instance, upon finding one's three-year-old child dipping toilet paper into the toilet and spreading them around the bathroom, a typical response from an exhausted mother cleaning child's messes all day long might be, "Why did you do this? Look what you have done! You've made another mess for mommy!" A better approach is to control one's exasperated tendency, take a deep breath, and ask, "What are you doing?" or "What did you do in the bathroom?" followed by questions designed to cause the child to realize he is having lots of fun, but having fun in an inappropriate way. After asking "what," the three year old will typically respond by telling you exactly what they have done; whereas, he would likely shrug his shoulders and say "I don't know" if mother had asked, "Why?" Changing the emphasis from "why" to "what" much more effectively facilitates the strategy of establishing responsibility and correcting behavior rather than simply punishing wrong behavior or reacting to wrong behavior in a way that does nothing toward bringing about a change of mind in the child.

In cases involving older children the principle still holds true, although in some cases "why" might more often be a legitimate question *after* one has asked "what" when determining details of the incident. For instance, suppose a teenage son hands his dad a speeding ticket he has received. The dad looks at the ticket, and in exasperation demands to know why his son was speeding. The teen will tend to shrug and mumble, "I don't know." Dad isn't establishing responsibility by approaching it in this manner. Better if he begins by asking, "What did you do?" (I was speeding.) "What is the speed limit in this area?" (45 MPH) "It would appear that you chose to go 65 MPH when you knew the speed limit was 45 MPH, is this correct?" (Yes) "Do you have any idea why the posted speed limit is 45 MPH is this area?" (No) "Let's see if we can come up with a few reasons. Did you notice any houses on the street?" (Yeah) "Who lives in the houses…How long do you believe it takes to stop the car when it is going 65 MPH…could you stop in time if a child ran into the street…a car backed out of the driveway…what would happen if you hit a child going this speed?" The idea is to ask questions that will prompt the teen to rethink his decision to speed, and then consider

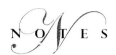

the consequences had an accident occurred as well as the consequences for disregarding the speed limit and being stopped by an officer, thus establishing responsibility. From there, the parent simply provides instruction with regard to how the teen will pay for his ticket, what sins the teen privately needs to ask God to forgive him for, and what the breach in parental trust will cost him with regard to using the family car in the near future. Notice the Dad did ask a why question, but it was in the context of getting details only after the Dad asked the question "What" in order to compel the child to verbalize his specific offense. Had the Dad followed the "Why would you do such a thing?" route in an attempt to determine unimportant details of the incident, the conversation would have taken a completely different course, most likely ending with a completely different, and less productive, result.

If a specific household rule has been broken, ask your child to tell you specifically what rule he has *chosen* to disobey. Ask your child if he knows what element of his behavior was sinful. (Example: If the offense is talking in church, the child needs to understand that talking is not what is sinful. Talking in disregard of others is selfish and therefore sinful. Or, if the offense is breaking a window, the broken window isn't the issue since accidents resulting in damage are a part of life. The issue is how the window broke—such as disobediently throwing a ball in the house after being told to take it outside.) This is an important aspect of discipline if your objective is to address heart issues rather than outward behavior alone. Children tend to follow the letter of the law rather than its intention in much the same way the Pharisees attempted to find ways around God's laws by ignoring the fact that sin originates in the heart, not in the action that comes from the heart. Always address the origin of the offense, not just the offense itself.

2. **Ask** your child what you said would happen if he did this.

3. **Clarify** what your child did wrong and what right thing you want him to do instead. (See put off and put on principle explained in chapter twelve.)

4. **Carry out** discipline and/or give instructions exactly how he is to make right his wrong. This might include such things as making arrangements for restitution if he broke something or asking forgiveness if he has wronged someone, closing the door properly if he slammed it, or asking a question respectfully if he had been rude or inappropriate. Always insist your child do what is right regardless whether he feels like it or not. Ask the child if he will obey or ask the child if he is willing to do the right thing. If he says no, additional instruction and/or discipline is necessary.

5. **Reaffirm** complete forgiveness, love, and fellowship as soon as the matter is closed. Pray with him when this is appropriate, and allow him to pray if he desires. Never force him to pray or seek God's forgiveness. Provide careful instruction, but encourage him to talk with God and seek His forgiveness on his own, in private. As much as possible and as soon as possible, you should encourage your child to respond to God willfully and spontaneously.

Reasons You May Be Screaming at Your Children

- It has become a habit for you to react to irritating situations rather than to act.
- You've become frustrated or fearful with your inability to control your children.
- You are not disciplining your child consistently or Biblically.
- Your tolerance level is too low and your action level too high. This happens when you tolerate problems that should have been taken care of immediately. Finally you can't take it any more and thus react by blowing up.
- Your expectations for your child are unrealistic.

What You Can Do To Stop Screaming

1. *Separate your personal problems and disappointments from your children.* Perhaps you are emotionally low because of your monthly cycle, tired, or experiencing personal problems unrelated to your children. These are times when it will be crucial to exercise more self-control, not excuse the lack of it because the situation you face is difficult. Remember that the consequences are serious when you habitually vent your anger on your children. Every parent becomes angry and frustrated with children at times, but not every parent reacts to that anger in a sinful and destructive way. Those who keep themselves under control have made self-control, rather than screaming, a habit. Remember that temperance, or self-control, is listed as part of the fruit of God's Spirit and is the by-product of our daily relationship with Christ.

2. *Establish respect and parental control with your children.* Be willing to take on the many battles required to maintain respect and control. Don't allow your child to ignore your commands. Doing so only teaches him not to take your instructions seriously and increases disobedience. Reduce your commands to those you are willing to enforce. Develop consistency in the way you discipline your children, knowing that children develop habits of behaving appropriately just as they do habits of behaving inappropriately.

3. *Take the time to establish guidelines and carry out the consequences.* Threats and screaming may temporarily stop behavior, but it absolutely does not change behavior. Anger never has and never will work the righteousness of God or transform a rebellious heart into one that willingly obeys. Right action is what is needed, not wordy reaction. After clearly defining both the boundaries and the consequences, carry out the consequences without arguing or procrastination. Give no second and third chances. Be both calm and deliberate. If you will continue to methodically act instead of scream, you will find you have less to scream about.

4. ***Check your expectations.*** Preceding almost every outburst of anger is the thought, "But he should have…" or "He shouldn't have…" We all have things we should or should not do, but we all occasionally fail. Be certain your expectations are reasonable and based on an accurate understanding of children. Anticipate and accept the problems you will inevitably have to work through with your children. Remember that the way you think before you experience angry frustration with your child will ultimately determine how you will respond to him. Practice godly love and forgiveness.

Conflicts Aren't All Bad

Confrontations conducted with an attitude of humility and love is a necessary and constructive part of learning to get along together and learning how to appropriately communicate with one another. It is important that your children have opportunities to observe a godly and controlled way of disagreeing and resolving conflicts because children ultimately do whatever they see, either good or bad.

To some extent, it is constructive and profitable for children to see Mom and Dad disagree and resolve conflicts Biblically and lovingly. It is NOT constructive to openly discuss matters that children are not yet emotionally able to handle or understand, or are not appropriate matters to share. It is also NOT constructive and profitable for children to observe Mom and Dad behaving in a disrespectful, petty, selfish, or uncontrolled manner. When this occurs, be sure the children also observe Mom and Dad acknowledging their behavior as sinful and seeking one another's forgiveness. Children are greatly blessed when parents display humility in this way, and they will imitate it in their future relationships and marriage.

Remember that your goal is to encourage your children to solve their own conflicts and disagreements without your intervention as much as possible. Therefore, it is preferable to try to supervise more than intervene as they grow older. However, any failure to abide by predetermined "ground rules" must be acknowledged and forgiven.

Learning how to disagree properly helps children learn how to live, for conflict resolution is a skill that will benefit them in every area of their future life. Take the time to learn and teach it. Your family life will be happier for it!

The following are helpful books that will provide added help and instruction in dealing with family conflicts:

The Heart of Anger – Lou Priolo

Family Guide to Peacemaking – Ken Sande

Why Am I So Angry – Debi Pryde

Lesson 8

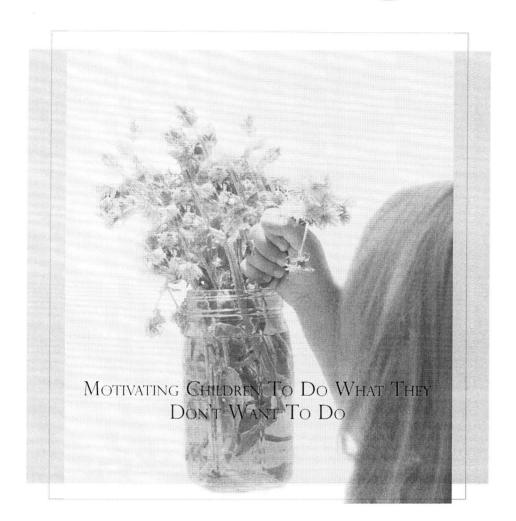

Motivating Children To Do What They Don't Want To Do

Behold, I set before you this day a blessing and a curse; a blessing, if ye obey the commandments of the LORD your God, which I command you this day: and a curse, if ye will not obey the commandments of the LORD your God.

Deuteronomy 11.26-28a

The LORD hath appeared of old unto me, saying, Yea, I have loved thee with an everlasting love: therefore with lovingkindness have I drawn thee.

Jeremiah 31:3

Key THOUGHTS

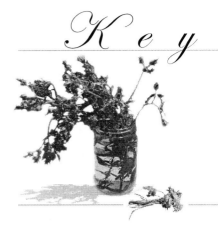

Children are motivated when they are given the tools they need to achieve. These tools include such things as encouragement, acceptance, teamwork, and help. They will be motivated to the degree that they

1. Desire the benefits of responsible choices.
2. Fear the consequences of foolish choices.
3. Desire to please God with their choices out of love for Him.

Discussion Problem

Johnny is ten years old and is an average to below average student. He hates homework and does not enjoy school. Reading is especially hard for him. Therefore, he is embarrassed when it's his turn to read out loud in class. He is also beginning to have difficulty with math.

Johnny's teacher has a large class and doesn't spend much time with children who have difficulties. Besides, she believes Johnny is a discipline problem; and she doesn't want to invest time in him. Recently she sent a note home expressing her frustration to Johnny's parents. She reported that Johnny was not cooperating in class. She had to scold him frequently. In addition, he is also failing to bring homework back to class.

When Johnny's mom and dad read the note, they hotly lectured Johnny and threatened to ground him for the rest of the school year if he doesn't do his homework or gets into trouble just one more time. The next day, Johnny's mother refused to let him play after school until he got his homework done. As usual, he dawdled and fidgeted while his mother continually barked at him and threatened him to get it done. By dinnertime, everyone was thoroughly upset and exhausted; and the homework was not finished.

After reading lesson eight, use the principles you learn to discuss the problem Johnny's parents and teacher have with Johnny. What could be the root of Johnny's outward behavior problem? What do you think of Johnny's teacher's attitude? Have Johnny's parents handled the situation wisely? Do you believe they have disciplined him properly and reasonably? How could Johnny's parents be contributing to Johnny's frustration and lack of motivation? What could his mother do differently?

Bible Study

1. In Proverbs 8:32-33 Solomon gives a motivation (blessed/happiness), to children along with a command to _____.

2. Proverbs 23:26 tells us that Solomon invites his children to _____ his _____ as a help in teaching them how to live.

3. From 1 Kings 2:1-3 we learn that David gave instructions to Solomon to be _____ and keep _____ and _____ so that he might _____ (a motivation).

4. According to 1 Chronicles 22:11-13, David planted the idea of needing _____ in his son's mind before Solomon asked God for wisdom and an understanding heart when he became king.

> *"We should seize every opportunity to give encouragement.*
> *Encouragement is oxygen to the soul."*
> George Adams

Motivation in the Real World

Wouldn't it be heavenly if children made their bed every morning, just because they loved to do it? Or washed dishes because the dishes needed to be washed? Or did their homework because they loved acting responsibly? These things may happen in a mother's dreams; but in the real world, children don't make their bed if they don't have to. They don't fight for the privilege of washing dishes. Nor do they do their homework because they're striving to learn responsibility.

The truth is that children do not naturally do unpleasant tasks on their own. They need inspiration and motivation of some kind in order to develop a desire to obey and achieve when obeying and achieving are not exciting or fun. If parents completely entrust a small child to feed the family pet without any oversight, the poor animal will likely starve to death. Leave the task of cleaning the refrigerator to a junior high son without ever enforcing compliance or uttering a commendation and within a few short months, you will likely have all kinds of fuzzy green things growing inside. A child does not naturally start out self-disciplined. Rather, he learns the art of self-discipline gradually over a period of time.

The younger the child, the more he will require direct supervision, inspiration, and restrictive discipline in order to motivate him to behave responsibly and productively. Habits that a young child is forced to develop in childhood become integrated into his personality as a natural spontaneous response only as he matures. Children tend to become self-disciplined to the degree parents are self-disciplined enough to enforce a disciplined life upon their children while they are young and can withdraw their control as they grow older.

A parent's goal is to prepare his child to live responsibly, as God defines *responsible*, without the necessity of parental force or enticements. Yet this can only occur if parents teach their children how to make wise decisions and prepare their children in such a way that they are able to gradually transfer parental control and decision making to the child. Children tend to be motivated toward self-discipline as they are given corresponding privileges; and when they realize to the degree they are able to govern and motivate themselves, they do not need a parent to do so for them. The adolescent's natural desire for autonomy as they grow older propels them toward assuming increased personal responsibility when parents are willing to relinquish control appropriately as the child demonstrates competence.

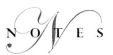

Children require this process of maturity before they will consistently do what is right simply because it is right, or work for rewards when they are delayed, or govern their own life without outside restriction imposed on them. In fact, children do not typically emerge from childhood into adulthood perfectly self-disciplined or motivated by spiritually mature passions. Usually this growing process continues throughout their young adult lives well into their mature adult years as God uses means other than parents to discipline and motivate a person who is grown.

The parent who believes he must sternly control and govern every move his child makes throughout his entire childhood fails to understand the importance of working to develop the child's desire and ability to govern and motivate himself. Instead of producing a grown child who is able to make good choices and handle adult freedom, he produces a child who is crippled in his ability to live a disciplined life without constant outside stimulation or restriction to motivate him. These children often rebel against the restraints of childhood as they grow older and naturally desire more freedom. On the other hand, passive children may simply remain overly dependent on others to motivate them or make decisions for them while others suffer bouts of lethargy and depression as a result of their undisciplined and unmotivated life.

Abraham Lincoln once stated that a democracy could not long survive if its citizens were not able to govern their own lives responsibly. Likewise, a family will not enjoy any amount of harmony or peace if its individual members do not develop the desire and ability to govern their own lives in a way that pleases God, simply because they want to, not because they have to.

The work of motivating and inspiring children to obey and achieve involves three basic areas of his thinking.

1. The child's desire to acquire the benefits of achievement and obedience—what he believes those benefits are and what he must do to obtain them.

2. The child's fear and dislike of the consequences of disobedience and lack of achievement—what he believes those consequences are and what he must do to avoid discomfort.

3. The child's heart attitude towards God and his desire to do right or wrong—what he believes about God's character, promises, personal involvement in his life and the manner in which he is held responsible for his belief and willful unbelief.

Desire for Benefits

Children are motivated as they realize that obedience and achievement have pleasant rewards that are possible for them to attain. Perhaps you will recall the story of a farmer who could not force his mule to go forward, no matter how hard he beat him with a stick. He pleaded, poked, pulled, and prodded; but the mule stubbornly refused to yield to the will of the farmer. Eventually, the farmer thought of an idea. He grabbed his fishing pole from the barn and attached a carrot to the pole so it dangled from the end. Then he got back on his mule and held the fishing pole out in front of the mule, tantalizing him to walk forward in an effort to grab the carrot. While the mule stretched his neck to bite the carrot in front of him, the farmer gently whacked him from behind with the stick. At last the mule was sufficiently motivated to move and continue moving so long as the carrot was dangled in front of him and the stick was applied, when necessary.

Notice that the farmer didn't dangle a fish, an old boot, or a piece of cheese to entice the mule. He deliberately chose a carrot because he knew the mule loved carrots. Good parents recognize the benefit of using desirable "carrots" in the work of motivating children, particularly while they are young. For instance, a toddler will not be induced to babble by the prospect of a straight "A" toddler report card for good behavior and exceptional effort. He *will* be highly incited to please his parents with coos and giggles if they respond with exuberant smiles and enthusiastic clapping. Try this same maneuver with a teenager, however, and he would sooner cringe with embarrassment than be encouraged to pursue good grades.

Given a choice, a four-year-old will typically choose a new bicycle over a check for $1,000. Wait ten years, and he'll gleefully go for the check. Try again when he's an old man anticipating the realities of heaven and he'll likely find enjoyment giving the check to a worthy cause rather than accepting it for himself. Age and spiritual maturity drastically change our childish perceptions and motives. Paul acknowledged this transformation in his comparison of human maturity with spiritual maturity. He said, "When I was a child, I spake as a child, I understood as a child, I thought as a child; but when I became a man, I put away childish things" *(1 Corinthians 13:11)*. Paul reminds us that we do not have the understanding or mental capacities of spiritually mature adults when we are children. As children, we are delighted and motivated by childish things. Only as we grow in wisdom, understanding, age, and maturity do we lose the motivations of childhood and become motivated by things that have eternal significance.

Many parents, in their efforts to instill mature, intrinsic motives in their children reject the idea of using anything but the most spiritually mature motivations to encourage their children. Such children are often made to feel guilty if they work harder to win something such as a promised outing with a friend than to simply win the approval of God. Yet these same children are limited in their understanding and have not grown spiritually enough to value the abstract promise of God's approval with the same enthusiasm as the immediate and tangible reward of an outing. These well-meaning parents need to realize that children see through the lens of childhood and only broaden their vision as they mature. We must patiently teach children about spiritual rewards and motivations, but at the same time, we must recognize the practical value of utilizing good things to make obedience and achievement enjoyable, attainable, and desirable. As they grow, they will gradually begin to recognize the value of spiritual things and will gladly put aside childish motivations for that which is better.

Properly applied, motivational carrots can be an invaluable aid to motivation and training. It is far better to motivate a child to obey, and even *help* him obey, than to attempt to force a child to obey against his will or ability if it is not necessary to do so. Of course, it is important to discipline a child when he refuses to obey. However, refusals to obey are fewer when a child is encouraged to comply with a parent's wishes through the use of kindness, loving encouragement, and a fun-loving sense of humor. The two-year-old having a hard time sitting still in the airport lobby will benefit if a sensitive parent leads him by the hand to a window and engages him by pointing out planes. Barking out a harsh command and ordering him to sit still or be spanked isn't likely to elicit desirable behavior.

If children willfully and defiantly disobey, it is most appropriate to apply promised consequences. However, parents too often use spankings and harsh consequences as a first line of defense rather than attempting to encourage willful obedience *first*. Children who are engaged in singing fun songs on a long car ride aren't as likely to fuss with a sibling or whine in their car seats from sheer boredom. Isn't singing until you're hoarse better than keeping things subdued with threats you will stop the car if they don't behave? It is easier to get children to pick up toys when you make a game out of it rather than threatening dire consequences if they don't clean. And why not spend some time admiring the clean room with your child so he more fully enjoys the internal pleasure of accomplishment and orderliness. Today he may only clean the room because he can't go out to play until he does, but with the right kind of encouragement, tomorrow he may clean it for the simple pleasure of accomplishment.

So you want your teenager to bring his friends home with him more often? Instead of lecturing him or presuming he has some kind of rebellious motive, try making your home a pleasant place for teens to hang out. Young people love to congregate at homes where they are made to feel welcome, where adults are happy to share some pizza and equip their yard with a basketball net or other such "toys" that teens find irresistible. You say your teen doesn't appreciate the work you do to keep his clothes washed, cleaned and ironed? Why not gradually assign his laundry as his responsibility? Start with making the youngest children put away folded clothes. When this is an established routine and the child is capable, teach him how to separate his clothes appropriately, and then get him washing and drying his own clothes and ironing his own clothes by high school. Once it is a well-established routine for your children to do their own laundry, they will greatly appreciate it if you help them out now and then by ironing an item when they are pressed for time. You have just made something that was once expected a "carrot" that is now greatly appreciated. Giving your children everything they want and catering to their every whim are good ways to demotivate them, not motivate them. Rather than becoming more thankful, indulged children become more demanding.

The use of warnings and spankings may ultimately be necessary, but they are required far less when parents begin by approaching their children with understanding and kindness. Parents who are reasonable in their requests and pleasant in their

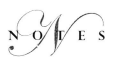

manner of motivating children enjoy far more cooperation and enthusiasm than parents who attempt to force obedience without any effort on their part to make obedience as reasonable and pleasant as possible. Forcing children to obey endless, petty commands simply because you want to establish your authority causes them to regard you with contempt rather than respect. It is immensely better to keep restraints as invisible as possible, commands as few as possible, and discipline as pleasant as possible.

Put yourself in your child's place and remember what delighted and motivated you as a child their age. Chances are you still remember the names of adults who entreated you with kindness and made it easy for you to do the right things. Which teachers did you outdo yourself for? The ones who pointed out every mistake and failure while ignoring what you did right, or the ones who found the things you did correctly and overlooked the petty things you did wrong? How would you react if your child's teacher sent a note home to report the kind things your child was caught doing, rather than a rule that was violated? More importantly, how would such a gesture encourage and motivate your child to practice kindness more often? If you are not commending your child at least twice as much as you are correcting, you are commending too little and correcting too much.

Remember that God Himself draws us to obey with loving kindness and is not the least bit hesitant to describe the rewards and benefits of loving and obeying Him. God comforted Jeremiah by saying, "Yea, I have loved thee with an everlasting love; therefore with lovingkindness have I drawn thee" *(Jeremiah 31:3)*. In *Romans 2:4* we are told that the goodness of God leads us to repentance. In *Psalm 68:19* we are reminded that the Lord "daily loadeth us with benefits." Solomon, in *Ecclesiastes 3:13*, acknowledges that our ability to enjoy the good of all our labor is the gift of God. Paul cannot adequately convey the greatness of God's rewards for those who love Him and simply says, "Eye hath not seen, nor ear heard, neither have entered into the heart of man the things which God hath prepared for them that love him" *(1 Corinthians 2:9)*. Over and over throughout the Scriptures God motivates and encourages His children with immediate and future rewards. God's carrots are exactly what our hearts long for, and unlike the farmer who dangled a carrot in front of his mule, God offers carrots that are attainable as well as desirable.

> *If you are not commending your child at least twice as much as you are correcting, you are commending too little and correcting too much.*

Fear of Consequences

In the story of the farmer and the mule, he not only used the reward of a carrot, but also wisely applied the stick of painful consequence when necessary. A young child will not be sufficiently motivated for long by the promise of a reward or the enjoyments of completing a task. If learning, obeying, or working isn't immediately gratifying, an individual requires a healthy fear of the consequences that will befall him if he does not apply himself to these unpleasant tasks.

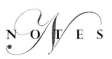

In the real world, rewards are rarely immediate. Therefore, adults must learn to work for delayed benefits in both long-term and short-term endeavors. Mature individuals work for the pleasure of future achievement, a paycheck on Friday, retirement at age sixty-five, and the acquisition of pleasurable items as his funds are gradually increased. The Christian tithes, knowing his investment is being stored in heaven. He gives to missionaries, knowing the harvest of souls is ongoing. Hard work brings a sense of satisfaction and peacefulness at the end of each day, but rarely at the beginning. Acquiring the discipline necessary to get started requires the hope of future enjoyment and the fear of future consequence.

A man works not only because working has great benefits, but also because failing to do so has many unpleasant consequences. If he does not work, he cannot make a house payment and thus will lose his home. He cannot afford to buy clothing, enjoy recreation that costs money, or indulge in a dinner out. He will soon face the grievous oppression of bill collectors. His car will be repossessed, and he will become dependent on others to get him around. Not working is *not* a pleasant choice to make. Both the rewards of working and the fear of the consequences of not working motivate one to work. The process of teaching children to be self-disciplined must include both the carrot (reward) and the stick (fear of consequences or chastisement).

If a five-year-old comes to kindergarten having learned no fear of consequences, he will often be extremely difficult to motivate. His teacher may try enticing, pleading, and threatening him; but he will not apply himself to learn. Why? Because learning is not always fun. Sometimes learning is hard, unpleasant work, which is not immediately rewarding. The child with *no fear* will not be able to sustain any degree of discomfort, but he will develop the tendency to demand only pleasant and instantly gratifying activities. A child will not naturally choose to do right because later it will be good for him. He must be taught and disciplined in order to believe some things are worth avoiding and other things worth waiting and working for.

Children gradually learn delayed gratification as they are given opportunities to exercise patience and wait for something desired, as well as given opportunities for more quickly attainable rewards. If, during the wait your child loses interest, you have likely exceeded his ability to sustain motivation for a delayed reward. Try gradually lengthening time until the gratification is given, while at the same time discussing the less tangible but equally enjoyable benefits of working and waiting. Point out that God made us in such a way that we are happy when we work, etc. When children earn money by working, teach them how to save for short term as well as long-term items, and how to set aside a tithe. Then give them freedom to use the rest as they wish. Allow children to experience the disappointments of wanting instant gratification so they will develop the desire to save for something bigger, etc. Teaching your child to play games where he is required to wait his turn, concentrate, or sustain effort helps him acquire the ability to patiently wait for the rewards of his labor. But do not spare him the discomfort of quitting too soon or the consequences of being unwilling to wait. The discomfort teaches him just as much as the reward.

Children tend to pitch a fit every time an adult says, "no," unless they have been taught to deny their impulsive desires because they fear the chastisement of mom and dad. Children are not likely to deny themselves unless they see an advantage in it. A child's immature mind cannot possibly understand the long-range consequences of self-willed behavior or the long-range rewards of responsible behavior. Because of this limited understanding, he stages a war of wills when asked to do something he does not like. Mom and dad need to win a decisive victory and enforce nonnegotiable obedience.

Teaching a child a healthy fear of the rod of correction provides a short-term, understandable motivation to avoid wrong behavior and submit to good behavior. In junior high, I did not go to school because I enjoyed it or thought going was a good idea. I hated going to school during that time in my life and did not enjoy studying. When classmates encouraged me to skip classes with them, I didn't say no because I believed ditching was unwise or because I had developed a healthy fear of God. I refrained from skipping classes because I knew if my dad found out, I would be disciplined.

As an adult, I see the benefits of school and the foolishness of skipping classes. I have acquired a mature motivation for studying. Yet in childhood, I could not possibly understand the long-term consequences of such foolish choices. If my parents had chosen to simply allow me to suffer the natural consequences of my choice, it would have been disastrous. I did, however, understand the short- term painful consequences my dad would deliver if I indulged my self-will. Consequently, I refrained from skipping school. At the same time, mercy played a part in my developing conscience and sense of responsibility when my mother expressed understanding with the difficulty I was having and sat down to help me each day with my assignments. I still remember the essays she helped me write, and how we laughed as we thought of funny new lines to add. Both the loving encouragement and the proper fear kept me on the right course when my natural inclination would have been to rebel and yield to temptation.

A little child who has *not* been taught to fear immediate consequences or chastisement will be unteachable and unmoldable. Because he is immature, he will not understand the long-term consequences of his self-will. Therefore, any attempt to motivate him with warnings or scare-stories will prove ineffective. In fact, threatening will probably alienate him further and make matters worse. Most likely he could care less about earning a college scholarship years down the road. He also doesn't care if he doesn't have enough money later to buy the bike his Dad is encouraging him to save for. He wants something now because his childhood shortsightedness is only geared for instant gratification at this stage of his development.

Unless a child learns when he is young that unpleasant consequences always swiftly follow foolish behavior, he will tend to grow up believing that the world (Mom and

Dad included) owes him a living. He will tend to believe it is *unfair* for his parents to demand he work to pay his debts and one day he will likely become an adult who is labeled *unmotivated*. As baby Christians, we learn to fear the consequences and chastisement that follow our foolish, rebellious choices. Repenting and making restitution with those we have wronged is not pleasant, but is necessary if we are to learn to control our words and actions. Likewise, when a child breaks a window, deliberate or otherwise, he must assume responsibility and be made to pay for the window to the degree he is able. When a teen gets a ticket for speeding or failing to stop at a stop sign, he must be taught to accept responsibility and pay for his own ticket whether he was violating a traffic law deliberating or accidentally. When children lie and cheat, they must be made to ask forgiveness from the one they wronged, including their teacher. If a child steals, he must return the item and/or pay for it as well as ask forgiveness. He will also need to accept whatever chastisement the judicial system imposes. To keep from overwhelming him, you might need to provide him with work to enable him to pay his debt or encourage him rather than lecture him. But shielding your child from experiencing hardship and consequences will only cripple him emotionally and teach him that he cannot cope with life and should not have to suffer consequences or hardship of any kind.

A child's age and level of maturity must be taken into consideration so the consequence does not overwhelm the child or cause despair, but the consequence should not be taken completely away from him. For instance, if your small child is required to go to someone to make a wrong right, it might be helpful for you to go with him and provide encouragement. Or if your child is having difficulty in math, you wouldn't want to take away all playtime since exercise is needful for his physical and emotional well-being. However, using a portion of time he might be playing to take him to a tutoring service so he can succeed in math would be a good way to mitigate the consequence with encouragement. It is a grave mistake to protect a child from feeling the consequences of his foolishness, choosing to lecture him instead. Better to forego the lecture and let him feel the pain of his error. Sparing him from pain and freeing him from current consequences only sets him up for failure and devastating pain in the future.

If we are God's children, we *will* be disciplined and chastised when we rebel. According to *Hebrews 12:5-15*, this chastisement is not punitive but beneficial to the future of God's child. At the moment, it may be grievous to both Father and child; but in the future, it produces behavior that results in great joy and many benefits. We, like our children, initially avoid sin and do what is right because we fear the consequences of disobeying. But as our Heavenly Father encourages us and we mature in our understanding of His loving character and wise management of our lives, we begin to avoid sin because we love Him and want to please Him with our whole heart. *Proverbs 16:6b* tells us that, "By the fear of the LORD men depart from evil." Just as we fear the consequences of putting our hand in a fire, we should also fear the consequences of sin. Only then do we learn to depart from evil for more mature reasons. When our spiritual understanding is developed, we avoid sin not only because we fear it, but also because we love righteousness and love pleasing God. Until then, much patience and encouragement need to be coupled with chastisement.

Key to a Child's Desire To Do Right or Wrong

We are able to train animals to behave in predictable ways by repetitiously reinforcing correct behavior with a reward and wrong behavior with an unpleasant response. If we could do the same with children, parenting would be immensely easier. But because children are created human beings who have been given a nonmaterial dimension that the Bible refers to as "the heart," they are far more complex and difficult to train than a household pet. An animal utilizes its brain but does not have the capacity to discern or perceive spiritual things, engage a moral conscience or exercise deliberate volition that is governed by weighing personal desire and belief. The God-given nonmaterial heart of man is more than just the mechanism with which we think and reason. It is the very essence of our character and being, the meeting place of God's Spirit with man's spirit, and the laboratory in which desire and belief are weighed and acted upon. Sometimes, no matter how much children are *conditioned* to act in a certain manner, they do not cooperate because they simply do not *want* to cooperate. The heart is able to derail what the mind has been conditioned to do.

Many a parent has been perplexed when the threat of certain unpleasant consequences and the promise of certain desirable rewards do not produce compliance or a change of attitude or character. Even the most ungodly can be trained to act in culturally acceptable or moral ways while the heart remains wicked and unchanged. People routinely obey laws for fear of punishment or love of personal benefit, making civil order in an ungodly society possible. While civil order may be the goal of society as a whole, it is not the goal of Christian parenting. We want more than compliance. We want a transformation of the *heart*, which is the real command center of every human being.

When the heart is changed in such a way that its motivations, desires, and beliefs are willingly conformed to those that are in harmony with God, punishment and reward become nonessential. The focus *automatically* moves from pleasing self toward pleasing God, making the fear of personal discomfort or the benefit of personal gain a side issue rather than a driving force. It is impossible for a human being to do what is right for purely righteous reasons until he is first given new life in Christ. Until he believes the gospel and receives the gift of salvation, he is dead spiritually and cannot begin to respond to God by faith any more than a dead person can respond to the living. "But without faith it is impossible to please him; for he that cometh to God must believe that he is, and that he is a rewarder of them that diligently seek him" *(Hebrews 11:6).*

What one believes regarding the gospel opens the door of salvation and makes the heart a habitable place for the Holy Spirit of God to dwell. Once the Lord Jesus has taken up residence, the ongoing work of reorienting desires and beliefs begins—to the end that the newborn child of God is conformed to be like Christ. The Bible reminds us "even a child is known by his doings, whether his work *be* pure, and whether *it be* right" (Proverbs 20:11). A little child has the capacity to believe and receive Christ as his Savior from sin. He has a will and heart of his own, just as every adult. He is not a blank slate, an empty computer program, or a pet, which merely needs to be conditioned to respond. Children are unique individuals who have the capacity to believe and to *choose* to do right or wrong, to be transformed by the work of God, to grow in their ability to think and reason, to understand the Scriptures and respond to them.

When the heart is changed in such a way that its motivations, desires, and beliefs are willingly conformed to those that are in harmony with God, punishment and reward become nonessential.

The Bible refers to man's heart over six hundred times, making a clear distinction between man's heart and man's mind or capacity to think. So important is the heart to behavior that God commands us to *keep* our heart, or prepare our heart, for out of it are the issues, or decisions of life *(Proverbs 4:23)*. The Bible explains that all actions and words originate in our heart, for our heart is the place where we weigh information, decisions, thoughts, and desires before we act on them. Our emotional responses also originate in our heart and are produced in response to what we perceive and how we perceive it in relation to our beliefs and desires. What we are in the quiet recesses of our heart is what we really are. Therefore, our primary goal is not to make our children *act* good, but to inspire our children to believe and respond to God's truth so that His power will transform them to *be* good. Rather than teaching our little ones to pray, asking God to help them try harder to be good, we ought to teach them to pray, asking God to grant them the desire and ability to believe and obey His Word so it can change their hearts and make them good.

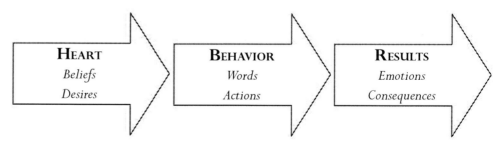

When we deal with the problem of motivating our children, we must deal with far more than rewards and consequences. We must reach the heart of our child as well as his mind. A child's brain can be conditioned, but his heart must be touched by the love and truth of God. The vehicle through which a parent is able to communicate God's truth and spark a child's desire to obey is the vehicle of love. All that a parent does to train, motivate, and discipline his child is to be clothed in the kind of sacrificial love that has its basis in a parent's right relationship to Christ. The Bible teaches us that such love is the very attribute of God's nature that draws us to Christ and causes us to love and respect Him as well as to repent of our sins. "Herein is love, not that we loved God, but that he loved us, and sent his Son to be the propitiation for our sins…We love him, because he first loved us" *(1 John 4:10,19)*.

We know and believe the love that God has toward us only as we hear it through His Word and grow in our knowledge and understanding of Him. Both children and adults are partakers of Christ's divine nature through the knowledge of Christ and through the exceeding great and precious promises He has given to us in His Word *(2 Peter 1:2-4)*. Your child's heart will never be transformed apart from the Word of God and the Spirit of God. Therefore, these ought to be the treasures most valued in your home and that which gives you prime delight.

Children need people who care enough to invest time and effort to love and understand them and to teach and demonstrate the love God has toward them. These are the people who touch them dearly and spark the fires of godly change. Because the human heart longs for genuine love, it gravitates toward anything that promises loving acceptance; and it responds to anything it interprets as love. The greatest motivation known to man is love. It is no wonder, then, that God places such importance on loving one another; and in particular, that mothers and fathers learn to sacrificially love their children as Christ loves His.

Things That Motivate Children To Obey and Achieve

Use the acrostic E-A-T to remember that children are motivated by encouragement, acceptance, and the knowledge they a part of the family "team."

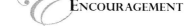

ENCOURAGEMENT   **A**CCEPTANCE   **T**EAMWORK

Encouragement

Romans 15:2-3—Let every one of us please *his* neighbour for *his* good to edification. For even Christ pleased not himself; but, as it is written, The reproaches of them that reproached thee fell on me.

Galatians 6:10—As we have therefore opportunity, let us do good unto all *men*, especially unto them who are of the household of faith.

Proverbs 15:23—A man hath joy by the answer of his mouth: and a word *spoken* in due season, how good *is it*!

Children are encouraged when . . .

- Parents patiently guide them through their fears and insecurities.
- Parents express approval regularly.
- Parents point out the good instead of always noticing bad or imperfect actions.

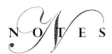

- Parents notice the little improvements and fan the sparks with expressions of enthusiasm and joy.
- They know God desires them to be happy and secure.

Acceptance

2 Corinthians 10:8—For though I should boast somewhat more of our authority, which the Lord hath given us for edification, and not for your destruction, I should not be ashamed:

1 Peter 4:8—And above all things have fervent charity among yourselves: for charity shall cover the multitude of sins.

Children feel accepted when . . .

- They know they are loved sacrificially.
- Their parents take an interest in their interests.
- They know they have value. Parents communicate this most by investing time in their children's lives and taking an interest in the details of their lives. Parents teach God's acceptance by teaching children the meaning of God's forgiveness and grace and by teaching them God loves them enough to know such details as the number of hairs on their heads. Children must know God accepts them on the basis of their relationship to Him through salvation *(Ephesians 1:3-6).*
- Parents openly express appreciation for their children's God-given individuality and do not express exasperation or condemnation for their imperfections.
- Parents set reasonable limitations and exercise nurturing authority.
- They know God does not ever react to them with disgust or rejection, but is always ready to love, forgive, restore, and help them.

Teamwork

1 Corinthians 1:10—Now I beseech you, brethren, by the name of our Lord Jesus Christ, that ye all speak the same thing, and *that* there be no divisions among you; but *that* ye be perfectly joined together in the same mind and in the same judgment.

Hebrews 10:24-25—And let us consider one another to provoke unto love and to good works: not forsaking the assembling of ourselves together, as the manner of some *is*; but exhorting *one another*: and so much the more, as ye see the day approaching.

Psalm 68:6—God setteth the solitary in families: he bringeth out those which are bound with chains: but the rebellious dwell in a dry *land*.

Children feel like they are part of a team when . . .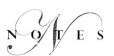

- Parents create an atmosphere of family unity and cultivate the awareness they are on the child's team, rooting for his success. Parents who create an "us-against-them" attitude in the home destroy the powerful motivation of team spirit.
- Parents use play as part of the training. Play encourages children to be enthusiastic about learning and being with parents.
- They know parents are willing to work together with them so they will succeed.
- Parents use consistent, controlled, deliberate discipline and training to help their children do right.
- Parents recognize their children's contributions and strengths and work to develop them.
- Parents are sensitive to their children's limitations and use short-term goals, which are attainable and not overwhelming.
- They know God is interested in them personally, and has made them unique and given them everything they need in order to fill a special place in His plan.

Restoring Lost Confidence and Zeal

When children have lost their confidence and zeal ...

- Relax your expectations temporarily until your child gains more confidence and mastery.
- Make success easy. One key to motivation is eliminating fears of failure. Make success attainable so you can give your child a string of successes to build his confidence and taste for achievement.
- Give your child the tools he needs to achieve (perhaps a tutor if he needs help in math, or experiences that will encourage him to learn a new activity).
- Keep the process of learning light and happy.
- Introduce new concepts gradually in the most non-threatening manner possible. Relax a child's anxiety by giving him only small sections of new material and setting small goals. This will help him develop confidence to try new things, risk failure, and achieve. He must first learn that he *can* succeed before he *will* succeed. Success breeds more success.
- Realize that the absurdity or silliness of a child's fears in no way lessens the sorrow and torment they cause the child. Be understanding; never belittle a child's fear.

Page 163

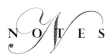

Personality Affects Motivation

A child's personality and individual interests will affect what motivates him. Carefully observe the things your child delights in most, what interests him, and what he talks about most frequently and eagerly. Note the boxes that most apply to your children.

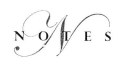

Outlets your child may use	Performing/ Interacting	Leading/ Achieving	Negotiating/ Solving	Expressing Emotion/ Creativity
Games your child may enjoy	Games of chance, group games, games using speaking or interaction	Strategy games which are highly competitive and challenging	Quiet games, games using personal skill	Games of logic, puzzles
Sports that your child may like	Interactive sports	Competitive sports	One-on-one sports	Non-competitive sports
Toys may interest your child	Toys that make noise, that have moving parts, that allow the child to pretend	Toys that challenge, that imitate a real thing, that allow the child to win	Toys that are rhythmic, that stimulate thought, that can be played with alone	Toys that stimulate creativity, that are cute, musical, or art related
Books your child may enjoy	Books that are funny, that have happy endings, that are science fiction	How-to books, success stories, motivational biographies	Picture books, books with interesting facts, mysteries	Story books, emotional books, novels
Hobbies that may interest your child	Exciting, fun hobbies involving interaction with others	Achievement-oriented hobbies that produce a finished product or goal	Self-absorbing hobbies that engage reasoning skills	Creative hobbies that provide outlets for creative expression
Rewards that are most desirable to your child	Enjoy playing together, desire to be with people and friends	Enjoy competing together, desire to earn privileges	Enjoy fixing something together, desire to please	Enjoy making something together, desire for emotional attachment
Correction that may be effective for your child	Require child to sit still in a quiet place	Remove child from competition and activity	Remove toy that is causing a problem	Send playmate home

Lesson 9

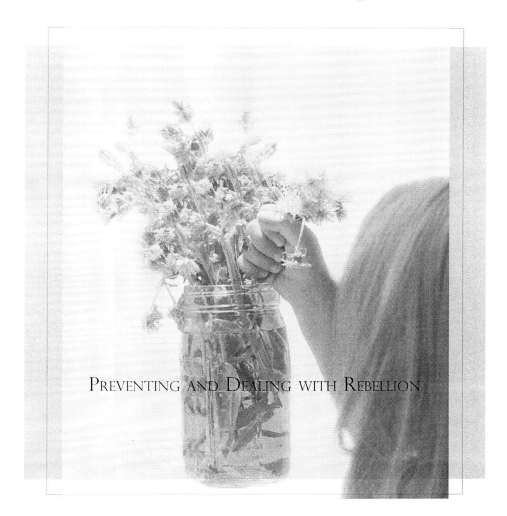

PREVENTING AND DEALING WITH REBELLION

Fathers, provoke not your children to anger,
lest they be discouraged.
Colossians 3:21

And Samuel said, Hath the LORD as great delight in burnt offerings and
sacrifices, as in obeying the voice of the LORD? Behold, to obey is better
than sacrifice, and to hearken than the fat of rams. For rebellion is as
the sin of witchcraft, and stubbornness is as iniquity and idolatry.
1 Samuel 15:22-23a

Key THOUGHTS

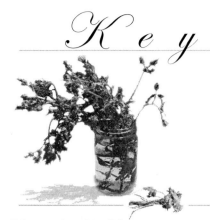

Rebellion is the end result of a progression of wrong thoughts and conclusions that often begin at a point when the child experiences injustice or confusion. In order to reverse rebellion, parents will need to use consistency when it is appropriate to chastise and reward. However, parents also must make diligent effort to remove what is feeding rebellion and implement things that encourage obedience. If parents have been hypocritical or have committed offenses against their children, they must acknowledge these, repent, and ask forgiveness from both God and those involved if they are to be effective in their attempt to restore their rebellious child.

Discussion Problem

Eleven-year-old Melissa is independent and outspoken. She is an average student, is overweight, and has no specific interests or talents. Recently she has begun applying layers of make-up and wanting clothes that make her look sexy. Melissa's mother Judy doesn't seem to be having any impact on her daughter. They fight constantly. In heated arguments, Judy tells Melissa she's stupid, a slob, and a failure like her cousin.

Melissa has not been a particularly compliant or sweet-spirited child, but neither has she been openly defiant or hateful, until recently. Melissa's parents fight and argue regularly, even though they are active church members who are well respected in their congregation.

Judy is openly rebellious toward her husband's authority and has long resented his desire for more conservative standards in the home. In some ways, Melissa's parents are restrictive and willing to make demands for obedience. However, their restrictions tend to be petty, inconsistent, or more for show than a Biblically based limitation. Their demands for obedience are likewise vague and inconsistent. The children have successfully manipulated them for years. Often they have sided against others on behalf of their children without objectively reviewing all the facts.

After reading lesson nine, use the principles you learn to discuss the possible reasons for Melissa's rebellion. What are the contributing factors? How is Melissa sinning against the Lord and her parents? How are her parents sinning against the Lord and Melissa? What can be done to resolve the situation?

Bible Study

1. From 1 Samuel 2:12, 22-25; 3:13, what error on Eli's part contributed to his sons' rebellion? _____
   _____
   _____

2. According to Genesis 19:14, 30-38, Lot's children did not listen to or respect him. Why might this have been so? _____
   _____

"Never despair of a child. The one you weep the most for at God's mercy-seat
may fill your heart with the sweetest joys."
Mary Blakely

Kids Are a Lot Like Horses

A well-trained horse readily submits to the will of its trainer and responds to the slightest cues. Shifts in the rider's weight, a touch on the neck or a hand, a nudge of the leg all communicate commands the horse immediately recognizes and obeys. A willing horse can be controlled without bit or heavy bridle, whips, or spurs. A mere look can be sufficient to guide him if his will is thoroughly yielded to a trainer who exerts dominance in a kind and gentle way. Such a horse is a pleasure to ride and delight to own, but his obedience doesn't come cheap. A lot of time and effort is invested to bring a feisty young colt like this to the place where he easily responds to the will of a rider. Submission is not natural to him, and he will resist it with a tenacity that discourages all but the most patient and persistent trainers.

Early in the training the young horse is made to circle a small ring compelled by the trainer who wields a whip and a lead rope. In his rebellion, the young horse circles with his head and eyes toward the outside of the ring away from the gaze of his supposed "tormenter." The experienced horse trainer isn't the least bit perturbed by such behavior because he understands the character of the horse and simply proceeds to control him as he is made to circle around and around the ring. Sometimes the horse stops and kicks or lowers his head and shakes it vigorously as if he is asserting his independence in spite of the predicament in which he finds himself at the moment. The trainer smiles because he knows it is all part of the process, and just continues urging the animal to obey. He wins one small battle at a time, never overworking the horse and never quitting too soon before he's won a decisive victory. Repetitiously the trainer resumes the exercise day after day until gradually the horse begins to comply and ceases resistance. Only when the colt turns his head toward the inside of the ring and begins watching the trainer does he know he has won the horse's trust and subdued his will sufficiently to proceed.

Parents often have no trouble at all comparing their children to wild horses who are none too anxious to have their wills conquered by love or anything else threatening to end their independence. Every parent experiences the effects of rebellion to some degree or another because all children come equipped with a natural human tendency to bristle under authority and want their own way, much like the unbroken colt. In fact, every misery that sin brings can be traced back to human self-will and pride. All human beings, including parents, desire the right to govern their own lives and naturally resist God's authority every bit as much as a wild young horse resists being governed by a trainer. The will must be subdued with love, patience, repetition, control, consistency, kindness, and inclusive authority. Some horses are broken without the use of much force, some more quickly than others, some easier than others. The same is true with children—their wills must be confronted and given opportunity to obey He who has the right to rule, or be faced with painful consequences.

God intends for parents as well as children to obey Him and willingly submit their wills to Him, for He has full ownership of His creation and has the right to govern and control our lives. He is not a cruel owner. He is benevolent and kind with none but the very best intentions for His own. Only an obstinate and ungrateful creature would dare to defy His authority and resist His will, and yet we who are His children often do just that. God entreats us with kindness and persists in His work. He tells us, "I will instruct thee and teach thee in the way which thou shalt go; I will guide thee with mine eye. Be not as the horse, or as the mule, which have no understanding; whose mouth must be held in with bit and bridle, lest they come near unto thee" *(Psalm 32:8-9)*.

Even as the trainer compels the horse to follow him, he himself must yield his will to the wishes of the horse's owner. God is the owner, but parents are the designated trainers commissioned to subdue the wills of their children and bring them into compliance with His will. A good horse trainer never gives a command and then asks the horse if he wants to obey. He doesn't give a command and then say, OK? Nor does he meekly suggest the horse obey or plead with the horse to obey. He does not give a command he cannot enforce, or is not willing to enforce, because to do so would send the wrong message to the horse and subvert his objective. When his authority is challenged, the trainer patiently but firmly meets the challenge and wins a decisive victory. He doesn't give the horse confusing commands, nor change the cues he is working to make second nature. He has clear-cut goals and progressively moves toward each one, gradually, patiently.

Sometimes rebellious children learn to resist, renounce, and disobey Mom and Dad's authority because Mom and Dad demonstrate open resistance, criticism, and disobedience to the authority God has placed over them. Parents who do so are like a horse trainer who is inconsistent in the commands he uses to train his horse or disobedient to the wishes of the owner. Mothers unwittingly teach their children to rebel when they refuse to obey their husbands, criticize others in leadership, refuse to submit to correction of any kind, or resist legitimate authority. Fathers teach their children to rebel when they do not submit to God's Word, do not love and respect their wives, disobey the laws of our government, or disregard others in leadership. Parents who fail to demonstrate submission to others, and open support for authority, actually *teach* their children to resist their *own* authority. They are like a horse trainer who undermines his own training with his own inconsistency. Children, like horses, will only excel to the degree the trainer does his job well and obeys the wishes of the owner.

Why is rebellion compared to the sin of witchcraft and stubbornness to idolatry *(I Samuel 15:23)*? Because the ruling desire of those who practice witchcraft is to possess power and authority that rightly belongs to God alone. When we resist God's sovereign authority and attempt to rule our own lives in God's place, we also attempt to assume power and authority over our own life that rightly belongs to God alone. The sin of idolatry is similar. It involves exalting something above God, of giving one's allegiance and love to something or someone other than God Himself. Stubbornness also exalts self above God and insists on satisfying self even at God's expense. To rebel is to disobey, resist, or renounce the authority to which one owes allegiance. As we seek to deal with our children's tendency to rebel against our authority, may we be ever mindful of our own responsibility to submit to the rightful authority of our Lord Jesus Christ.

Preventing Rebellion
1. Removing that which prevents a child from developing obedient and responsible behavior.
2. Implementing what is needful and helpful to help a child develop obedient and responsible behavior.

Removing the Impediments

Before your child will respond to your efforts to love and encourage him, you must be willing to remove anything that hinders and prevents him from wanting to obey or respect you. This might include changing or resolving problems in your own life, which contribute to your child's discouragement or rebellion. It might also include replacing rebellious friends, associations, music, or activities that encourage rebellion against godliness and parental authority.

Children are extremely susceptible to becoming whatever they are around. They imitate what they see and hear including the sassy, stubborn behavior they see on television or that they hear friends using. Attitudes are formed by whatever occupies our thoughts and minds. The content of conversations with friends, video games, school lectures, television, and any other source of mental input all contribute to our mindset and subsequent outward attitude and actions. "For as he thinketh in his heart, so is he" *(Proverbs 23:7)*. If you are to win the war with rebellion, you must be willing to take great care to steer your child away from any influence that hinders the development of a godly, obedient attitude. This includes, of course, what you yourself say and do and watch. Parental fighting, discontent, faultfinding, and anger will be mirrored in the way children live their lives. And what parents do in moderation, children often do in excess.

Implementing Encouragements

Removing those things that impede the development of good behavior is only effective if a parent also implements those things that encourage good behavior. Remove your child from rebellious friends, but provide good friends who know how to have fun in acceptable ways. (This would include your friends as well.) Refuse to allow ungodly music, but provide lots of happy music that encourages a love of things that are pure and good. Remove activities that lead to an ungodly lifestyle or interfere with family or church activities. But do not neglect to replace them with activities that are interesting, wholesome, and fun. Control or eliminate television watching, but go out of your way to provide desirable activities that will fill that time.

Make certain the Christian leaders who influence your child are not angry, hateful, or contentious. Avoid self-righteous and arrogant Christians who major on petty external issues. But do not neglect to deliberately choose those who emphasize the more important issues of the heart. Choose a youth group and Christian school that are producing happy, enthusiastic teens who are excited about serving the Lord. Do not look for perfection or size; look instead for Christian love and humility. Sometimes it helps to watch the seniors who are graduating and ask yourself if these are the kinds of young people you want your child to emulate.

Instead of always saying, "Don't do that," make it possible to say, "Let's do this." Instead of emphasizing what your children cannot do, emphasize what they can do. Make the effort to fill your home with lots of laughter and fun, steering your children toward "what is better," not just away from what is bad. In chapter one, we discussed the instructions given to parents in *Psalm 78* as to what they are to teach in order to prevent children from becoming stubborn and rebellious. May I remind you that the major emphasis is on teaching what is good, not teaching what is bad. God commands parents to teach their children to praise the Lord, to marvel at God's strength, and to remember the wonderful works that God has done. Be sure the environment you set in your home is one of thankfulness, centered on the blessings and joys of the Lord. If you will start your day with a smile, singing sincere praises to the Lord, you will find it sets the pace for the entire family. Morning battles are very hard to stage in an atmosphere of love and praise.

Begin Where God Begins

No loving parent wishes to handle a rebelling child in ways that will make matters worse or be of no value. We all want our efforts to be blessed and profitable for our children. Perhaps you are a parent who has come to the place where you can readily admit that you are spinning your wheels and getting nowhere fast. Or perhaps you are wondering why the efforts of so many sincere parents seem to be for naught, or why even the sweetest of children in the most ideal circumstances sometimes begins to challenge authority in ungodly ways. There are many reasons why a child might rebel, but God's power will resolve none of them unless those who are confronting the rebellious child willingly begin where God begins. Before a parent's efforts to deal with rebellion can possibly be blessed by God or produce real change, he must be willing to follow God's order prior to engaging in a confrontation.

The prevailing principle of confrontation is that those who confront another examine their own hearts first. Painful as it might be, the light must first illuminate our own heart and reveal its flaws before we can successfully illuminate the sins of a rebelling child's heart.

We cannot see clearly enough to cast the mote out of a brother's eye unless we first cast the beam out of our own *(Matthew 7:3-5)*. The Scriptures tell us that before Ezra stood to instruct Israel, he prepared his heart to seek the law of the Lord, and to do it *(Ezra 7:10)*. Israel repented under Ezra's instruction and put away their sins, but only after Ezra prayed and confessed the sins of the nation. Nehemiah also confronted Israel with sin and saw them humble their hearts and repent with great sorrow. He too began by confessing his own sin first *(Nehemiah 1:4-11)*. David, after confessing his own sin and seeking God's forgiveness, prays that the joy of God's salvation would be restored to him and then follows this by saying, "Then will I teach transgressors thy ways; and sinners shall be converted unto thee" *(Psalm 51:13)*.

Every parent, no matter how godly, is able to make a list of personal flaws and weaknesses in their parenting. All parents sin, just as all children sin. Those who believe otherwise demonstrate the absolute truth of this statement, for a refusal to admit the obvious would be profoundly arrogant and proof enough of it. To say one is without need of improvement or without sin of any kind would represent either blatant deception or the most pernicious sort of self-deception. When Solomon declares, "reproofs of instruction are the way of life," he speaks not only to youth, but to adults as well *(Proverbs 6:23)*. The Bible warns, "he that refuseth reproof erreth" *(Proverbs 10:17)* and "he that trusteth in his own heart is a fool" *(Proverbs 28:26)*. We all need exhortation, reproof and instruction in order to keep ourselves following God's ways because our sinful hearts are prone to wander and prone toward being blinded by error. Sin, by its very nature is deceitful and able to harden our own hearts when any one of us ceases to hear instruction (See *Hebrews 3:13*).

We cannot refuse God's instruction and then expect God to bless our instruction to our children. If we refuse to humble ourselves we cannot expect God to produce humility in them—and humility is precisely what is necessary in order to conquer attitudes of rebellion toward authority. If ever we needed God's help and grace, it is in the matter of raising our children, for no parent is perfect enough to merit God's blessing or wise enough to produce a godly child without God's grace. Several times the Scriptures state that God resists (is opposed to) the proud, but gives grace (all God's blessings undeserved) to the humble *(James 4:6; 1 Peter 5:5; Proverbs 3:34)*.

No parent facing the difficulties of a rebellious youngster wants God to be against him. Our powerlessness to change the heart of our child should bring us to our knees to confess we can do nothing apart from God. We desperately need His help. We need not bother praying and crying to God for help with our rebelling child if we will not humble ourselves to deal with problems God's way, or humble ourselves to identify and confess our own sins first. God's ears are deaf to such a parent's cry.

For those parents who are willing to approach their children's rebellion on God's terms and willing to examine their own hearts first, God is ready and willing to hear and forgive *(Psalm 86:5)*. Pray as David did, "Search me, O God, and know my heart; try me, and know my thoughts; and see if there be any wicked way in me, and lead me in the way everlasting" *(Psalm 139:23)*. Thankfully, God is not demanding perfection from parents—but He does demand truthfulness; and He does demand humility. A parent's humble willingness to admit failures and forsake sin opens the door to God's forgiveness and blessing. Very often it also opens the door through which rebellious children humble themselves and repent of their rebellion. By dealing with your own sins first, you are demonstrating for your children the same humility God desires for them. Humility not only elicits God's blessing and grace, it works to soften the rebelling child's heart. The sins of parents often provoke and discourage children, as well as cause them to excuse their own sins. On page 202-203 is a worksheet that is intended to help parents determine possible areas where they have sinned knowingly or unknowingly. Go through it carefully and mark those areas where you recognize you need to make changes in your life.

Laying the Groundwork for Peace

After considering the possibilities, ask your child's forgiveness for sins you have committed against him as well as against God, keeping in mind sincere confession produces respect, rather than disrespect, as some would suppose. Beginning this way fulfills Paul's instructions to the spiritually mature Galatians who were told to restore others who had been overtaken in a fault in a spirit of meekness (humility), considering themselves, lest they also be tempted *(Galatians 6:1)*. Before your child will willingly respond to you, you must right your wrongs against him, demonstrate a life consistent with your words, and live worthy of your child's trust and respect. This requires time and patience, so do not expect instantaneous results. Do what is right because it is right, not as a manipulative means to get the response you want from your child. Focus on what God is doing in your life right now, and how He is using this difficult situation to provoke change in you as well as in the life of your child.

If you are sincerely willing to know how you might have committed an offense against your child, it will require you to allow him a chance to express his perception of your wrongs against him, not just express your perceptions of wrong. This is a tough thing to do, because quite typically the rebellious child expresses himself in an angry and disrespectful manner. Regardless whether your child's anger stems from legitimate or imagined wrongs against him, let your child know you are going to listen to him patiently without interrupting *except when he becomes disrespectful and hateful*. Let him know ahead of time that you will stop him if he becomes disrespectful and that you will ask that he reword the remark, but as long as he will honor this condition you will listen patiently. THEN DO SO.

Do not demand that your child speak without emotion and do not correct his angry tone. Now is not the time to deal with his anger—it is a time to listen and consider what truth and validity are in your child's words and what events have provoked his bitterness. Sometimes the problem will come bubbling to the surface immediately if the child believes the parent is sincere in his efforts to understand him and see the problem through his eyes. Other times the child's remarks will be vague or misguided, in which case it is often wise to listen and not respond immediately so as not to incite an argument when emotions are on edge. If this is the case, let your child know you have listened carefully and need some time to think over what he has said. Then, set a time within twenty four hours (preferably less) to get back with him and give a response.

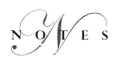

It is possible your child senses an offense has been committed against him but lacks the maturity or knowledge that would enable him to articulate it well. Look for such problems and encourage your child or reword them, asking your child if this is what he means. Do not presume to know what your child means or what your child is thinking. This is a sure way to discourage and incite your child's frustration (anger). Give him the same respect you wish to have and ask if such and such is what he means, or if such and such could be possible. Again, do not be distracted by his immature or offensive manner, rather, look beyond his immaturity to discover facts you can work with and respond to appropriately. Do not accept blame merely to appease your child. This would be just as dishonest as refusing to accept responsibility for a genuine offense. But do not neglect to acknowledge error where you have been wrong. You may need to redefine accusations into Biblical language. For example, he may wrongly accuse you of "yelling" at him. It may be that you spoke to him with unkindness or in a tone of anger, and he is interpreting it as "yelling." In this case, you would ask his forgiveness for speaking unkindly or being rude or impatient, but you would not ask forgiveness for "yelling."

Once you have dealt with the major issues that have caused or contributed to your child's attitude, you will want to work at establishing a relationship in which offenses and problems are resolved quickly and effectively. Your child needs to know you will listen and respond if you have genuinely sinned, but you will also confront him and deal with offenses when they cannot be overlooked. The book *Peacemaking for Families* by Ken Sande is an excellent resource in learning how to reconcile wrongs and resolve problems in a spirit of love. I also highly recommend the little booklet by Jay Adams called *How To Overcome Evil*. This booklet is a practical exposition of *Romans 12:14-21* and is a powerful reminder that a Christian possesses different means with which to overcome offenses. You may also find help in chapters 3, 4, 10, and 11 from *Secrets of a Happy Heart*, the first book in the Titus 2 Series, or the book called *Why Am I So Angry*.

Wisdom Conquers Rebellion

In the Bible, one is called a fool who acts contrary to sound wisdom and follows his own inclinations. It is very close to, if not sometimes synonymous with a person we might refer to as a "rebel," which is one who disobeys, resists, or renounces a legitimate authority. Certainly, a rebellious person is foolish and lacks wisdom. He is self-willed and reasons according to what he desires at the moment. If what God desires or some other human authority desires agrees with a rebel, he may comply, but he resists when it runs contrary to his own will.

Foolish behavior is inherent to a small child who naturally follows his impulses without weighing his actions. He starts life will little understanding as to what is acceptable or what is not. The capacity to reason only develops over time as a child develops physically and is disciplined and taught how to choose right behavior. Much foolish behavior in children is not in itself a rebellious defiance against authority. Rather the foolish behavior sometimes represents the child's immature ability to discern a wise course of action or the impulsiveness of his childish nature. For instance, suppose an 8-year-old child fills a bag with sand and climbs to the top of playground equipment to drop it on the head of his friend passing below. The child giggles as he climbs, imagining the bag of sand spilling on his playmate like a water balloon. When the bag of sand knocks his friend to the ground unconscious, he is stunned but immediately senses he has done something wrong. Mothers quickly arrive on the scene, and emotion-backed words begin to fly. "What were you thinking? How could you do this? Don't you realize how heavy a bag of sand is? You could have killed him! Go to your room and do not come out until your Dad comes home!"

In the father's outrage and embarrassment, he administers a spanking without so much as inquiring what was on his child's mind when the child plotted his dastardly deed. To emphasize the seriousness of the offense, the parents restrict him to his room for a week and take away his bike. The child, meanwhile, does not know if his friend is hurt, or how badly he is hurt. He feels miserable about what has happened and grieves that he has caused his friend pain. He sits alone in his room, his emotions vacillating between sorrow for what he has done and anger that his intentions are being portrayed as a rebellious and vicious act. He cries himself to sleep because his friend is no longer allowed to play with him, and he has no way to resolve or undo what has happened.

Enough incidents like this one and such a child will likely begin a downward spiral from foolish childish behavior to full-blown rebellious behavior. It is right that the parents be understandably concerned, but they have wrongly misjudged their child's motives and reacted on the basis of fear rather than sound judgment. Ironically, the parents' behavior is as foolish and unwise as that of the child. Not only have the parents failed to discern what actually prompted the incident, they have wrongly accused the child of rebellion, judged the motives his heart, and aroused guilt without providing a way to resolve the guilt. They have administered discipline for rebellion when there was no rebellion and wrongly used rejection as a means of emphasizing the seriousness of the act. To further impress upon their son the consequences of his action, they take away something he loves, thus unwisely prolonging the incident and insuring their son's resentment. They do not identify a sin the child has committed, a means to resolve that sin, or a means to express sorrow and seek forgiveness from his friend. This foolish disciplining is a sure recipe for future disaster.

This boy has certainly done something foolish and impulsive that had serious potential for harm. His motive, however, was no different than it was when he hurled water balloons at his birthday party during a parent-supervised water balloon war that included the same friend. The sand bag incident provided a good opportunity to teach the boy a basic physics lesson that would help him learn the distinction between a balloon filled with water and a bag filled with sand. It would also be an incident that would stick in his mind as something that could cause serious harm to someone unintentionally. The incident would have provided an opportunity to teach the lesson of taking responsibility for accidents, even when no malicious intent was involved. This boy should have been allowed to help his friend, to hold the ice bag, to express his sorrow, and ask forgiveness. Handled correctly, the parents could have used the event to teach many life principles that would no doubt have been remembered for a lifetime. It even presented an excellent occasion in which the offended child could learn the concept of forgiveness. Instead, both children will remember the event as bitter evidence that parents are unjust and unloving.

Let's consider a different example. A ten-year-old girl decides to walk a mile from home to a shopping center to buy a candy bar for her younger sister while her parents are away from home working. The younger sibling was sad about a failure at school, so the older child thought using her own money to buy the candy would be something that would cheer her up. Knowing she wasn't supposed to leave the house, she waited until her teenage sister was on the phone to slip out the door and head for the store undetected. However, to get to the store, she has to walk through a rather notoriously rough part of the neighborhood where many drug dealers hang out. An hour later, the teenage babysitter realizes the child is not in the house and begins to question the other children. At that moment, the ten-year-old returns from her shopping excursion, bag in hand, and presents it to her little sister.

An angry older sister alternates scolding while phoning the mother to report the violation. In no time, the mother arrives home, quite visibly upset, and proceeds to hunt down her now weeping daughter who is curled up in a chair in the family room. Throwing down her purse and waving her arms in anger she begins an hour-long discourse on the dangers of walking through the neighborhood, the stupidity of the child's actions, and the insensitivity shown to the older sister. This produces more weeping from the ten year old interspersed with angry justifications for her actions. Finally the mother grabs her daughter by the arm and leads her to the bedroom where she administers a spanking and then stomps off to the kitchen to make dinner in a now tense and angry household.

Again, the mother reacted out of fear for her daughter's safety and anger that she ventured outside. In her understandable concern about danger, she ignored the real offense and used her anger to emphasize the horror she felt and insisted that her daughter not leave the home. Her daughter, meanwhile, does not comprehend the danger. She doesn't understand the wicked potential of the "nice" people she passed along the way, nor does she comprehend the scope of the danger she put herself in. In her childish and foolish way of thinking, her mother sounds unreasonable and from her perspective, irrational. She reasons that her intentions were good and unselfish and her mother's rule unreasonable and harsh, given the explanation she has received about dangerous people. Furthermore, she is resentful that she received a spanking for what she interprets as an unselfish and kind act toward her younger sister.

This child's assessment is dead wrong, but is exactly what the mother communicated in the manner she handled this problem. The offense that ought to have been addressed was deliberate rebellion toward a rule the mother had clearly instituted and warned would result in certain consequences. The children had been told not to leave the home for any reason. The fact that the child employed sneaky means to exit the house proves she knew she was disobeying. Clearly, this constitutes rebellion toward authority. It would have been right for the mother to convey her concern for the safety of her child and explain the potential for harm in a serious, but not angry tone. It would have been right for the mother to acknowledge that being willing to spend her own money for her sister and being concerned for her well-being is indeed commendable and loving. But it was not right to spank the child for anything other than her disobedience.

This mother missed an opportunity to teach her daughter that she is required to obey regardless whether or not she agrees with the mother or understands all the reasons her mother has established this rule. This would have helped hone the child's skills in reasoning Biblically and gone a long way in preparing her to obey God, even when it isn't clear why He gives a certain command. What the mother actually missed was an opportunity to teach her child godly wisdom and the ability to discern right from wrong. Instead of curtailing future rebellious behavior, this mother actually fertilized the seeds of full-blown teenage rebellion and insured future battles that will only get worse.

In dealing with rebellion, parents must have the wisdom to discern whether or not the child's behavior represents childish foolishness, true rebellion, or both. If they do not, they will undoubtedly misapply discipline, fail to deal with true rebellion appropriately, and provoke their children to continue in their childish foolishness rather than grow in wisdom. Dealing with and preventing rebellion requires parents to give particular attention to the development of wisdom in their child, which entails the right application of Scripture to life's problems. Wise parents look at what underlies behavior, not just at the outward behavior itself. Like the horse trainer who patiently subdues a horse's immature exuberance and impulsiveness, the wise parent must work toward encouraging spiritual maturity in his children in incremental steps, utilizing every real life event as hands-on classroom experience that teaches how to apply knowledge in practical ways.

For this, we need wisdom that only comes as we learn the Word of God, pray for God's gracious gift of wisdom, and open our eyes to the marvelous opportunities we are given (quite regularly) to teach and model wisdom to our children. "How much better it is to get wisdom than gold! And to get understanding rather to be chosen than silver! He that handleth a matter wisely shall find good; and whoso trusteth in the Lord, happy is he. The wise in heart shall be called prudent; and the sweetness of the lips increaseth learning. Understanding is a wellspring of life unto him that hath it; but the instruction of fools is folly. The heart of the wise teacheth his mouth, and addeth learning to his lips. Pleasant words are as an honeycomb, sweet to the soul, and health to the bones" *(Proverbs 16:16, 20-24)*.

> *Dealing with and preventing rebellion requires parents to give particular attention to the development of wisdom in their child, which entails the right application of Scripture to life's problems.*

When children grow spiritually they develop the ability to discern evil and weigh actions. They grow in their ability to reason and spot those who use deception and unBiblical arguments in order to justify wrong doctrine. Wise children grow in their ability to act responsibly, as God would define *responsible*, and develop a Biblical rationale for their actions. Wisdom, knowledge and understanding are the antidote for foolishness and rebellion. "Wisdom then is the principal thing; therefore get wisdom: and with all thy getting get understanding" *(Proverbs 4:7).*

A Wise Parent According to James 3:17-18

But the wisdom that is from above is first **pure**, then **peaceable, gentle,** and **easy to be intreated**, full of **mercy** and **good fruits, without partiality,** and **without hypocrisy**. And the fruit of righteousness is sown in peace of them that make peace.

- *Pure*—Free from moral corruption; free from impure motives
- *Peaceable*—Free from private feuds or quarrels; undisturbed; not agitated
- *Gentle*—Not rough or harsh; soothing
- *Approachable*—Accessible; easy to come near; easy to talk to
- *Merciful*—Exercising mercy and compassion; tender; unwilling to cause pain; not cruel; disposed to pity offenders and to forgive their offenses and forbear punishment that is deserved
- *Good fruits*—Outworking of Spirit-filled life gained through diligent relationship with Christ; benevolent; bears fruit of the Spirit; endeavors in Christ-like service to others
- *Impartial*—Fair; not biased in favor of one party more than another; unprejudiced; equitable; just
- *Without hypocrisy*—One who is genuinely virtuous and godly, not simply assuming the appearance of virtue and godliness; one whose life is consistent with the profession of what one believes and exhorts in others

Stop and Evaluate

Are you ready to see how you're progressing in your ability to wisely discern good and evil? Following is an exercise that works best in a group discussion. If you are studying this book alone, see if you can't round up a few friends or family to join you. After reading the story aloud (go ahead, give it some drama!), stop and discuss your impressions with others in your study by answering the following six questions. You will find answers at the end of this lesson that you can refer to after you have made your list.

1. What emotions do you believe you would have experienced during this lecture?
2. What is wrong with this lecture?

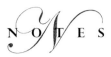

3. What scriptural violations are involved?

4. What serious spiritual problems and sins are revealed in this speech?

5. How is this speech like some parent's lectures to their children?

6. If you were a rebellious child, how would a lecture like this make your relationship with parents worse?

Discernment Exercise - The Teacher's Meeting

Suppose you are a Christian schoolteacher. You have worked hard all week, bringing work home, staying up late preparing lessons, and answering phone calls from parents. You are barely making minimum wage but consider the financial sacrifices worthy of your calling. Still, there are many personal things you are doing without so you can make it on your salary and the bills are weighing heavy on you. Friday has finally arrived and you are looking forward to getting a full night's rest and enjoying some time with your family. Before heading home, however, you make your way to the school conference room where the administrator will conduct a weekly teacher's meeting. After a few brief preliminary remarks, the principal proceeds with a lecture that is animated with angry gestures, pulpit pounding, and facial scowls. He continues to berate the weary staff with the following comments.

"You are causing a terrible spirit in our school. You call yourselves Christian leaders, but you do nothing but waste time. I saw one of you drinking a cup of coffee when you should have been in class. Another one of you was walking out in front of the building instead of fulfilling your responsibilities in the classroom. This is a blatant refusal to obey authority. You have no respect for the rules and no regard for the money parents are paying you to educate their kids. You ought to repent of your selfishness and laziness. If you can't control yourself, you have no right to be a part of this school. Really, it's nothing but raw rebellion. And your rebellious spirit is ruining our school. I even heard one of you laugh when the pastor was preaching. And don't think I didn't see the note that was passed either. What utter spiritual apathy and disrespect for the man of God! What kind of an example are you providing for our kids? They look up to you, and you are letting them down. I doubt you have any love at all for these kids. You certainly don't appreciate them. In fact, your rebellious spirit is contaminating everyone around you. God considers rebellion so heinous that He compares it with devil worship. Do you want to go down as a devil worshiper? Don't think God won't hold you responsible for your lousy attitude. You are headed for big trouble with a capital T. God is going to take His hand off of your life and let you fall flat on your face. If you don't get with the program, you are going to make a mess of your life; and you'll have only yourself to blame. God has put me in your life to tell you the truth. I know it hurts, but you need a good dose of reality. Just remember, you can never say that no one warned you."

Suppose some of the principal's statements had some measure of truth to them, and you did harbor ill feelings toward him or other school personnel. Would this speech have turned your heart toward God or inspired you to want to resolve the problems you were dealing with? Even if your heart was pure and without fault, this speech would have done nothing but sow resentment and discouragement. Had you begun with ill feelings it would no doubt have only made those feelings seem justified, diminishing any desire to interact with the principal or attempt to please him. Quite likely, you would have been making plans to submit your resignation and withdraw from such an oppressive environment at the soonest possible opportunity.

The Downward Progression of Rebellion

Obedient children do not undergo a metamorphous in the night and awaken one morning rebellious, although some days you may wonder. All children express sinful rebellion when they disobey their parents or assert their own will throughout their growing up years, but most often children are quickly brought under control through love and consistent discipline. When love and discipline do not produce a change, and rebellion becomes a character trait rather than an occasional problem, you can be certain there is more going on under the surface than can be seen in the obstinate behavior of a rebellious child. Unraveling the tangled cords of rebellion becomes much easier when we understand its starting points and natural progression. Becoming more aware provides invaluable insight for those who are raising children who have not yet exhibited evidence of full-blown rebellion. If rebellion can be intercepted in its beginning stage or prevented altogether, parents and child alike can avoid much heartache.

Self-Centered (Sinful) Nature

Because the human heart is naturally self-willed and sin itself is an expression of rebellion towards God's authority, the human nature alone is sufficient enough to begin the progression of rebellion. The human heart is "deceitful above all things, and desperately wicked; who can know it?" *(Jeremiah 17:9)*. Children are capable of sinfully responding to life in such a way as to blindly choose the path of rebellion— with or without offenses committed against them by anyone. Because children begin life with a bent towards self-gratification, all that is necessary to insure they grow up rebellious is to do nothing about it. Parents who ignore or respond inappropriately to a child's self-will unwittingly fan the sparks of full-blown rebellion. What may be easily ignored in the early years gradually smolders until it explodes into a raging fire in the teen years.

The sinful heart of man changes the way he responds when mistreated. When human beings experience injustice and heartache, they are far more prone to react in anger than in the way Christ responded when He was mistreated. The Lord Jesus was sinless, and perfectly submitted to the will of the Father. Therefore, when he was mocked and ridiculed by others, He was able to refrain from returning hateful comments with flawless faith. When He was abused and mistreated, He, being perfect, did not threaten retaliation in return. Instead, Jesus committed Himself to God who judges righteously and left revenge to the Father alone *(1 Peter 2:22-23)*. We are able to respond in this way only as God's Spirit transforms our human nature and works a miraculous change in us. Certainly, it is not the typical way human beings respond to mistreatment. The naturally "me-centered" child is even less able to restrain his childish impulse to hate and retaliate when he is wronged. Because children are both immature and naturally sinful, hitting back when they are hit and calling names when they are called names most often characterize their response.

Seasoned believers who are confident in God's love and happily growing in their faith develop an inner strength that sustains them in time of trouble. Children are little lambs that are too young to have grown sufficiently strong enough to withstand the dangers of this world. They need protection and special care in order to become mature. Because children lack the spiritual framework in which to deal sufficiently with trials, they tend to become discouraged easily and are less able to overcome disappointment and injury. A child's anger or rebellion can usually be traced back to a hurtful incident or incidents that were never fully resolved. "The spirit of a man will sustain his infirmity; but a wounded spirit who can bear?" *(Proverbs 18:14)*.

Distress or Hurt

Children quite naturally pick up an attitude of persecution if they do not understand why they are being treated in a particular manner. Because they are more self-centered, they often imagine they are being rejected, mistreated, or dealt with unfairly when in fact they are not. When they *are* genuinely rejected, mistreated, or dealt with unfairly, they are most sensitive to it and almost immediately perceive and react. Whether the injustice is real or imagined, it in no way lessens the reality of its torment or its eventual outcome if it is not resolved. If someone who understands children does not talk it out and sort through what's real and imagined, children are capable of assuming the worst and responding in very self-destructive ways.

Family disputes and problems that are not resolved wound a child and cause much inward distress. Children of divorce are its most innocent victims and often get lost in the trauma of their parent's disputes and cruelty toward one another. Some grieve well into their adult years and most do not come through the divorce unscathed. Constant fighting between Mom and Dad or tensions in the home are capable of causing illness in children as well as serious behavior problems. Sometimes siblings have conflicts that are squelched but not resolved. These also give rise to bitter feelings that can progress into rebellion.

Childhood is a time when children develop questions that deeply disturb them and require answers. When parents dismiss these questions as silly or unimportant, a child is wounded. Children are prone to develop fears and anxieties that need to be patiently addressed and resolved. Instead, some parents treat their children's fears with contempt or disinterest, making matters worse. Even when children resolve fears on their own or through other means, they remember the parent's insensitivity and are wounded by it. Children who have sincere difficulties learning or keeping up with their peers academically especially need parental compassion and involvement. The trials of childhood are remembered—so are the ways adults responded to those trials.

There are many ways children can be deeply wounded while they are away from the protective care of parents, but perhaps one of the most potentially damaging is through an experience with sexual molestation. It is noteworthy for parents to be aware that more children are molested by other children than by adults, and most children who are molested by adults are molested by adults the parents love and trust, or by a parent himself. Most victims feel unable to confide in their mothers for a variety of reasons. Mothers are often abused wives, viewed by the child as offering no protection. Many victims believe their mothers knew and condoned the abuse by their silence or unwillingness to separate themselves from the abuser. As children grow older, they often place more blame on the mother, whom they believe did not protect them, than the family member who molested them. For this reason, mothers often become the major targets of a wounded child's resentment.

Children who have been abused or molested may become abruptly withdrawn; seem confused; excessively fearful; extremely compliant or extremely rebellious; or may display extreme changes in typical behavior or personality. The premature arousal and exploitation of the sexual abuse victim, whether male or female, causes guilt and intense shame over the sexual acts. The very manner in which a molester manipulates a child emotionally and enforces the child's compliance as well as secrecy produces an enormous load of guilt and confusion in the child's heart. Pedophiles develop strong rationalization mechanisms and are almost always EXTREMELY defensive when confronted with any evidence of their sin. Their ability to lie and manipulate is *extremely* convincing. When confronted, a pedophile will commonly attempt to alleviate his guilt with passionate protests of innocence and will go to great lengths to portray his victim as seductive and vile. The abuser becomes highly skilled at minimizing his actions, rationalizing them, and blaming others—including his victim. This in itself is a powerful precursor to despair that so often propels a child toward eventual rebellion.

Once a child has been physically used, the offender will typically employ guilt tactics, pressure, threats, or blackmail to maintain control and further involve himself with the child. The molester will most commonly enforce secrecy in one or more of three ways. He will use *fear*, such as threatening to harm a beloved pet or the mother, by warning the child that no one will believe him or by threatening to kill himself if the child discloses the secret. A second means is the use of **seduction**. The molester develops an emotional attachment with the child that causes the child to experience pleasurable sexual sensations that he or she will begin to crave, even though the child experiences extreme guilt and confusion at the same time. Lastly, molesters often use ***bribery***, providing privileges or things the child greatly desires and threatening to take them away if the child does not cooperate.

A victim's problems may develop in three general areas. He or she may suffer with ***unresolved guilt*** - resulting in an inability to discern proper responsibility, acceptance of false guilt, self-inflicted pain and suffering. Premature sexual arousal often leads to strong sexual desires that cannot be righteously resolved outside of marriage, which leads to further guilt, feelings of despair, and confusion. Second, molested children likely experience the effects of a ***betrayal of trust*** by someone they respected, resulting in development of fears, resentments, or the inability to participate in establishing healthy relationships with others. Third, molested youngsters often suffer with feelings of ***alienation*** (being alone and different), resulting in depression, anger, or confusion.

Children who are rejected or believe they are rejected, children who are abused or used for adult sexual gratification, children who are subjected to things that violate their conscience, and children who experience other such unresolved conflicts and problems all produce deep wounds that are difficult to see immediately. Sadly, the wounded child is most vulnerable to suffering that easily transforms into anger, bitterness, and despair.

Bitterness and Despair

A child does not know how to resolve complex problems without being taught how to do so. He will initially attempt to solve problems using childish reasoning and methods. When this fails repeatedly, he typically slides into hopelessness and becomes bitter. If he has been made to believe lies, he may become confused, but will not likely have the maturity to recognize or reject them, further adding to his sorrow or confusion. Because a child's nature is to trust and believe what he is taught, wicked people are able to easily exploit his innocence in order to use or manipulate him into agreeing or complying with them. When this happens, children often believe their situation is hopeless, that no one would believe them, and that no one can help them. As the child grows older, he becomes less gullible and develops the strength and maturity to view the mistreatment more accurately. Many youngsters seem to be unaffected by wrongs committed against them while they are very young, but become very angry as they become older and remember what was done to them.

Unresolved guilt is one of the deadliest problems that give rise to eventual rebellion. When a child intuitively knows he has done something wrong but does not know how to seek or receive God's forgiveness, he will secretly harbor fear and guilt that will progress into bitterness and despair. If the child believes he has done something wrong when in fact he has not, the result will be just as profound as if he did. He cannot easily distinguish between real and false guilt and does not possess the knowledge and understanding, let alone the confidence, to reject false guilt. This is one reason why Christian parents must identify that which is God's law and that which is parental preference, and must deal thoroughly and Biblically with issues that produce guilt. Guilt that occurs because we have truly violated God's law is intended to bring us to a place of repentance and restored fellowship with God. Guilt that is produced for any other reason is to be rejected as false.

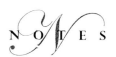

Parents who heap on the guilt as a means of controlling their children do unspeakable harm.

It is not wrong to establish household rules that forbid actions that are not sins. It is, however, wrong to teach children that a violation of preference is sin. A Christian school may institute a rule that forbids wearing a certain article of clothing, not because the clothing choice is sinful, but because it is not deemed conducive to the school's objectives. School personnel who enforce the rule need to make certain the student who violates the rule is deliberately choosing a course of action contrary to the authority he is under, then they must emphasize that he is being disciplined for disobedience, not for wearing the forbidden clothing. This is not a clothing issue, but an authority issue. Parents and school administrators who fail to make this kind of distinction and instead label such rules as sins may win compliance in the younger years only to be faced with major rebellion against spiritual things in years to come.

Parents who heap on the guilt as a means of controlling their children do unspeakable harm. God did not make us in such a way that we can withstand unresolved guilt without serious consequence. Parents who threaten little children by telling them God will not love them or God will punish them with sickness, etc. are misrepresenting God and committing a wicked offense against a child. A child's unresolved guilt, real or false, eats at him and torments him, causing havoc both mentally and physically. When a child's attempts to find relief fail, he will invariably give up and become bitter and angry. It is a dangerous thing to misuse parental authority in order to manipulate children with guilt. We are given a severe warning by God that whoever "shall offend one of these little ones which believe in me, it were better for him that a millstone were hanged about his neck, and that he were drowned in the depth of the sea" *(Matthew 18:6)*. A child who believes on Christ has witnesses in the courts of heaven that will testify against parents who mistreat him. Christ warns, "Take heed that ye despise not one of these little ones; for I say unto you, that in heaven their angels do always behold the face of my Father which is in heaven" *(Matthew 18:10)*.

Parents must teach their children how to repent of their sin and find assurance of God's forgiveness. When parents ignore sin or do not resolve it through forgiveness, that sin has the potential of causing many problems for the child. This is one reason parents should avoid using prolonged chastisement. Except in rare cases with older children, it is far better to deal with disobedience swiftly. Chastisement should end quickly and completely. When the chastisement lasts a long time, it appears to the child that you are holding the offense over the child's head. Parents who hold a grudge or regularly bring up forgiven offenses of the past are not only acting in an ungodly manner; they discourage their children and set the stage for anger and future rebellion.

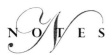

Anger and Frustration

By the time a child's problems and conflicts reach the point of becoming outward expressions of anger, he has likely developed the habit of nursing his wounds, mulling over offenses, thinking obsessively about what's bothering him, and harboring grudges and resentments that are reviewed in the hidden corners of his heart continually. His inward focus on himself and his problems eventually makes him a walking bruise. He will likely howl with pain at the slightest bump and use it as an occasion to vent the angry tension that his introspection builds inside his mind.

The angry child is not usually a problem solver. When problems arise, he merely reacts in protest; for his experience has taught him that they bring pain, not resolutions. Because he typically interprets the difficult events of his life as rejection, he tends to treat others the way he believes he has been treated. He becomes increasingly more unforgiving, unloving, self-absorbed, and resentful. Because he has not known the peace that forgiveness and God's love brings, he does not forgive or love easily. Interpersonal relationships crumble under the tension he produces, further adding to his anger and torment. Anything that prompts him to experience guilt is viewed with disdain. He has not learned how to resolve guilt caused by sin or guilt caused by a misguided conscience; therefore, he manages it by blaming others, denying it, justifying it, or rationalizing.

Some children manage to hide their anger and more blatant rebellious activity until they graduate from high school and begin to leave home. Others let their resentments simmer at a slow boil, building up steam gradually over time. Their preferred manner of expressing resistance is to become lethargic and uncooperative. They are the eye rollers, the quietly sarcastic commentators, and masterful arguers.

Rebellion

As the habits of anger progress, they will drive the child to find outlets to express his hidden rage. He will often pick fights with siblings, refuse to cooperate, lose interest in school, and start becoming more open and bold in his defiance. Music that challenges authority and defies decency appeals to him. Outrageous clothing, offensive words, stubborn refusals to comply, and heated arguments often become commonplace. Shocking people with his words and actions may become a way to express his resentment and derive a perverted form of pleasure in being able to exert control in his life. Usually, he has no interest in spiritual things, particularly if he views spiritual activity as something that confines, condemns, and rejects him. He often associates spiritual things with people who he recognizes as hypocritical, hateful, or self-righteous.

Some youngsters will turn to drugs or alcohol in order to experience moments of relief and peaceful calm, exuberance, or confidence induced by the drug. They are typically shortsighted teens that do not comprehend the ways the drugs will complicate problems further. At this point, however, the rebellious youngster is quite often inwardly giving up and adopting an "I don't care" attitude. His private

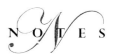

world is void of hope and filled with sorrow. He gravitates toward other young people who relate to his mindset and offer him acceptance. Sexual exploits often become another way to cope with his growing unhappiness or bolstering his sagging ego. Even more dangerous, however, is the tendency this young person has toward considering suicide as a means of retaliating against the illusive enemies of his mind and quieting the torment that robs him of real joy. Having no healthy respect toward God, self-murder seems a reasonable solution.

Christian parents often make the mistake of challenging a rebelling child's salvation (You couldn't possibly be saved and act like this!) or presuming the child is a believer on the basis of a prayer the child repeated when he was young. Both extremes have the potential to do great harm, either by accusing him unjustly and adding to his fears, or by removing doubts of his salvation when the doubts are a genuine result of having never truly repented of his sin or put his trust in Christ. Never presume to know the heart of your child—even angels restrain themselves from drawing that assumption. It is possible for a child who has truly been redeemed to become rebellious. Being a believer only adds to his conviction and torment because he cannot repeatedly sin against the Lord or rebel against His claim on his life without consequence. In time, he may repent and be drawn back to Christ.

It is also possible for a child to believe he is safe from the torments of hell because he said a prayer, and mother insists he is saved when, in fact, his heart is unregenerate and dead spiritually. It would be disastrous to assure such a child when he needs to question his own salvation. Do not attempt to persuade him that he is or is not saved. It is best to take the position that you cannot know his heart and can only discern from his behavior that there is something seriously wrong in his life spiritually. It might be wise to let him know you see no evidence at the moment that the Holy Spirit lives within him and encourage him to examine his faith. But do not be so presumptuous to make an emphatic pronouncement regarding his salvation one way or another unless the child himself has stated that he does not believe and is not saved. In such a case, take him at his word and entreat him as you would any lost person.

Older Rebellious Children

As a child grows older, his defiance tends to become increasingly more difficult to control or resolve. When children are young, they are like a young tree that can be bent and redirected fairly easily. As the tree grows, it is less bendable and takes much more patience and care to get it growing in a different direction. When it reaches maturity, however, the tree no longer bends at all. At this stage, change is only possible when the tree is broken. This is not to say the parent breaks the "tree," but reality is that the parent must now realize his own efforts to change the child will likely be firmly resisted. In such a case, parents can be encouraged that their prayers on behalf of their child have not lost their power and their love is as powerful as it ever was. It does mean that you will need to change the way you deal with your child, recognizing that allowing him to leave home to pursue his own way may be the only means by which his will is broken and he returns in repentance. Use the story of the prodigal son's father as a pattern as to how you should respond. Let the child go, but do not give up on him. Watch and pray, keep the door open, and be ready and willing to forgive the moment he turns back home in repentance.

Do not allow a grown and rebellious child to control you or demand you support him financially, particularly when he is unwilling to work or live in your home peaceably. Many parents get caught in the trap of believing they must continue to house and feed their grown child so he does not "end up on the streets" or worse. Rather than protect your child, you are merely enabling him to continue an irresponsible life at your expense. Your son or daughter might not repent of his foolishness in any other way than to be broken by his own sin or the consequences rebellion inevitably brings. He has refused your discipline and authority, but that does not mean he has escaped God's discipline or authority. God uses means to bring us to repentance. In childhood, our parents are God's primary tools; but in adulthood, the tools merely change. Your rebelling child will eventually be confronted with a greater authority and more painful discipline than anything he experienced at home. Do not interfere with God's work. Be compassionate, be loving, and be kind—but do not jump in to spare your child painful consequences he actually needs.

Things to remember when dealing with older rebellious children:

- Explaining "why" or giving "lectures" rarely, if ever, brings about an apology such as "Will you forgive me for shouting or treating you unkindly?" Hoping an angry child will "understand" and comply if you explain, beg, or give more is a futile attempt!

- An angry child will be angry no matter what you give him, and no matter how carefully you try to reason with him. Being "more" of anything generally will not work because the child's anger does not originate in something anyone else is or is not doing, but arises out of his own self-centeredness, attitude of superiority (pride), and fears of rejection, failure, or guilt. He yells and accuses, not because something is wrong, but because he wants to feel powerful, wants to dominate, or wants to intimidate and manipulate others in order to get something he wants. This is why reasoning with an angry child is so fruitless an effort. Many things might trigger a temper outbreak or affect its intensity. He will typically be sensitive to changes, failures, or fears of inadequacy. He usually has not developed skills that help him resolve problems or communicate effectively. He talks, but he has a hard time listening.

- An angry child is filled with inner tension that he releases when he blames and accuses others, hurts others, or acts in aggressive or destructive ways. When the child successfully causes someone else to pity him or accept blame, he feels justified for his anger. When he is able to get others to accept blame, or accuse those he is blaming, he is able to convince himself that someone else provoked and caused his anger; therefore, he is not responsible for his anger. Often someone else *will* be guilty of some small fault that is used by an angry child to justify his outbursts. The fault is usually blown up out of proportion so much that it is obviously unreasonable—to everyone, that is, except the angry child. This does not faze the angry child nor cause him to "see" how unreasonable he is being; for if he admitted that someone or something did not cause his anger, he would have to face the reality that he himself is the problem; and this is precisely what an angry child will fight with all his might to avoid. To admit wrong would mean he would lose his justification for blowing up and would not have the freedom to release the angry tension that builds up within him, at someone else's expense.

Things to do when dealing with rebellious children:

- Firmly and clearly set limits on what you will and will not tolerate from your child.

- Deal with each angry and sinful response as it happens, not later after the fact. Do *not* deal with issues that happened earlier or issues that might happen in the future. Always deal only with what is happening RIGHT NOW!

- Call the child's attention to the fact that he is acting in a sinful and angry way. Do not threaten or bargain with him by saying, "If you do this, I'll do that…" Rather, *authoritatively* state the fact that you will not accept angry outbursts, (or unkind words, etc.) Always identify specifically what he is doing or saying that is unacceptable. Then tell him flatly, STOP IT! Look your child right in the eyes, stand, or sit erect. Do not whine or argue or plead! Mean what you say, and say what you mean! Then say no more!

- Leave the room when the angry child resorts to manipulative responses such as pouting or withdrawing in silence. Do not be bothered or manipulated into responding to his immaturity or silent treatment tactics to get a response from you. Ignore him! Go get busy doing something.

- When your child begins to argue or angrily challenge something you've said, DO NOT continue to argue. While it is fine to express a differing view, it is absolutely unacceptable if he does not express his views and opinions in a *respectful* and *godly* manner. Do not get pulled into an argument or attempt to correct his effort to refute or misconstrue something you've said. Again, say firmly, "STOP!" then REPEAT your original statement without attempting to explain what you said or meant.

- DO NOT make attempts to defend yourself if your angry child accuses you of ridiculous acts, etc. Say firmly, "STOP accusing me, NOW." Make a flat statement letting the child know that you are not ruffled by his irrational accusation and "he knows better than that."

- DO NOT accept sarcastic humor that is a disguised put down or act defensively if he tells you he was "just joking." Instead say, "Do you feel more important when you laugh at me (or put me down, or speak to me rudely)?" Then LEAVE the room calmly and redirect your attention.

- If you ask your child a question, and he responds with an accusation or a statement designed to divert you or distract you from your question, DO NOT RESPOND TO THE DIVERSION statement! Instead, repeat your question firmly. Say firmly, "STOP trying to change the subject." Then repeat it again until he answers it.

- You must not respond to his denials of wrong doing by trying to explain how he hurts you or others. Disregard statements like, "I don't know what you are talking about"; "You just don't have a sense of humor"; "You're crazy"; "You're making things up"; "You're getting upset at nothing"; or "I never said that." ***Do not pay attention to such words at all!*** Do not try to analyze, understand, or reason with the abusive words of an angry child. You are not going crazy. The problem is in the heart of the rebelling, abusive child. If you get caught in the trap of doubting your perceptions and accepting blame, you will not have a chance to deal with this kind of abusive, angry behavior in a constructive or effective way.

- An angry adult child will often engage in sarcastic criticisms, treat your efforts or concerns with contempt or disgust, make light of your views, undermine your authority or dignity, and laugh or scorn when you are experiencing pain or make some mistake. These and other equally destructive tactics all reveal the abusive and angry child's cruelty and attempts to fixate on the failures of others in order to satisfy his own unreasonable whims. He blames others for his own sin in an effort to manage his own guilt when he does not want to face his sin or deal with it. Often, he is cruel as a means of taking vengeance into his own hands for wrongs that were committed against him in childhood, or that he believes were committed against him.

- If you have committed real offenses against your child, it is very, very important that you deal with your sin by acknowledging the painful effects your sin has had upon others, accepting full responsibility for your actions, and asking your child's forgiveness. Once you have done this, DO NOT continue to apologize to your child or allow the child to continue expressing his outrage over the offense. If he forgave you, remind him that forgiveness means he will leave it in God's hands to correct you; he will not bring it up again; he will not dwell on the offense; and he will restore full fellowship. If he refuses to forgive, remind him that refusing to forgive others results in emotional torment *(Matthew 18:34-35)* and puts him in great spiritual peril.

Angry children want to believe they are angry because of wrongs others have committed against them. This is a form of self-deception that allows the child to excuse his behavior in an effort to assuage guilt. DO NOT cave in to his self-pity. This will only encourage him to continue blaming others for his sinful anger and selfishness. On the other hand, do not minimize or excuse sinful wrongs that have been committed against the child. Acknowledge them and call them wicked. Offer understanding with regard to the ways they have wounded the child. Explain that calling such offenses sin and recognizing them for what they are is righteous. Taking vengeance upon offenders that belongs to God alone or responding with anger and rebellion toward God is a sinful response that will only alienate a child from God's fellowship, which is the only means of finding comfort that can heal his wounded heart. Remind him how God views the mistreatment of a child and how He has promised to deal with it in His time and in His way *(Romans 12:19; 1 Thessalonians 4:6,8)*. At the same time, God is able to work in such a miraculous way that even such wickedness can be turned around for good in the victim's life if the child will but trust Him and turn to Him for help. God "healeth the broken in heart, and bindeth up their wounds" *(Psalm 147:3)*.

In Conclusion

When our children are young, we vaccinate them in order to prevent childhood diseases that have a devastating impact on their physical health, thus sparing them from harm. Christian parents who understand the perils of the sinful human heart are given the means to "vaccinate" their children against spiritual diseases that are capable of destroying a child's spiritual health and well-being before he is even grown. Our children are better able to deal with life's trials when we obey God's commands to love our children, to treat our children with gentleness and understanding, to protect our children from those who would undermine their budding faith, and to train our children to know and love the Scriptures. Above all, we inoculate our children when we model a healthy relationship with the Lord Jesus Christ and teach our children how to appropriate God's love and forgiveness and how to "come boldly to the throne of grace to obtain mercy and find grace to help in time of need" *(Hebrews 6:16)*. Insisting on our child's respect and obedience, training them to deal with offenses humbly and honestly, and deliberately teaching them how to obtain God's wisdom in order to resolve life's problems and trials all strengthen and equip our children to withstand the fiery darts of the devil. No loving parent would think to send his child out to play in ten-degree weather without a coat to protect him from the cold. May we never send our children out to play in a world filled with perils of every sort without the protection of God's wisdom, knowledge, and understanding. *Dangerous Parenting Detours* by Walt Brock offers valuable insight into how parents lead their children down the wrong road toward rebellion.

How Parents Discourage Their Children

Colossians 3:21—Fathers, provoke not your children to anger, lest they be discouraged.

Parental Anger and Pride

____ Marital conflicts, shouting, tension, threats

____ Reacting to everyday problems with anger, bitterness, and criticism

____ Disciplining in explosive anger and rage

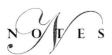

____ Refusing to acknowledge their own wrongs while demanding that children do

Parental Neglect

____ Not meeting your child's legitimate needs (not his demands)

____ Not understanding your child's difficulties and encouraging him

____ Not listening to your child; or regarding his thoughts and ideas unimportant

____ Not making it possible for your child to develop special interests of his own

____ Not disciplining consistently with love and firmness

____ Not setting and enforcing reasonable limits and restrictions for your child

____ Not investing adequate time in your child's life

____ Not keeping your promises

Injustices - Offenses Committed against a Child by a Parent

____ Favoritism, taking pride in one child's accomplishments over another

____ Humiliating your child by such things as scolding him in front of others, making fun of his failures or physical characteristics, or calling him demeaning names

____ Over-disciplining or physical abuse

____ Sexual exploitation or failure to protect your child from sexual exploitation

____ Unreasonable, unrealistic expectations and demands

____ Arbitrary, confusing, or harsh rules and restrictions

____ Blaming, unjust accusations, or drawing conclusions without listening to child's side of story or investigating all the facts

Parental Hypocrisy

____ Professing godliness publicly while living in ungodly ways privately

____ Privately criticizing church members while publicly treating them with kindness

____ Demonstrating a lack of genuine love for God

____ Showing no zeal or faith in God's promises

____ Disrespecting God's commandments

____ Being apathetic towards church attendance or responsibilities

____ Neglecting family's needs while caring for the needs of others

____ Over-involvement with church work while neglecting home and family

____ Complaining or rebelling against rules or restrictions

____ Refusing to respect or submit to authority

____ Dishonesty, lying to cover up failure, exaggerating

____ Criticizing spouse to win child's sympathy

NOTES

Answers For Discussion Problem on page 189

What emotions do you believe you would have experienced during this lecture?

- Would you have been glad to be there or would you have wanted to get up and walk out?
- Would you have sensed that the principal loved you, or that he was disgusted by you?
- Would his speech have made you love or despise him?
- Would you have felt respect or disrespect toward him?
- Would this have made you want to confide in him or come to him with a personal problem or would it have convinced you he was the last person in the world you would ever confide in?
- Would this have provoked a defensive attitude, or a tender submissive spirit?
- Would you have felt angry about, or appreciative of his assessment?
- Would this little "pep" talk have left you feeling encouraged or discouraged?
- Would this talk have made you want to work harder at being responsible or give up trying to please?
- At any time during the "speech" do you believe you would have felt led to repent?

What is wrong with this lecture?

- He started out with the pronoun *you* and made a sweeping accusation.
- He berated you as Christian leaders.
- He falsely accused *all* of you of wasting time.
- His speculation was made into fact.
- He did not investigate the coffee incident or the walk outside. Had he done so, he would have learned that your class was having music, and you were on a legitimate coffee break and that the teacher walking across the front of the building was hurrying to the restroom.
- He falsely accused you of having no regard for parent's sacrifice and totally disregarded your personal sacrifices on behalf of the students and parents.
- He attributed your apparent failure as a serious character flaw of irresponsibility and a willful refusal to obey authority.
- He judged your heart and motives, which God forbids us to do.
- He condemned you for your apparent failure with absolutely no effort to discover truth, correct, or build up your faith.
- He misjudged your behavior and exaggerated it to the point of labeling it *rebellious*, a sin worse than witchcraft.

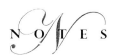

- He wrongly attributed all school failure to you and declared you responsible for whatever is wrong.
- He falsely accused you of laughing disrespectfully during a sermon when in fact you were laughing because of something funny in the sermon.
- He assumed the note seen passed was devious even though he did not see what was written.
- He accused you of spiritual apathy and used derogatory terms to further condemn you and support his supposed "right" to be angry with you.
- He created a sense of guilt to manipulate you into agreeing with him.
- He used unjustifiable fear as a motivation to change behavior.
- He grossly misrepresented God and God's attitude toward you.

What scriptural violations are involved?
- No self-evaluation first—in violation of *Matthew 7:2-5; Romans 2:21-23*
- No effort to determine truth before confronting—in violation of *Proverbs 18:13*
- Condemning (judging) another—in violation of *Matthew 7:1*
- Raising a false report—in violation of *Exodus 23:1*
- Falsely accusing another without cause—in violation of *Proverbs 24:28*
- Misrepresenting God—in violation of *Leviticus 19:11*
- Desirous of God's curse upon another—in violation of *Job 31:30; Psalm 38:16*
- Using vengeance to "punish" others—in violation of *Romans 12:19*
- Using malicious words to confront others—in violation of *Ephesians 4:31*
- Using evil to overcome evil—in violation of *Romans 12; 1 Peter 3:9*
- Using hatred to express outrage—in violation of *Titus 3:3*
- Withholding mercy—in violation of *James 2:13*
- Lack of love for brothers and sisters in Chris—in violation of *1 John 3:10; 4:20*
- Abuse of authority—in violation of *Colossians 3:21; James 3:1; 2 Corinthians 10:8*
- Failure to provide a godly pattern—in violation of *Titus 2:7; Philippians 3:17*
- Failure to handle the Word of God carefully—in violation of *2 Corinthians 4:1-2*

What serious spiritual problems and sins are revealed in this speech?
- Lack of mercy, love, forgiveness, patience, self-control, humility, understanding—or in other words a *lack of spiritual fruit.*
- No correct application of truth = no wisdom

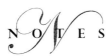

How would the following Scriptures apply to this lecture?

- For, brethren, ye have been called unto liberty; only use not liberty for an occasion to the flesh, but by love serve one another. For all the law is fulfilled in one word, even in this; thou shalt love thy neighbor as thyself. But if ye bite and devour one another, take heed that ye be not consumed one of another. This I say then, Walk in the Spirit, and ye shall not fulfill the lust [desires] of the flesh. For the flesh lusteth [wars] against the Spirit, and the Spirit against the flesh; and these are contrary the one to the other; so that ye cannot do the things that ye would....*But the fruit of the Spirit is love, joy, peace, longsuffering, gentleness, goodness, faith, meekness, temperance*....Let us not be desirous of vainglory, provoking one another, envying one another.... *Galatians 5:13-25*

- ...The diseased have ye not strengthened, neither have ye healed that which was sick, neither have ye bound up that which was broken, neither have ye brought again that which was driven away, neither have ye sought that which was lost; but with force and with cruelty have ye ruled them. *Ezekiel 34:2*

- That no man go beyond and defraud [oppress] his brother in any matter; because that the Lord is the avenger of all such, as we also have forewarned you and testified. He therefore that despiseth, despiseth not man, but God, who hath also given unto us his Holy Spirit. *1 Thessalonians 4:6,8*

Lesson 10

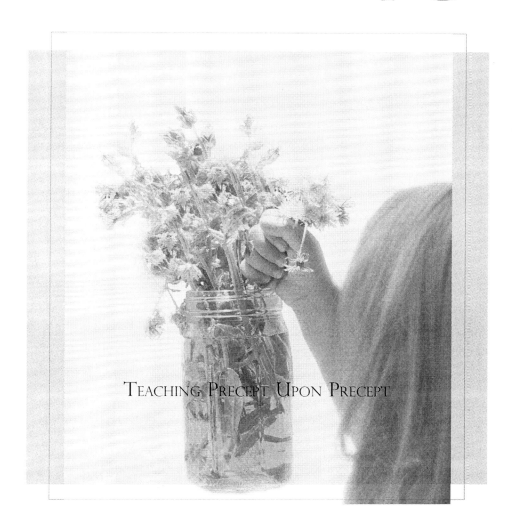

Teaching Precept Upon Precept

Whom shall he teach knowledge? And whom shall he make to understand doctrine? Them that are weaned from the milk, and drawn from the breasts. For precept must be upon precept, precept upon precept; line upon line, line upon line; here a little, and there a little.
Isaiah 28:9-10

But continue thou in the things which thou hast learned and hast been assured of, knowing of whom thou hast learned them; and that from a child thou hast known the holy scriptures, which are able to make thee wise unto salvation through faith which is in Christ Jesus.
2 Timothy 3:15

Key Thoughts

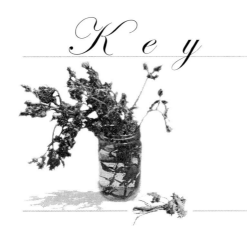

"Train up a child in the way he should go, and when he is old he will not depart from it" (*Proverbs 22:6*). This verse is not only a command given by God to parents, but also a prerequisite to the promise of God's blessing on the lives of our children. Training involves a deliberate process of teaching and educating through patient instruction and repeated practice.

Discussion Problem

Four-year-old Kari is keenly interested in what other people are doing. She wants to know why her Grandpa smokes cigarettes and why that lady "doesn't have much clothes on." Kari asks "why" continuously and is very eager to learn explanations for everything. Whatever her mother would tell her, Kari would accept; but her mother isn't interested in taking time to explain. Her mother and father don't believe their children need to know the reasons behind their actions and beliefs, but should concentrate on merely obeying and conforming to their wishes. Kari's older sister, Linda, is thirteen years old and becoming very rebellious. She tells her girlfriends how silly her parents' rules are and is already talking about leaving home as soon as she's eighteen.

After reading lesson ten, use the principles you learn to discuss the possible reasons Linda may be rebelling against her parents' wishes. How could Kari's parents be wrong in their dealing with Kari's question? What misconceptions may be contributing to their children's attitudes? Why should Kari's mother take more time answering questions or teaching her children?

Bible Study

1. According to Exodus 13:8-16, we can infer that children learn when they are given a visual _____ of God's ways and purposes.

2. In Deuteronomy 4:9-10, we read that God wants parents to be transparent, honest, and descriptive about God's work in their lives as a means of _____ their children to love and respect God.

3. Deuteronomy 6:6-9 explains that God wants parents to freely talk about _____ and how it applies to everyday situations and problems as things come up in family life day by day.

"My mother was the source from which I derived the guiding principles of my life."
John Wesley

Precept upon Precept

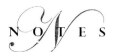

It has been said that life is made up of many small events. Most big changes in our lives occur as a result of many little decisions, rather than a few major decisions. Every achievement, every building, every big event, and every person are built little by little, hour upon hour, one day at a time. We become what we are as a result of common day-by-day decisions and events, most of which go unnoticed and are seldom remembered as significant when they occur.

In ancient Israel, women would spend countless hours at a loom, weaving threads of carefully prepared wool into tapestries that would then be used for garments or home furnishings. A piece of fabric could only be made by tightly weaving one thread at a time, one on top of another, over and over, until the fabric began to expand and take shape. One thread hardly appeared to make a difference. Even several threads seemed an insignificant accomplishment. The task required perseverance and vision in order to keep a woman repeating the painstaking process of weaving hour after hour, day after day, one tiny thread at a time, until a large enough piece of fabric was finished.

In Isaiah's day, God rebuked Israel because they did not take seriously the prophet's efforts to painstakingly teach them God's truth, one precept at a time. Isaiah used the vivid example of women weaving one thread at a time (or line, as it is called in the *King James Version*) in order to make a whole piece of fabric. He compared the method the prophets were using to impart the knowledge of God to the way young children are taught. Isaiah tells us that the prophets were consistent and persevering in their preaching and teaching.

Prophets taught a little at a time, building one concept on another, in order to help the people of Israel understand God and grow strong. The prophet's efforts were compared to the weaver who is dedicated to weaving one thread at a time. The comparison holds true for a mother or father who teaches their children skills and good behavior one little concept at a time.

Isaiah 28:9-10 says, "Whom shall he teach knowledge? And whom shall he make to understand doctrine? *Them that are* weaned from the milk, *and* drawn from the breasts. For precept *must* be upon precept, precept upon precept; line upon line, line upon line; here a little, *and* there a little." Good teaching or parenting is not accomplished in big chunks. Rather, a teacher must be willing to patiently teach one concept at a time, building one thought upon another until the knowledge and character of his student develops and noticeably begins to change to reflect the teacher's hard work. Because the effects of good parenting are not instantly noticeable, many parents foolishly assume that an investment of their time and influence is not crucial to their children's welfare. These parents also fail to realize how all their *little* angry words and *little* selfish indulgences add up and affect their children's personality, confidence, and spiritual health.

In *Proverbs 14:1*, God compares building the relationships and lives of family members to building a house. He says, "Every wise woman buildeth her house: but the foolish plucketh it down with her hands." A wise woman quietly and painstakingly builds the people who make up her home. Like the weaver, she adds one little thread at a time, knowing that eventually her patience and hard work will pay off. A foolish woman does not recognize how her selfish disregard for the way she conducts her life and vents her anger damages her family. She carelessly tears her family members apart, one little incident at a time, one day at a time, until there is nothing left standing that would resemble a happy home or family. It didn't "just happen." She pulled her home down one brick at a time until it simply collapsed. A bowl left under a dripping faucet doesn't fill quickly. One drip of water hardly seems to make a difference, but one drip of water at a time, dropping slowly and methodically from the faucet will eventually fill the bowl until one drop will cause the water to overflow the edge.

Again in *Deuteronomy 6*, God presumes parents are spending time with their children and instructs them to make use of common daily-life incidents to teach God's love and care. First, the parents are instructed to love God with all their heart and soul and might. Then they are told to impart the knowledge of God's truths as opportunities arise throughout each day. *Deuteronomy 6:6-7* says, "And these words, which I command thee this day, shall be in thine heart: and thou shalt teach them diligently unto thy children, and shalt talk of them when thou sittest in thine house, and when thou walkest by the way, and when thou liest down, and when thou risest up." God is not instructing parents to use such conversation as a time to scold children or incite them to "tune out" or become resentful. Wise parents would never use the Bible as a weapon. Rather, God is instructing parents to engage in conversation that draws a child into discussion and causes him to marvel at God's wisdom and love. When discussions about God take place from the earliest years of childhood, it is a natural part of everyday life that children accept and enjoy. Begun later, it may seem awkward to children at first, or may seem that parents are lecturing or scolding. Parents saved as adults will want to be especially sensitive to the way abrupt changes in family life can affect older children, and be careful not to overwhelm their children in their zeal to establish a Christian home.

Children are not taught the most meaningful principles of life in times of formal family instruction as much as they are by example and by little instructions and comments woven throughout the day. Teaching children a little here and a little there accomplishes far more than instructing them in large doses. This truth functions whether you are teaching them common-sense facts of life, instructing them on how to do a task or project, preparing them for their future, or explaining God's truths. The majority of instruction should be given indirectly in small doses, so as not to produce resistance or overload them with information. To be most effective, it must also be mixed with enjoyment and given only as a child is ready for the truth.

Sometimes parents produce powerful impressions indirectly through such things as the music they play or allow in their home, the way they have fun, or the importance they place on faithfulness to the local church family. People who converse within earshot of children also make lasting impressions, good and bad. Little ears are

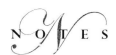

The most effective way to teach children about the ways and love of God is all the time, little by little, as the family performs the duties of a normal day.

listening, and little minds silently reason as Mom and Dad talk together in the car, throughout the day, or on the telephone. The greatest family devotions are not always carried out at a specific time and place, even though daily or weekly family devotions can certainly be a source of great encouragement and strength to a family. The most effective way to teach children about the ways and love of God is all the time, little by little, as the family performs the duties of a normal day.

Parents teach most effectively when they demonstrate how to meet daily trials and perplexities in godly ways. The way we handle life's trials and the explanations and reasons we give for our faith influence the hearts of our children. Yet it is not enough just to live our faith—we must give reasons for what we believe if we expect to make a lasting imprint on their hearts and minds. Experiences make permanent impressions like a handprint in wet cement when we connect what God has said in His Word with the way we are choosing to respond. For instance, we might explain to our children that we have a calm assurance our problems are a normal part of our earthly experience and never occur without God's watchful care because God said "there hath no temptation [trial] taken you but such as is common to man; but God is faithful [He cannot lie], who will not suffer [allow] you to be tempted [tried] above that ye are able; but will with the temptations also make a way to escape, that ye may be able to bear it" *(1 Corinthians 10:13)*. We respond with confidence knowing God will always help us when we call upon Him because He said, "Call upon me in the day of trouble; I will deliver thee, and thou shalt glorify me" *(Psalm 50:15)*. We are not ruffled when afflictions come because God said, "Many are the afflictions of the righteous; but the Lord delivereth him out of them all" *(Psalm 34:19)*.

Examples of "Little-by-Little" Teaching

"Mommy is making cookies for Mrs. Wilson next door even though she is a mean lady because God tells us the only way to overcome evil is with good. Would you like to help me take them to her and see how she acts then?" *(Romans 12:21)*. "Mommy isn't upset that Aunt Susie didn't say thank you because Jesus said He never forgets our work and labor of love when we serve others for Him" *(Hebrews 6:10)*. "Daddy is studying the Bible so he can be wise and know what God wants Him to do. He wants to be like the man who built his house on a rock, not like the one who built his house on sand. Do you remember what happened when the storms came and rained on those two houses?" *(Matthew 7:24-25)*. "Son, I'm so thankful that God has given you the grace to refrain from reacting in anger even though your friend was unfair in the way he treated you. God is pleased too, because He said that the man who is slow to anger and able to rule his own spirit is stronger and greater than the man who is able to govern a city or a country" *(Proverbs 16:32)*. "God hears the prayers of little children just as much as the prayers of mommies and daddies. Would you like to see where God tells you that?" *(Exodus 22:23; 1 Samuel 3:10; Matthew 19:14)*. "Let's play a Bible game. Who can find the five alls in the thirty-fourth chapter of Psalm? These are the promises that are helping your mother and I remember not to worry even though Daddy doesn't have a job right now."

Results of "Little-by-Little" Teaching

Needless to say, establishing a happy Christian home requires both commitment and a considerable investment of time and effort. Furthermore, the home will only become spiritually strong if it is built with the specific materials that God has provided. "Through wisdom is an house builded; and by understanding it is established: and by knowledge shall the chambers be filled with all precious and pleasant riches" *(Proverbs 24:3-4)*. Parents are able to build a godly and stable home only as they lean on God's wisdom, understand and practice God's ways, and invest time to deliberately teach their children how to live by principles found in God's Word. The results may not always appear to be immediate as mom and dad patiently build, brick upon brick, here a little, there a little. Slowly the foundations and framework are established as parents learn and then put into practice Biblical principles. Finally, the home takes shape; the rooms are decorated and filled with precious things; and it stands strong as an oasis from the storms of life, a place of refreshment, fellowship, and joy. No amount of money or worldly honor can compare with the happiness such a home brings as the years go by.

The mother and father who learn God's wisdom will, in time to come, rejoice and enjoy the fruits of their labor. Many mothers through the centuries have been encouraged to persevere in their devotion to the welfare of their families by the promises that are given in *Proverbs 31:25, 28, 30-31*. "Strength and honor are her clothing; and she shall rejoice in time to come. Her children arise up, and call her blessed; her husband also, and he praiseth her. Favor is deceitful, and beauty is vain: but a woman that feareth the LORD, she shall be praised. Give her of the fruit of her hands; and let her own works praise her in the gates." God provides promises for fathers who are faithful to Him as well. He tells us, "The just man walketh in his integrity; his children are blessed after him" *(Proverbs 20:7)*. And, "Mark the perfect [mature] man, and behold the upright; for the end of that man is peace" *(Psalm 37:37)*.

Growth Is a Gradual Process

Can you imagine a father sending his three-year-old son out to mow the yard, trim the hedges, and spread the fertilizer? Or a mother handing her six-year-old daughter the car keys and telling her to drive herself to the mall and buy a dress? What teacher would distribute a college level calculus book to her fourth graders and expect them to be ready for their first calculus test the following day? No reasonable adult has any problem understanding such requests would be downright absurd, not to mention illegal or insane. Yet many responsible and loving Christian parents often expect the equivalent from their children spiritually. Many parents seem to forget that spiritual growth, like physical growth, is a gradual and learned process. For instance, the ability to understand spiritual concepts, deny self, give for mature motives, obey from the heart, or persevere in difficulty characterize Christian maturity, not the new babe in Christ. A child is not necessarily sinning simply because he has difficulty understanding and applying spiritual concepts and perspective.

We are told that although Jesus was the Son of God, "yet learned he obedience by the things which he suffered" *(Hebrews 5:8)*. As a youngster, Luke records that "Jesus increased in wisdom and stature, and in favor with God and man" *(Luke 2:52)*. If Jesus, the perfect Son of God needed to learn such things as obedience through things that he suffered, should we then expect our *imperfect* little children to learn such things as unwavering obedience immediately simply because we demand them to do so? Such an expectation would be absurd and lead to certain discouragement of the child, not to mention untold misery to the parent who entertains such a notion. Learning to obey willingly for mature motives comes only as a parent invests many hours teaching, disciplining, encouraging, warning, correcting, practicing, explaining, and chastising. This holds true whether we are training our children to be unselfish, to trust in God's care, love others, exercise restraint, discipline their thought life, forgive, suffer persecution, endure hardship, or exercise the many privileges of believers saved by grace. Children who read the Scriptures without careful oversight and instruction can become confused, for some things are hard to understand and easy to misunderstand without help. Peter tells young believers who face this same danger to "grow in grace, and in the knowledge of our Lord and Savior Jesus Christ" *(2 Peter 3:18)*.

Children grow physically as they are fed good food, beginning with mother's breast milk. The eager newborn roots for his mother's warm breast as soon as his tiny cheeks are stroked or pressed against her body. At first he needs assistance finding the nipple, but once he tastes his mother's milk, he begins to crave it whenever he senses hunger. It doesn't take long before he becomes quite adept at locating his food. First the baby tastes; then the baby develops a strong desire. In the same way, our children develop a strong desire for the things of God and the Word of God only when they first taste how good God's love is. Peter compares new believers to newborn babies and tells them to "desire the sincere [uncontaminated] milk of the word, that ye may grow thereby; if so be ye have tasted that the Lord is gracious" *(1 Peter 2:2-3)*. A child's "first tastes" of the Lord's gracious and loving nature need to be deliberately cultivated and encouraged in order for the child to grow in his desire for spiritual truth. Children cannot grow spiritually enough to digest soft foods and meat unless they have first been taught that God is good.

In many ways, the growth process in our own Christian life parallels the growth process in our children's lives. We grow in grace one step at a time, little by little, not instantaneously. Christian maturity is not accomplished in one revival meeting or at one crisis-point in our life. God does not give us instant knowledge or instant godliness. We mature spiritually a little at a time, one event at a time, one little success at a time, with one piece of understanding built upon another throughout

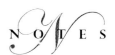

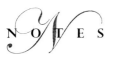

the years. Sometimes big changes occur in our lives, but most often change occurs in small advancements.

Jesus used many means to convey spiritual truth and build his disciple's faith in the years they were being prepared for future ministry. When Peter was invited to walk on water but then became afraid, Jesus stretched out His hand to pull him up and said, "O thou of little faith, wherefore didst thou doubt?" *(Matthew 14:31)*. Jesus was pleased with the faith Peter *did* demonstrate, but commented that he had *little* faith—not "no" faith—then proceeded to increase Peter's faith and understanding a little at a time with each new incident and challenge. Years later Peter was able to write with perfect understanding that believers become partakers of Christ's nature by appropriating the promises of the Bible, mastering one building block of the faith after another. "And beside this, giving all diligence, add to your faith virtue; and to virtue knowledge; and to knowledge temperance; and to temperance patience; and to patience godliness; and to godliness brotherly kindness; and to brotherly kindness charity" *(2 Peter 1:5-7)*.

Building Blocks of Spiritual Growth

2 Peter 1:5-7—And beside this, giving all diligence, add to your faith virtue; and to virtue knowledge; and to knowledge temperance; and to temperance patience; and to patience godliness; and to godliness brotherly kindness; and to brotherly kindness charity.

	GROWTH IN NEW BELIEVER	GROWTH IN CHILDREN
LOVE	Ability to respond to God out of love, serve out of motive of love, and give of self to others out of love for them.	Ability to be unselfish, giving, and obedient out of love instead of being motivated by fear or chastisement.
BROTHERLY KINDNESS	Willingness to forgive and love others sacrificially for Christ's sake.	Ability of child to put himself in another's place and get along with other's; yielding his own rights when necessary.
GODLINESS	Holiness;Godliness; ability to produce spiritual fruit.	Child's spiritual understanding and qualities governing his own life;internalized convictions.
PATIENCE	Ability to perservere in the Christian life in the face of opposition.	Child's ability to perservere, acquire self-discipline; increased attention span.
SELF-CONTROL	Putting into practice all that is learned; becoming responsible; denying self.	Child's ability to control and deny his self-willed nature.
KNOWLEDGE	Continuing understanding of doctrine and all God wishes us to know through the Scriptures in order to live the Christian life.	Ability to learn basis for family rules, limitations, morals.
VIRTUE	Moral excellence; character; inner attitude which is a result of yielding to God's control and leadership.	Seeds of attitude sown as parents establish authority and control; child learns to yield to them.
FAITH	Initial trust, confidence, and reliance on Gospel and love of Christ.	Initial trust in mother; confidence and dependance on her love and care.

NOTES

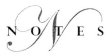

Biblical Methods of Instruction

1. Use Repetition

Children easily forget new concepts. This requires a parent to prepare to cheerfully and patiently teach the same concept over and over and over again in order to engraft it into his child's heart and life. The younger the child, the more repetition will be required. Yet even older children and adults learn through repetition. In noting how Jesus taught His disciples, you may recognize that He often taught the same principle using different means and different situations. Wise parents will seek to do the same.

2. Be Gradual

Children are easily discouraged when adults give too much information too quickly. What and how much information to give depends on the child's age, maturity level, and present ability. A four year old cannot assimilate what a fourteen year old can. Parents set their small children up for failure and destruction when they expect them to deal with temptations, opposition, or confusing concepts before the children have the understanding and ability to resist or cope. A good farmer protects young, tender vines from storms and adverse conditions until they have grown sufficiently to withstand the elements. Children must be protected and gradually taught in the same way.

3. Build a Little at a Time

Everything a little child is allowed to see, hear, or experience forms his tastes and molds the desires he will pursue as a young adult. Music he hears as a toddler will contribute to the musical choices he will make as a teenager. The kind of friends he has been provided as a toddler will form the basis for his taste in friends as a teenager. Books and television programs from childhood will each add a deposit to his bank of understanding, which he will draw upon throughout his life as he makes decisions and chooses a particular course of action. Every experience, incident, influence, impression, and piece of knowledge is foundational to his character and direction.

4. Incorporate Instruction throughout the Daily Routine

Setting children down and lecturing them accomplish little more than teaching children how to quietly endure and tune out a parent's concerns. It is far more effective to teach little lessons throughout the day, in short increments, and in ways that make the lessons enjoyable, rather than tolerable. To "train up a child in the way he should go" *(Proverbs 22:6a)* is to educate a child. When a parent educates, they impart knowledge in ways that evoke an enthusiastic response in our students. As much as possible, children need explanations and reasons behind a parent's actions and choices.

Lack of communication causes young children to become fearful or irritable, while a lack of communication in older children causes resentment and misunderstanding of the parent's wishes. "Because I said so" may silence questions, but it will not help a child who needs ideas and reasons to believe and choose the way he should go. Never let a child distract you, argue with you, or put off obeying you by asking "why." But do tell him you'll be glad to give an explanation *after* he's obeyed, whenever it is possible to do so. Even better, learn to educate and explain to your children why and what you're doing without them ever having to ask.

5. Control Good and Bad Influences

Children are natural imitators. In spite of all a parent's best efforts to teach otherwise, children will still act like their parents or whomever they are around a great deal! Children pick up speech patterns, habits, priorities, attitudes, beliefs, ways of handling disappointment, and irritation from those they are around. Without any effort at all, children unconsciously pattern themselves after whomever and whatever they observe, especially when they like whom they watch. The actions and words of those your child respects have a powerful influence on the development of his interests, desires, and character. This is precisely why advertisers spend millions of dollars on split-second television advertising that targets children. Showing a favorite actor eating a name brand candy bar for a fraction of a second has been shown to dramatically increase sales immediately afterward.

Little children are by nature receptive to whatever they are told. This permits parents the opportunity to rightly influence and teach their children while they are very young and moldable. However, the danger is that it also allows parents and others to easily influence children in a harmful way. Children are not yet able to readily discern evil, nor will they have the understanding or maturity to reject errors or accurately sift through the influences that could be good or harmful to them. Parents must do the sifting for their children even while they teach their children how to discern good and evil for themselves. This, of course, presumes that parents have grown spiritually enough to be skillful in the word of righteousness and have exercised their senses long enough to be able to discern both good and evil according to *Hebrews 5:14*.

Every Christian is responsible to protect and provide for God's littlest lambs, but how much more do Sunday school teachers, Christian school teachers, family members, pastors, and others also have the greatest impact on our children. Even so, parents are the gatekeepers of their children's hearts and minds and must be responsible to guard who comes in and who goes out. Just as you wouldn't think of unnecessarily exposing a baby with compromised health to a nursery worker with full-blown flu symptoms, neither should you unnecessarily expose an impressionable child to anything or anyone whose attitude can forever infect your child's life. The apostle Paul was able to exhort others to follow him to the degree they followed Christ, knowing people need such examples. "Brethren, be followers together of me, and mark them which walk so as ye have us for an ensample" *(Philippians 3:17)*.

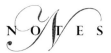

Promises and Warnings

God promises many good things to those who flee wrong influences, and warns of heartache to those who do not. Those who choose wise companions become wise, but those who choose the rebellious as companions are destroyed, according to *Proverbs 16:13*. Wrong influences result in much heartache. Consider the story of Jehoshophat and his wife who associated with unsaved friends. Their child married the unsaved child of their friends and brought untold heartache to himself, his family, and his nation. Consider Lot's children, who were allowed to assimilate into the world and learn the ways of the world. They rejected God and mocked Lot when he tried to warn them to flee. Consider the story of Dinah, Jacob's daughter who went after the wrong kind of fun with the wrong crowd and was sexually violated as a result. Consider Eli's children who were so unrestrained by their father that they preferred the world to God's laws and were destroyed as a result. And finally, consider David's children who were indulged and lacked parental instruction and involvement. They grew up to bring devastating heartache and rebellion to David as a result. The Bible says, "But Amnon had a friend...." and goes on to describe the influence Amnon's friend had on Amnon to do evil. God tells us of these and so many more that were influenced by friends who led them astray. Do not underestimate how much your child is taught by his friends and those who have an entrance into his life.

- Who are your children's friends?
- Where do your children receive advice?
- Who and what entertains your children?

Scriptural Truths about Things and People That Influence

2 Corinthians 6:14-18—Be ye not unequally yoked together with unbelievers: for what fellowship hath righteousness with unrighteousness? And what communion hath light with darkness? And what concord hath Christ with Belial? Or what part hath he that believeth with an infidel? And what agreement hath the temple of God with idols? For ye are the temple of the living God; as God hath said, I will dwell in them, and walk in *them*; and I will be their God, and they shall be my people. Wherefore come out from among them, and be ye separate, saith the Lord, and touch not the unclean *thing*; and I will receive you, And will be a Father unto you, and ye shall be my sons and daughters, saith the Lord Almighty.

1 Corinthians 15:33—Be not deceived: evil communications corrupt good manners.

2 Timothy 2:21—If a man therefore purge himself from these, he shall be a vessel unto honor, sanctified, and meet for the master's use, *and* prepared unto every good work.

Isaiah 59:1-3—Behold, the LORD'S hand is not shortened, that it cannot save; neither his ear heavy, that it cannot hear: but your iniquities have separated between you and your God, and your sins have hid his face from you, that he will not hear.

For your hands are defiled with blood, and your fingers with iniquity; your lips have spoken lies, your tongue hath muttered perverseness.

1 John 3:21-22—Beloved, if our heart condemn us not, *then* have we confidence toward God. And whatsoever we ask, we receive of him, because we keep his commandments, and do those things that are pleasing in his sight.

Scriptural Truths about Things and People To Avoid

Avoid those who hate God.
2 Chronicles 19:2—And Jehu the son of Hanani the seer went out to meet him, and said to king Jehoshaphat, Shouldest thou help the ungodly, and love them that hate the LORD? Therefore is wrath upon thee from before the LORD.

Avoid those who are angry.
Proverbs 22:24-25—Make no friendship with an angry man; and with a furious man thou shalt not go: Lest thou learn his ways, and get a snare to thy soul.

Avoid those who are foolish.
Proverbs 13:20—He that walketh with wise men shall be wise: but a companion of fools shall be destroyed.

Proverbs 14:7—Go from the presence of a foolish man, when thou perceivest not in him the lips of knowledge.

Avoid those who cause division and strife.
Romans 16:17-18—Now I beseech you, brethren, mark them which cause divisions and offences contrary to the doctrine which ye have learned; and avoid them. For they that are such serve not our Lord Jesus Christ, but their own belly; and by good words and fair speeches deceive the hearts of the simple.

Avoid those who are froward.
Proverbs 22:5—Thorns and snares are in the way of the froward: he that doth keep his soul shall be far from them.

Note: A *froward* person is perverse. He persists in error. He is self-willed and stubborn. *Webster's 1828 Dictionary* defines *froward* as "not willing to yield or comply with what is required; unyielding; ungovernable; refractory; disobedient; peevish."

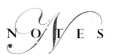

Avoid those who are evil.

Psalm 26:5—I have hated the congregation of evil doers; and will not sit with the wicked.

Proverbs 12:26—The righteous is more excellent than his neighbor: but the way of the wicked seduceth them.

Proverbs 24:1—Be not thou envious against evil men, neither desire to be with them.

Ephesians 5:6-7—Let no man deceive you with vain words: for because of these things cometh the wrath of God upon the children of disobedience. Be not ye therefore partakers with them.

Ephesians 5:11—And have no fellowship with the unfruitful works of darkness, but rather reprove them.

Avoid those who follow the world's philosophies.

Jeremiah 10:2—Thus saith the Lord, Learn not the way of the heathen, and be not dismayed at the signs of heaven; for the heathen are dismayed at them.

Romans 12:2—And be not conformed to this world: but be ye transformed by the renewing of your mind, that ye may prove what is that good, and acceptable, and perfect, will of God.

Galatians 5:7-9—Ye did run well; who did hinder you that ye should not obey the truth? This persuasion *cometh* not of him that calleth you. A little leaven leaveneth the whole lump.

Colossians 2:8—Beware lest any man spoil you through philosophy and vain deceit, after the tradition of men, after the rudiments of the world, and not after Christ.

James 1:27—Pure religion and undefiled before God and the Father is this, To visit the fatherless and widows in their affliction, and to keep himself unspotted from the world.

James 4:4—Ye adulterers and adulteresses, know ye not that the friendship of the world is enmity with God? Whosoever therefore will be a friend of the world is the enemy of God.

Avoid those who teach false doctrine.

Exodus 23:32-33—Thou shalt make no covenant with them, nor with their gods. They shall not dwell in thy land, lest they make thee sin against me: for if thou serve their gods, it will surely be a snare unto thee.

2 John 10—If there come any unto you, and bring not this doctrine, receive him not into your house, neither bid him God speed.

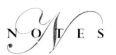

Avoid other Christians who love the world.

Psalm 1:1-2—Blessed *is* the man that walketh not in the counsel of the ungodly, nor standeth in the way of sinners, nor sitteth in the seat of the scornful. But his delight *is* in the law of the LORD; and in his law doth he meditate day and night.

1 Corinthians 5:9-11—I wrote unto you in an epistle not to company with fornicators: yet not altogether with the fornicators of this world, or with the covetous, or extortioners, or with idolaters; for then must ye needs go out of the world. But now I have written unto you not to keep company, if any man that is called a brother be a fornicator, or covetous, or an idolater, or a railer, or a drunkard, or an extortioner; with such an one no not to eat.

1 Corinthians 15:33—Be not deceived: evil communications corrupt good manners.

2 Peter 2:18—For when they speak great swelling words of vanity, they allure through the lusts of the flesh, through much wantonness, those that were clean escaped from them who live in error.

Making Instruction Most Effective

1. Before you give advice, take the time to listen and gain a clear understanding of your child's perceptions and feelings. Children listen most when they believe they are understood and when parents spend time listening to them carefully. Children often resolve their own problems in the process of talking about them when an adult is listening attentively. They often are seeking only to be understood, rather than being given detailed instructions as to what to do. Resist the urge to make things better immediately. Instruction and direction can be given without an abundance of words, and sometimes, with no words at all.

2. Follow the rule of saying the right thing, at the right time and in the right way. The right thing to say will always follow the rule of love—treating your child the way you would want to be treated if you were in his place. The best time to instruct is during happy times when you are able to teach in casual conversation, not when you are administering chastisements and never in front of your child's peers or siblings if the content is personal. The right way is with respect, not talking down to your child when you instruct him, not raising your voice, never using sarcasm or a tone of contempt.

3. Keep instruction very limited during times when emotions are tense. Our tendency as parents is to instruct or lecture in place of discipline or before we discipline. Lecturing is a poor substitute for discipline, yet parents continue to deceive themselves into believing it is constructive because an angry lecture *can* stop a behavior. What it *cannot* do is change the child's heart. Emotionally charged moments are usually the least likely time you will affect lasting change of a constructive nature.

4. Incorporate your training into everyday activities. Take advantage of life's natural experiences and problems by using them to illustrate Bible principles and common sense. Ask the Lord for living illustrations. Pray that He will open your eyes to the many possibilities in everyday life. Think of your children's spats and problems as opportunities to teach them how to handle and resolve problems properly. Thank the Lord when your children are caught in an offense as it provides an opportunity to correct and help them. The home is a miniature training ground for adult life!

5. Teach ahead so your child will have the information he needs *prior* to the time he will need it. Constantly seek to prepare your child for the next stage of his life. For instance, a fourteen year old who wants to learn how to drive will value his mother's driving instruction more than a sixteen year old who doesn't believe he needs it. Likewise, a little girl of ten will take advice on makeup more seriously than a girl of fifteen who thinks she knows all there is to know about make up. If you wait until the time when children need the advice, they probably won't take you seriously. You'll be more effective if you talk to them *before* it comes up.

6. Involve your child in family discussions and encourage him to draw right conclusions on his own whenever possible. Ask his opinion and how he came to that opinion. Encourage him to express his ideas and thoughts and commend him whenever you are able. Respond with delight every time he makes a wise decision or expresses a particularly insightful thought.

7. Use stories and books that illustrate good character and godly principles and are of interest to your child. Develop a desire in your child to identify with the protagonist in every story. Encourage your child to discuss books he reads, give his evaluations and opinions. *Honey for a Child's Heart* by Gladys Hunt is an excellent resource for identifying wholesome books of interest to each age group. It has a helpful section that provides guidelines you can teach to your children so they will learn how to identify objectionable elements and choose books wisely on their own.

8. When you teach or read Bible stories to your children, always provide practical applications that relate to your child.

9. Talk to your child while you're working around the house or running errands, explaining to him what you're doing and why. Make working together fun.

10. There are times when learning is more serious and less conducive to fun. It helps to conclude these times with something enjoyable that children can look forward to. For instance, making popcorn or other treats to eat during family devotions helps children associate it with something enjoyable. You will especially want Bible time to be a special time.

11. Spend *much* more time talking about virtues to be imitated than vices to be shunned. Familiarity with evil is never an advantage, even when it is described as something disgusting. If you dwell on the defects of others, your children will quickly learn to perceive people's faults more readily than their virtues.

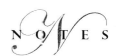

Children who are taught to detect every little fault and flaw in others become obnoxious and self-righteous. Sadly, if children become prideful, they often end up doing the very things they find wrong in others.

12. Teach your children to obey the same manners at home that you want them to use when visiting away from home. Don't allow your child to do anything at home that would embarrass you at someone else's home.

13. Without making it an issue whatsoever, keep your children in your company as much as possible by doing things with them and bringing them with you. Make your home the place their friends like to congregate. This will help in many ways. First, it will give you many more opportunities to guide and influence for good. It will give you insight in the way your children relate to others. It will prevent them from establishing wrong influences or becoming tempted through idleness. Children who are busy, involved in many interests, and experiencing a variety of excursions develop a happier outlook on life and better able to amuse themselves in constructive ways when they are older.

14. Teach your little children basic principles for conduct and convictions early. This will strengthen their character and help them resist future temptations. A child will more easily fall prey to sin if his desires are excited into action before he understands how to resist temptation. The child who knows exactly what's wrong with something before it comes up in his life will more easily resist evil suggestions when they do present themselves.

15. Remember that a silent influence and subtle lessons, which children do not consciously perceive, are always better than continuously calling attention to rules and prohibitions. Remember to teach your children why and how to say *no* rather than merely forbidding certain behaviors.

16. Use the word *no* sparingly, particularly in your child's preteen and teen years. When you have to forbid a desired activity or behavior, refrain from immediately barking out an "absolutely not" or an emphatic "no!" Instead, ask questions that will encourage your child to think about why his choice is wrong. Always try to get your child to make the right choice on his own, if possible. If you have to step in and say "no," do so by providing a Biblical reason. In some cases, it might be appropriate to suggest a better alternative and ask your child which choice he thinks is better. If he still doesn't catch on, tell him "No," but do not be "tyrannical!"

17. Teach your child that some choices are not a matter of right and wrong, but a choice between something better. For example, riding your bike is better than watching television. Going fishing is better than throwing rocks. Having friends over is better than being away from home. In making choices, it's helpful to sometimes ask things like, "Which outfit is *more* modest?" or "Which action is *most* kind?" or "Which activity is *most* wholesome?" Always, always replace the bad thing you forbid or take away with a good or better thing.

18. You'll have ample opportunities to say, "No," so look for opportunities where you can say, "Yes." It is a good general principle to say, "Yes" unless there is

some specific reason to say, "No." Any time your child wants to do something that's wholesome, support his desire even if it seems childish to you. At the same time, parents must always know the details and be willing to check to make sure there is appropriate supervision, etc. Remember, if you do not deliberately teach your child to love wholesome activities and provide them for him, then the world, as well as your child's schoolmates, will teach your child to love unwholesome activities. Once he develops a taste for the wrong kind of music, entertainment, and activities, he will find wholesome music, entertainment, and activities boring. Therefore, fill your child's life with good, happy people and activities.

19. Mothers need to take every opportunity to talk about their children's father in such a way as to cause them to love, respect, and appreciate him. Fathers need to do the same, always encouraging his children to respect and love their mother. Disrespect for the other parent ought never to be tolerated, for if you do, your children will use the "divide and conquer" tactic to cause division where there should be unwavering unity between parents. Children need both parents, and as many other adults and family members as possible, to agree on the same values. This reinforces your work as a parent. Your little child will one day grow up and need the counsel of his father or his mother. Parents who undermine their child's confidence in a mother or father find that the child usually ends up losing confidence in both parents. Let no man deceive you with vain words: for because of these things cometh the wrath of God upon the children of disobedience. Be not ye therefore partakers with them *(Ephesians 5:6-7).*

Lesson 11

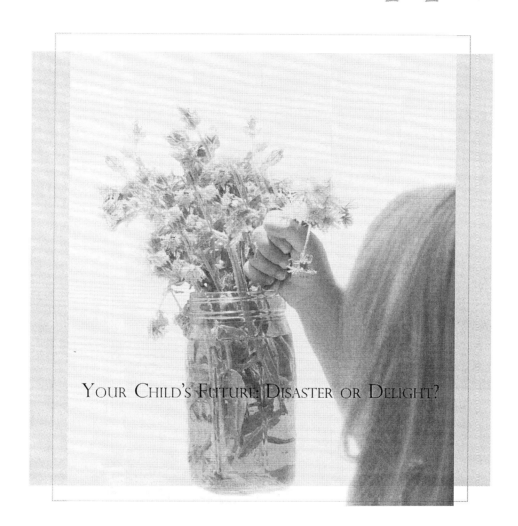

Your Child's Future: Disaster or Delight?

But as it is written, Eye hath not seen, nor ear heard, neither have entered into the heart of man, the things which God hath prepared for them that love him.
1 Corinthians 2:9

Thus saith the LORD, Behold, I set before you the way of life, and the way of death.
Jeremiah 21:8

Key THOUGHTS

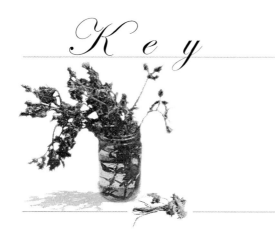

The salvation of a child involves the same work of God's grace and results in the same change of heart as the salvation of an adult. God saves a child from the penalty of sin, delivers him from the love of sin, rescues him from the habit of sin, and sets him free from the desire to sin. The great Baptist preacher Charles Spurgeon said, "It is the highest wisdom to pray for our children that while they are young their hearts may be given to the Savior." The most important thing a parent can ever do for his child is to lead his child to receive Jesus and love Him.

Discussion Problem

Fourteen-year-old Rhonda is often depressed and withdrawn. However, when she's with her friends, she perks up and shows enthusiasm. Other times she's moody and irritable, especially when she spends time alone. Her depression episodes began the week of a revival meeting after which she expressed a fear of not being saved.

Her mother assured her she was saved when she was four and told her not to worry about it. However, the depression episodes have continued for two years. Rhonda hasn't talked about her fears since that time, but her mother is beginning to wonder if she handled her daughter's concerns in the right way.

After reading lesson eleven use the principles you learn to discuss Rhonda's depression problem. What connection could there be between her depression and her doubts regarding salvation? Did her mother counsel her correctly? What could she have done different? What should she do now?

Bible Study

According to the following verses, what should a family devotion time include?

_____ Ephesians 5:19; Colossians 3:16

_____ Psalm 107:8-9; 1 Thessalonians 5:16

_____ Hebrews 4:16; James 5:16

_____ 1 Thessalonians 5:11

_____ Proverbs 23:12; Isaiah 38:19

_____ Galatians 6:10; Hebrews 10:24

"Adoption gives us the rights of children,
but regeneration alone gives us the nature of children."
Author Unknown

The Importance of Salvation and Spiritual Instruction

Years ago, two sisters who lived in a rugged area of North Dakota disappeared after heading home from school in a snowstorm. The path was already covered in snow as the girls began their one-mile walk back home after dawdling in the woods in search of rocks. With the wind and snow swirling madly about them, they could not be certain they were on the right trail. They zigzagged through the woods, hoping to find a familiar landmark but could no longer see even a foot in front of them because of the blinding snow and wind. Exhausted, they stumbled upon a hollowed tree and decided to crawl inside to escape the biting cold and wait for the storm to pass.

Meanwhile, the girls' parents spent a fretful night worrying about their daughters who they believed were still in the schoolhouse, unable to walk home in the storm. By morning, the wind had ceased its howling, and sunshine was beginning to glisten on mounds of freshly fallen snow. The father wasted no time preparing his horse for a journey to the schoolhouse to fetch his daughters. When he found the school locked and empty, fear began to grip his heart even as he tried to assure himself that the girls were safe and warm in someone's home. As the day wore on, however, his search became more frantic as others joined him to look for the girls. There seemed to be no trace of them until finally, at days end, someone came upon a brightly colored scarf tied to a branch in a tree. Digging madly, the father discovered his daughter's umbrella, and then uncovered enough snow from the fallen tree to see the lifeless form of his daughters huddled together inside, frozen to death. Both parents cried out loud with mournful gasps and wept bitter tears as they fell to their knees and tightly held their daughters. Such a needless tragedy was made all the worse because the girls were within yards of their own home when they made the fateful decision to crawl into the tree. So close to the safety and warmth of their home yet so blinded by the snow, they could not even see the lights of their home.

Losing their children in such a grievous way was a heartache these parents never fully got over. The knowledge that their children froze to death so close to home tormented them for the rest of their lives. Certainly, this was a tragedy no parent would ever want to experience. Yet as terrible as it was, this calamity pales in comparison to the tragedy endured by Christian parents who lose to death a grown child who has utterly rejected the gospel of the Lord Jesus Christ. Children who grow up in Christian homes and die lost are like those who die in a snowstorm just steps from the warmth and safety of home. But unlike those who die a physical death and enter heaven's glories to await a glad reunion with family, those who are lost enter the eternal torments of the damned without any hope of seeing their loved ones again. These are so blinded by sin they cannot see the light of home and die a senseless death in the very shadow of safety and deliverance.

Parents whose children reject Christ suffer the deepest sorrow of all when death robs the parents of any further opportunity to plead for their children's salvation or entreat them with Christian love. It is a hopeless sort of grief that brings a parent into the deepest depths of bitterness and regret. Even Job, in all his sufferings, did not have to experience the sorrows of a wayward child who wants nothing to do with the Savior. Job's sons and daughters were respected in the community and remained in fellowship with one another even after they were grown. His experience was unlike David's, who lost the heart of Absalom and felt the hatred of his own child's selfish treachery. Job knew the pain of losing his beloved children to death and being separated for a time, but he was spared the agonies of David who wept upon hearing of Absalom's tragic death and cried in his bitterness, "O my son Absalom, my son, my son Absalom! Would God I had died for thee, O Absalom, my son, my son!"

If David could, he would have loved the opportunity to go back and do things differently. He would have cherished another chance to be a more attentive father, more concerned for the souls of his children while they were still young and tender, less concerned about fulfilling the desires of his own flesh. But his chances were gone, and his opportunities to love and influence his son were abruptly ended. Only his regret remained, and in anguish of soul, he cried the bitter tears of a brokenhearted father powerless to change the eternal destiny of his own son. If Absalom's life has any worth at all, it is to serve as a warning to others who might yet be spared the regrets of David.

The Importance of a Parent's Prayer

In July of 1890, the mother and father of Arthur Layzell attended an evening prayer meeting that was being conducted on behalf of the congregation's children. One by one the parents entreated the Lord to save their children and plead with Him to work in their lives mightily. Attending the prayer meeting along with several other pastors was a Baptist preacher by the name of Charles Spurgeon. He was so moved with the sincerity and earnest desire so evident in the mothers' and fathers' petitions for their children that he decided to write to some of them, though he had never met them. Following are Spurgeon's words to a child of Christian parents who was yet unsaved. Remarkably, it was written when Spurgeon was very ill, just two years prior to his death. In it you will notice all the crucial elements of a sincere and loving, yet thoroughly truthful and moving presentation of the gospel directed straight to the child's heart. Some time after receiving this letter, Arthur did receive the Lord Jesus as his Savior. Years later, he gave the original copy of the letter to his son who cherished it as did his father.

> *Dear Arthur, you are highly privileged in having parents who pray for you. Your name is known in the courts of heaven. Your case has been laid before the throne of God. Do you not pray for yourself? If you do not do so, why not? If other people value your soul, can it be right for you to neglect it? See, the entreaties and wrestling of your father will not save you if you never seek the Lord yourself. You know this. You do not intend to cause grief to dear mother and father; but you do. So long as you are not saved, they can never rest. However obedient and sweet and kind you may be, they will never feel happy about you until you believe in the Lord Jesus Christ, and so find everlasting salvation. Think of this. Remember how much you have already sinned, and none can wash you but Jesus. When you grow up you*

may become very sinful and none can change your nature and make you holy but the Lord Jesus, through His Spirit. You need what father and mother seek for you and you need it NOW. Why not seek it at once? I heard a father pray, "Lord, save our children, and save them young." It is never too soon to be safe; never too soon to be happy; never too soon to be holy. Jesus loves to receive the very young ones. You cannot save yourself, but the great Lord Jesus can save you. Ask him to do it. "He that asketh receiveth." Then trust in Jesus to save you. He can do it, for he died and rose again that whosoever believeth in him might not perish, but have everlasting life. Come and tell Jesus you have sinned; seek forgiveness; trust in Him for it, and be sure that you are saved. Then imitate our Lord. …Yours will be a happy home, and your dear father and mother will feel that the dearest wish of their hearts has been granted them. I pray you think of heaven and hell, for in one of those places you will live forever. Meet me in heaven. Meet me at once at the mercy seat. Run upstairs and pray to the great Father, through Jesus Christ.

Yours very lovingly,

C.H. Spurgeon[1]

The greatest responsibility and privilege of parents is to pray for their children, earnestly entreating God's throne of grace that their children's hearts may be wholly given to the Savior while they are young. Yet too often, Christian parents fail to understand the seriousness of their children's conversion, assuming it is only a matter of leading a child in prayer rather than a miracle of God's saving grace that can only be wrought by the power of the Holy Spirit. Children can be led to repeat anything a parent wishes them to say, but parents are powerless to change the hearts of their children apart from the work of God. Prayer is the most important means through which a parent effects the life of a child, for there is no greater power in the world that is capable of enlightening a child's spiritual understanding than the Holy Spirit of God. "We have not," however, "because we ask not…" *(James 4:2)*.

How different is the life of one who is converted while still young compared to the life of one who is converted years later after suffering the devastations of sin and shame! Conversion saves a child from a multitude of sins. It accomplishes the same results as it does in the life of an adult and makes the hearts of children (as well as adults) a place where the Holy Spirit lives and works to produce the fruit of God's grace.

Toward the end of David's life, it would seem he became more involved in the life of his son Solomon than he had in the lives of his older children. Sometimes the failures and heartaches endured by young parents cause them to take more seriously the responsibility of shepherding children born in their later years. It is interesting to note that although the Scriptures record more prayers of David than any other Bible character, there is only one recorded in which he petitions God for a son or daughter. David asked God to give unto Solomon a perfect (wise) heart; to keep the Lord's commandments, testimonies, and statutes; and to build the temple for which he had prepared *(1 Chronicles 29:19)*. God wonderfully answered David's prayer, and we see the prayer of Solomon his son shortly thereafter when he, in turn, prayed, "Give me now wisdom and knowledge, that I may go out and come in before this people; for who can judge this thy people, that is so great?" *(2 Chronicles 1:10)*. There is no recorded prayer of Solomon for any of his children. God did record that both sons who came to the throne after him were disobedient and evil. In contrast, Job prayed for all of his children, and although they were taken home to heaven early, there is no indication they were anything but God fearing men and women.

The Conversion of Children

In the Gospel of Matthew, Christ provides a clear description of child conversion, its reality and its importance. In response to the disciples asking who would be the greatest in the kingdom of heaven, the Lord begins by calling a little child and setting him next to Him where all could see. The crowd was likely very surprised to see Jesus tenderly including a little child in his address. Certainly, it would have been an unusual gesture for a Rabbi who was highly respected among the most intelligent and influential men of Israel. Teaching little children was likely considered beneath their dignity, so it doubtless captured the people's attention when Jesus, the Son of God, drew a child to himself in their presence and said, "Verily I say unto you, Except ye be converted, and become as little children, ye shall not enter into the kingdom of heaven" *(Matthew 18:2-3)*. Jesus makes an astounding statement by saying conversion occurs on a child's level. Rather than the child having an adult experience, Jesus declares that the adult is to have a child's experience. People will often admit they are a sinner, but to be saved, one must become as a little child and admit we are a *helpless* sinner in need of a Savior.

Next Jesus told the disciples that they must humble themselves as the little child sitting next to Him if they wished to be great in the kingdom of heaven. "Whosoever therefore shall humble himself as this little child, the same is greatest in the kingdom of heaven" *(Matthew 18:4)*. I can imagine the disciples felt very uncomfortable, if not ashamed of their pride, when Jesus used a small child to describe the kind of humble and trusting faith that not only produces salvation but is most highly esteemed by God. No one ever receives the grace to be saved who doesn't come humbly to Christ. To come in humility is to come in utter dependence on Christ, with no self-sufficiency or self-righteousness. This kind of contrite, or humble, spirit that is so necessary for salvation is already in a child's nature.

Jesus then turns the people's attention toward considering His high regard for children and establishes the tremendous worth of a child to Him. "And whoso shall receive one such little child in my name receiveth me" *(Matthew 18:5)*. Those who place the kind of value on children that Jesus places on them honor Him and please Him, for to value and receive a child is to receive the Lord Himself. Certainly Jesus is making us see that the spiritual training of a child is of utmost importance to Him. Therefore, if we are concerned with pleasing Him rather than ourselves, we will give importance to the same things He esteems important.

The Lord further conveys His concern for the protection and care of children by beginning a solemn warning with the words, "But whoso shall offend one of these little ones which believe in me..." *(Matthew 18:6)*. To offend a child who believes on Christ is to oppress or in some way treat a child unjustly. Jesus has a claim on those children who believe the gospel and regards them as His own. Clearly, Jesus is implying that a child *can* believe in Christ, the gospel. *Believe* means "to rely on, trust, adhere to, receive." The consequences to one who would cause a child to stumble, or harm a child by taking advantage of one's authority over him, or by neglecting a child's salvation is incredibly severe. God declares that such a person deserves not simply death, but a horrible death. "It were better for him," Jesus warns, "that a millstone were hanged about his neck, and that he were drowned in the depth of the sea" *(Matthew 18:6)*. To be bound and thrown into the sea with a weight tied around one's neck would be a terrifying way to die. Yet Jesus is saying the consequence of abusing a child is *worse* than this. The helplessness and fear that one would experience if killed in this way lays upon the adult the kind of helplessness and fear a child experiences when he is mistreated, abused, or neglected by those who ought to be giving the utmost attention to his care and protection.

Again, Jesus gives a strong warning to adults, reminding them to use the utmost caution in the way they handle and regard children. He says, "Take heed that ye despise not one of these little ones; for I say unto you, That in heaven their angels do always behold the face of my Father which is in heaven" *(Matthew 18:10)*. To undervalue a child or overlook the fact that God takes special note when an adult in authority oppresses one who is so helpless is to miss God's evaluation and put one's own soul in great jeopardy. Regarding a child with contempt or failing to exercise patience and forbearance invites God's vengeance. Furthermore, God wants us to remember that the angels in heaven watch over God's littlest children, and they freely come and go from God's throne, no doubt giving a report of all they see.

The angels, who are ministering spirits to those who will be saved, give witness to the fact that children need salvation, for they too are lost in their sins. "For the Son of man is come to save that which was lost" *(Matthew 18:11)*.

Children come to Christ the same way adults do! There are *not* two gospels, one for children and one for adults. When the Bible refers to the *gospel*, it means the good news that God became a man, died in our place, paid the full penalty for our sin; that Jesus was buried and rose again; and that Jesus offers salvation as a free gift of His love, complete forgiveness, restoration of fellowship, and eternal life in heaven to all who will believe and receive Him by faith. The gospel alone is the power of God unto salvation. We must not leave anything out when dealing with a child's eternal soul.

Jesus then asks a question, provoking the disciples to regard children as part of the flock, to be sought and protected as sheep. "How think ye? If a man have an hundred sheep, and one of them be gone astray, doth he not leave the ninety and nine, and goeth into the mountains, and seeketh that which is gone astray? And if so be that he find it, verily I say unto you, he rejoiceth more of that sheep, than of the ninety and nine which went not astray" *(Matthew 18:12-13)*.

Then lastly, Jesus reminds his hearers that it is not God's desire that any child grow up unsaved, only to perish rather than inherit eternal life. "Even so it is not the will of your Father which is in heaven, that one of these little ones should perish" *(Matthew 18:14)*. It is possible for children to grow up, live successful lives by the world's standards, but ultimately perish. No child or adult can obtain God's forgiveness or salvation without coming face to face with the message of the cross: people's sin deserve death; but God in His mercy died in man's place and offers forgiveness to all who will believe.

No child or adult can obtain God's forgiveness or salvation without coming face to face with the message of the cross: people's sin deserve death; but God in His mercy died in man's place and offers forgiveness to all who will believe.

Teach Your Child How To Have a Personal Relationship with God

How Do I Start? When Is He Ready?

Parents begin building a solid foundation for their children's future understanding of God by teaching them truth about such things as who God is, what God made, His ability to see and know everything, His care and love for children, etc.. Parents especially need to teach their children to love the Bible because it is God's Word and answers our questions about Him.

As children begin to mature and develop a conscious awareness of sin and guilt, parents need to begin explaining what sin is, that all people sin, that sin makes God sad, but that God forgives us for sinning when we admit we've done something wrong and are sorry for our sin and then ask Him to forgive us. Children need to understand that God will forgive them and then treat them as though they never sinned. Do not bring up past offenses the child has committed in an effort to make him feel bad or guilty *once he's admitted he did wrong, been disciplined, and forgiven.* Parents need to model God's forgiveness by their own willingness to forgive.

When a child is old enough to recognize that he is a sinner and that sin brings dissatisfaction, he is able to understand salvation. Remember, every question deserves an answer. Listen. Be available. Be willing to talk and find answers for your child's spiritual questions. Let the child tell you that he wants to be saved. Never coerce a child into praying a salvation prayer. Never insinuate the child should be saved to please the parent, teacher, preacher, or friend. Never embarrass your child or push him into any spiritual decision. Above all else, pray for your child's salvation and for wisdom in dealing with the spiritual life and eternal destiny of your child.

Verses about God's Love for His Own: *Deuteronomy 33:12; Psalm 42:8-9, 14; Psalm 63:3; Psalm 103:4; Psalm 146:8; Proverbs 15:9; Isaiah 38:17; Isaiah 49:13-16; Isaiah*

66:13; Jeremiah 31:3; John 3:16; John 14:21-23; John 16:27; John 17:26; Romans 5:8; Romans 8:31-32, 39; 1Corinthians 2:9; Ephesians 1:3-6; Ephesians 2:4-5; 2 Thessalonians 2:16; 1 John 3:1-2; 1 John 4:9-10

How Do I Teach My Child about Salvation?

Begin to teach children the gospel message of the Bible in simple terms that they can understand. The gospel message must always begin with the fact of God's love. The child must know that Jesus is God, that He created us, that He knows us, and that He cares for us. Children, as well as adults, will need to understand the difference between sin and sins.

They need to know that being saved does not mean that one never again commits an act of sin; but that being saved means that a person's attitude about sin has changed. They need to know that sin is choosing to do what we want to do when God wants us to do something else.

Always use as illustrations the sins a child will relate to such as lying, kicking, biting, disobeying, selfishness, or displaying selfish anger. Explain that sin leads to unpleasant consequences. If parents have done well in disciplining a small child, he will understand this cause and effect easily. The consequence of sin leads to separation from God both now and eternally, for there is no sin in heaven.

Emphasize that God loves us even though we are sinners. God is without sin. Because God loved us, He left heaven, came to earth, and died in our place for our sin. God personally took our punishment for us. Explain that after Jesus died, He was buried; but three days later He came alive and now lives in heaven. Explain that we receive salvation as a free gift from God when we trust Him. A child must understand that such things as going to church and giving money can't save him. Only Jesus can save him when he believes or trusts in what Jesus did for him. Avoid using abstract terms that are confusing to children. A phrase such as "ask Jesus into your heart" will not necessarily be helpful. Instead, tell him what it means to trust Jesus to save him from the penalty of sin

See complete explanation of salvation on pages 244-246.

How Do I Help My Child Obtain Assurance of Salvation?

Teach the child to rely on what God says about His salvation. Preface assurance verses by reminding them "God *says* right here in the Bible…" If the child can read, ask him to read the assurance verses. Then you read and personalize the verses.

Ask, "What does God *say* in this verse?" Help or ask the child to memorize John 3:16 during the coming week. Read *Romans 10:13* and *John 3:16* substituting your child's name for "whosoever." Emphasize that the word *whosoever* includes anyone, even a child. Explain that although we sometimes might not *feel* saved, our feelings don't

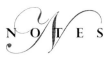

change what God *says* or what God has promised us. Our feelings are not always reliable, but we can always rely completely on what God says.

It may be helpful to give the illustration of a very nervous person taking his money to the bank and trusting the bank to keep it for him. It would be silly for him to then go home, worrying about his money. Ask, "Is the money safe even if he worries about it?" Explain that when the silly person is finally very sure that the bank is a safe place for his money, he will feel safe. However, the money is safe whether he is afraid or not. Read *2 Timothy 1:12* and *John 5:24* for additional help. Help your child remember this key point: Assurance and understanding come as we *believe what the Word of God says.*

Verses about Assurance: *Romans10:13; John 1:12,13; John 3:18; John 3:36; John 5:24; John 6:37; John 10:27-29*

After My Child Trusts Christ, Then What?

After your child accepts Christ, encourage him to tell someone as soon as possible that he has been saved. Have him verbalize to you in his own simple words what he has done. With very young children in particular, it is very helpful to make his salvation as memorable an occasion as you can so it will be easier for him to remember as the years go by. Treat it very seriously. Write down the date. Encourage your child to tell the pastor and other family members that he has asked Jesus to forgive him for his sins and trusted Jesus to save him.

Immediately after a child puts his trust in Christ for salvation, talk about the thousands of promises in the Bible that are specifically given to the child of God. (Christian bookstores commonly carry little books that list promises of God.) Show your child how some promises are unconditional, such as the promises the Jesus will never leave us or forsake us, while other promises are conditional upon our doing what God commands, such as the promise in *Psalm 50:15* where God promises to deliver those Christians who call upon Him (pray) in times of trouble. The child then learns, "God will deliver me when I pray." Following are verses of promises that are given when we do our part. Have your child complete the sentence for each promise.

God will _____ when I _____.

Verses about God's Promises: *Psalm 22:24; Psalm 34:4; Psalm 34:17; Psalm 72:12; Psalm 86:5; Psalm 28:7; Psalm 31:24; Psalm 54:22; Psalm 111:10; Psalm 112:1; Proverbs 3:5-8; Proverbs 16:7; Isaiah 26:3; Matthew 6:33; Matthew 7:7-8; John 3:18; John 8:31-32; Romans 8:28; Ephesians 6:8; Philippians 4:6-7*

Teach your child God's unfailing promises and begin building his faith in God's faithful character. A *Nave's Topical Bible* is an excellent resource for this purpose.

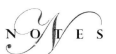

How Do I Teach My Child about Baptism?

If your child has never heard of baptism, or if he's struggling to grasp all you've been teaching him, don't try to explain too much for him to absorb in one day. If your child is old enough to understand he is a sinner in need of a Savior, he will likely be able to understand baptism if it is carefully explained in simple terms. Be sensitive to his fears, however, and his need to understand what you are instructing him to do. As soon as your child is ready to discuss it, explain what baptism is and why the Lord Jesus asks us to be baptized right after we are saved.

Be very certain the child understands that he is *not* saved by baptism. We are to be baptized after we have whole-heartedly believed in Jesus for salvation *(Acts 8:37)*. Explain that baptism tells a story. It tells that we believe Jesus died, was buried, and then rose again to live forever and ever. When we let the pastor dip us under the water, that pictures Jesus letting Himself be punished on the cross for our sins and being buried. When the pastor quickly brings us right back out of the water, it pictures Jesus coming out of the grave where He was buried. We can see the command to be baptized in *Matthew 28*, the example of baptism in *Acts 8*, and the meaning of baptism in *Romans 6*.

Baptism also tells another story. It tells how we once didn't care if we sinned, but now we have been saved. Since we now live with Jesus, and will keep living with Him forever, we choose not to love sin anymore. That's what the pastor means when he says, "saved to walk in newness of life." He means that since we are now saved, we now want to live our life so we can please Jesus.

Take the child to see people being baptized. After the baptism, let him see the room leading to the baptistery. Explain step-by-step how the people who are to be baptized get ready, and how the pastor helps them into the baptistery.

Finally, say to your child, "Will you tell me (or let a parent, pastor, teacher know) when you want to be baptized?" If the child agrees, ask, "Would you like to be baptized next week, or would you like to wait awhile?" If he responds, "I want to wait," do not try to persuade him or act disappointed. Resist the urge to make this decision for him. If you do, his baptism will not benefit him as it would if he alone made the choice. Say, "That's fine. I will be praying Jesus helps you to make that decision soon." Then leave the topic alone. Don't bring it up until the child does. Answer any questions he may have.

How Do I Teach My Child To Pray?

Teach children how God wants them to pray. Do not teach children that Jesus is a Santa Claus in the sky waiting to give them every toy they ask for. Teach them that Jesus sees and hears them all the time, even when they are thinking and not saying a word out loud. Children need to understand that God loves them and wants them to talk to Him every day. He especially wants to help them become good Christians. Tell them Jesus wants to know all about their problems. He wants to help them understand what to do so He can solve all their problems His way. Teach children to pray specifically for needs. Point out answers to prayer as they occur and then teach children to express thanks in every prayer. Also children should be sure they ask forgiveness for their sins when they pray. Teach children to be sure they aren't angry with anyone when they pray. If they are angry, parents need to teach their children how to deal with the situation causing their anger. Always pray as a family before meals. Avoid using nursery rhyme prayers or memorized prayers, for this will discourage children from learning to talk to God in their own words. Teach your child to memorize Scriptures about prayer, being careful to explain each of the passages he memorizes. Encourage teens to read books about Christians who understood the importance of prayer and the joys of answered prayer. Many of the leading Christian textbook companies such as Bob Jones Press and A Beka Book, carry several biographies and novels that will help inspire your children to pray.

Verses about Prayer: *Psalm 34:15-17; Psalm 145:18; Proverbs 15:8; Matthew 6:5-13; Matthew 7:7; Luke 5-13; Luke 18:1; Romans 8:26; Philippians 4:6; 1 Thessalonians 5:17; Hebrews 4:16; James 5:16*

How Do I Teach My Child To Love the Bible?

Teach children to *love* learning from the Bible. Always exalt the Bible. Help your child want to know what the Bible says to them. Encourage your child to begin memorizing verses that will help him in his daily life by memorizing with him and making Bible memory fun. *Never* underestimate a child's capacity to understand spiritual things and grow in faith as he learns from the Bible. *Let your children see you reading your Bible.* Always have your Bible open when you teach a Bible lesson. Share your enthusiasm and interest in the Bible.

As you read your Bible, look for passages of Scripture that you can explain clearly and then help your child apply those truths to their lives. Remember that children grow spiritually when the Scriptures are explained to them clearly. Merely reading the Bible to them or unwisely using it as a weapon when they disobey will not help. Make understanding the Bible an *enjoyable* experience. Encourage your children to underline and mark in their Bibles. This will help them focus their attention better and begin to master the skill of Bible application. Encourage children to look for specific kinds of verses—verses that encourage them, verses that help them get along with others, verses that would be good to memorize someday, verses that explain something important, etc.

- God's Word produces faith and confidence in God's promises: *Acts 17:11; Romans 10:17; 1 Thessalonians. 2:1; Ephesians 6:16; Hebrews 11:1,6*
- God's Word teaches us to fear the Lord: *Psalm 111:10; Psalm 24:14; Psalm 31:19; Psalm 112:1; Proverbs 16:6; Proverbs. 22:4*
- God's Word produces wisdom and understanding: *Proverbs 1:7; Proverbs 9:10; Proverbs 2:1-6; Proverbs 19:20; 2 Timothy 3:15-16*

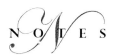

- God's Word enables us to live right: *Deuteronomy 29:29; Proverbs 6:20-23; John 6:63; 2 Timothy 3:16-17*
- God's Word makes our life successful: *Joshua 1:8*
- God's Word makes our life productive: *Psalm 1:2; Acts 20:32; Isaiah 55:10-11*
- God's Word keeps us alert to Satan's devices and prevent his destruction in our life: *Psalm 17:4; Ephesians 6:17; 1 Corinthians 10:11*
- God's Word contains power that will heal our distress and sorrows: *Psalm 107:19*
- God's Word keeps us from sinning: *Psalm 119:9,11; Proverbs 14:16,27*
- God's Word produces great peace in our life: *Psalm 119:165*
- God's Word enables us to confidently help others: *Proverbs 22:20-21; 2 Timothy 2:15*
- God's Word gives joy and happiness: *Colossians 3:16; 1 John 1:4; Rev. 1:3; Jeremiah 15:16*
- God's Word enables us to withstand the adversities of life: *Matthew 7:24-25*
- God's Word will motivates us: *Luke 24:32*
- God's Word will give us purpose in life: *Ecclesiastes 12:13; John 8:31-32*
- God's Word will reveal sin and error in our life: *Hebrews 4:12*
- God's Word will enable us to grow spiritually: *1 Peter 2:2*
- God's Word enables us to appropriate the promises of God and develop the nature of Christ: *2 Peter 2-4; James 1:21-23*
- God's Word will enable us to witness boldly: *Titus 1:9; 1 Peter 3:15*
- God's Word will make us confident Christians: *Ecclesiastes 8:1*
- God's Word will result in answered prayer: *Psalm 4:3; 1 John 3:2; John 15:7*

How Do I Teach My Child To Deal with Sin?

Your child needs to know that sometimes, even though we're saved, we will sin. Sin is like a sneaky lion, lurking in quiet places, ready to pounce when we least expect it. Sometimes sin clothes itself in what seems harmless and even delightful to us. To some degree, Christians hate sin and feel miserable when they engage in it. Explain that when we were saved, Jesus came to live right inside us, though we can't see Him or feel Him. Even though we can't understand how, Jesus can be everywhere all at the same time. Explain that Jesus (or the Holy Spirit, if the child is old enough to understand) helps us to know when we've sinned. He also helps us to do the things that will make God happy and us happy too. Christians need to pray that God will help them hate sin more and more.

When we know we've sinned, we are to come quickly to Jesus, tell Him our sin, and ask Him to forgive us for our sin and help us to hate our sin. When we sin we are still saved, but Jesus wants us to hate sin because it hurts Him and is never good for us. He always wants us to admit our sin to Him. Teach your child to memorize *1 John 1:9* and other verses dealing with forgiveness. Explain that *confess* means "to admit our sin or agree with God that what we did was sin." From *John 6:37* you can explain that Jesus doesn't go away when we sin. *John 10:27-29* will help explain that when we are saved, we will want to follow Jesus and listen to Him. Rather than teaching your child to "apologize" or say he's "sorry" when he sins against others, teach him how to ask forgiveness for specific ways he has sinned. This concept often needs to be modeled by parents.

How Do I Help My Child Deal with Guilt?

Our built-in "guilt" system alerts and protects us from emotional trauma and pain in much the same way our complex nervous system protects us from physical trauma. Without pain, we wouldn't know we were having an appendix attack, or whether or not our hand was resting on a hot stove. Pain alerts us to the problem so we can do something about it before the consequences are devastating. Likewise, our guilt "sensors" motivate us to do something about sin before sin brings devastation into out lives.

Guilt for genuine offenses against God is good for us when we resolve it Biblically. However, guilt can be extremely destructive if we attempt to resolve its discomfort by pacifying it, ignoring it, denying it, justifying it, drowning it out with pleasures, or punishing ourselves in an attempt to feel better. God has given a wonderful, specific plan that enables us to resolve *all* our sin and guilt and remove *all* its pain. When our guilt motivates us to come to the Lord Jesus Christ for salvation or forgiveness, we are able to find instant relief; but if we refuse to handle guilt God's way, our problems will snowball and cause great distress.

Ignoring a problem that is producing guilt in our children's lives is not merciful. Rather it is most unkind. *In a kind, loving manner* a parent should talk with the child about their guilt and the sin or misconception that is producing it. Provide discipline if necessary, and lead the child to accept God's forgiveness. Always provide reassurance of God's forgiveness. Teach your child Scripture verses about God's forgiveness. When we understand and believe God has forgiven us, we do not suffer with the mistaken notion that we cannot forgive ourselves. This process of teaching may be tedious, but it is extremely needful. When parents carry out discipline in a calm, loving manner and offer complete forgiveness as God does, children are relieved and happy. However, if parents allow guilt to fester and grow, children become irritable and most unhappy.

> *A parent is sinning if he treats a repentant child with alienation, repeated reminders of an offense, coldness, or any other antagonism that prolongs the guilt to satisfy the parent's anger.*

It is crucial that parents help their children avoid the effects of false guilt. Distinguish between household rules and parental preferences that are not sins and issues

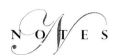

that are clearly defined as sinful in the Bible. Your child does not sin by violating a preferential household rule, but by rebelling against the parent's authority. A child must not be made to feel guilty for an offense that violates man's standards or expectations, or for an offense that someone else has committed. These things generate a false guilt that the child must reject. Sometimes children believe they are guilty for disharmony in their home, which has nothing to do with them. False guilt also troubles them for imagined offenses or for offenses others have committed against them. Parents need to be sensitive to this tendency in some children and help their children understand the difference between real and false guilt to avoid becoming unnecessarily distressed.

Parents must never use guilt as a means to control or manipulate their children. This extreme selfishness misrepresents God and constitutes an abuse of authority that God will judge. Parents must also recognize that God forbids any refusal to extend complete forgiveness to their repentant children. Again, God does judge such behavior. A parent is sinning if he treats a repentant child with alienation, repeated reminders of an offense, coldness, or any other antagonism that prolongs the guilt to satisfy the parent's anger. The consequence of such parental sin is often immensely destructive to a child's spiritual and emotional welfare.

Colossians 3:13b says, "even as Christ forgave you, so also do ye." We are to forgive as God forgives us.

- How does God forgive, and on what basis does He forgive? *Psalm 86:5; Proverbs 28:13; 1 John 1:9*
- How does God treat the unrepentant? *Luke 6:35; Luke 23:34; 1 Peter 2:22-23*
- How does God treat the repentant? *Psalm 32:1-2, 5; Psalm 103:11-13; Exodus 34, Isaiah 1:18; Isaiah 55:7; Hosea 14; Romans 8:1; Galatians 4:4*

How Do I Teach My Child To Treat Those Who Sin against Him?

First, we are to strive to overlook petty human frailties in a spirit of mercy and patience. *Proverbs 13:10; Proverbs 25:15; Psalm 130:3; Proverbs 19:11; I Thessalonians 5:14; Romans 12:18*

Second, we are to humbly confront those who cause divisions by specific sins, or who are bringing destruction upon themselves by sinning, with the motive of restoring them in a spirit of love and kindness. Those who are spiritual are those who are able to confront sin without regard for himself or herself, without anger and without a spirit of contempt or condemnation. *Galatians 6:1; Luke 17:3-4; Matthew 18:15-16; Ephesians 4:25*

Third, we are commanded to forgive from our hearts any who repent and consider the matter closed and forgotten, never to be brought against the offender again. *Matthew 18:21; Matthew 18:33-35; Ephesians 4:32*

How are we to treat those who *do not* repent? *Leviticus 19:18; 1 Corinthians 4:12; Exodus 23:4-5; Proverbs 24:17,29; Proverbs 20:22; Proverbs 25:21; Romans 12:20; Luke 6:27-34; Matthew 6:12; Mark 11:25; Romans 12:14; Romans 12:17,19; 1 Peter 2:20-22; 1 Peter 3:9; James 3:14; Hebrews 12:15; Ephesians 4:29-32*

How To Explain the Plan of Salvation

We are separated from God.

Our sins have alienated us from God.

Isaiah 59:2—But your iniquities have separated between you and your God, and your sins have hid his face from you, that he will not hear.

Romans 6:23a—For the wages of sin is death.

There are two kinds of death, physical and spiritual. Physical death is the separation of the soul from the body. The body dies, but the soul was created by God to live forever. Spiritual death is the separation of the person from God. People are separated from God by their sin nature. Should a person die separated from God by sin, he will spend eternity separated from God, because the wages of sin is eternal death in hell *(Revelation 20:14-15)*.

We are all sinners.

The awareness of our sinful nature causes us to feel guilty before God.

Romans 3:23—For all have sinned, and come short of the glory of God.

Romans 3:10—As it is written, There is none righteous, no, not one.

We need God.

We cannot resolve our guilt or end our alienation from God by good works or self-effort.

Romans 3:20—Therefore by the deeds of the law there shall no flesh be justified in his sight: for by the law is the knowledge of sin.

Romans 10:1-3—Brethren, my heart's desire and prayer to God for Israel is, that they might be saved. For I bear them record that they have a zeal of God, but not according to knowledge. For they being ignorant of God's righteousness, and going about to establish their own righteousness, have not submitted themselves unto the righteousness of God.

Titus 3:5—Not by works of righteousness which we have done, but according to his mercy he saved us, by the washing of regeneration, and renewing of the Holy Ghost.

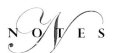

We have hope.

God loves us so much that He made a way for us to be reconciled to Him. He became the God-man Jesus and died in our place. His death paid the penalty for our sins.

John 3:16—For God so loved the world, that he gave his only begotten Son, that whosoever believeth in him should not perish, but have everlasting life.

Romans 5:8-9—But God commendeth his love toward us, in that, while we were yet sinners, Christ died for us. Much more then, being now justified by his blood, we shall be saved from wrath through him.

We can be forgiven.

We receive God's forgiveness when we repent of our sins, believe Jesus is Who He says He is (God), believe He died on the cross in our place for the penalty of our sins, believe that He rose again, and receive His offer of salvation and forgiveness.

Galatians 2:16—Knowing that a man is not justified by the works of the law, but by the faith of Jesus Christ, even we have believed in Jesus Christ, that we might be justified by the faith of Christ, and not by the works of the law: for by the works of the law shall no flesh be justified.

Romans 6:23b—But the gift of God is eternal life through Jesus Christ our Lord.

Romans 10:9-13—That if thou shalt confess with thy mouth the Lord Jesus, and shalt believe in thine heart that God hath raised him from the dead, thou shalt be saved. For with the heart man believeth unto righteousness; and with the mouth confession is made unto salvation. For the scripture saith, Whosoever believeth on him shall not be ashamed. For there is no difference between the Jew and the Greek: for the same Lord over all is rich unto all that call upon him. For whosoever shall call upon the name of the Lord shall be saved.

We are free from guilt.

When we confess that we are sinners who cannot save ourselves or make ourselves righteous by effort, we are freed from the guilt and condemnation that we deserve.

John 5:24—Verily, verily, I say unto you, He that heareth my word, and believeth on him that sent me, hath everlasting life, and shall not come into condemnation; but is passed from death unto life.

Romans 8:1—There is therefore now no condemnation to them which are in Christ Jesus, who walk not after the flesh, but after the Spirit.

Hebrews 10:17—And their sins and iniquities will I remember no more.

1 John 1:9—If we confess our sins, he is faithful and just to forgive us our sins, and to cleanse us from all unrighteousness.

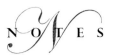

We are no longer separated from God.

When we trust Christ to save us, we are no longer alienated from Him in sin. Now He is our loving Father.

John 1:12—But as many as received him, to them gave he power to become the sons of God, even to them that believe on his name.

Romans 8:15—For ye have not received the spirit of bondage again to fear; but ye have received the Spirit of adoption, whereby we cry, Abba, Father.

Romans 8:35,38-39—Who shall separate us from the love of Christ? Shall tribulation, or distress, or persecution, or famine, or nakedness, or peril, or sword? For I am persuaded, that neither death, nor life, nor angels, nor principalities, nor powers, nor things present, nor things to come, nor height, nor depth, nor any other creature, shall be able to separate us from the love of God, which is in Christ Jesus our Lord.

We have a new destiny.

When we trust Christ to save us, we have a whole new identity, new purpose, and a wonderful new destiny.

1 John 3:1—Behold, what manner of love the Father hath bestowed upon us, that we should be called the sons of God: therefore the world knoweth us not, because it knew him not.

Ephesians 2:1-10—And you *hath he quickened*, who were dead in trespasses and sins; wherein in time past ye walked according to the course of this world, according to the prince of the power of the air, the spirit that now worketh in the children of disobedience: among whom also we all had our conversation in times past in the lusts of our flesh, fulfilling the desires of the flesh and of the mind; and were by nature the children of wrath, even as others. But God, who is rich in mercy, for his great love wherewith he loved us, even when we were dead in sins, hath quickened us together with Christ, (by grace ye are saved;) and hath raised *us* up together, and made *us* sit together in heavenly *places* in Christ Jesus: that in the ages to come he might show the exceeding riches of his grace in *his* kindness toward us through Christ Jesus. For by grace are ye saved through faith; and that not of yourselves: *it is* the gift of God: not of works, lest any man should boast. For we are his workmanship, created in Christ Jesus unto good works, which God hath before ordained that we should walk in them.

John 14:2-3— In my Father's house are many mansions: if *it were* not *so*, I would have told you. I go to prepare a place for you. And if I go and prepare a place for you, I will come again, and receive you unto myself; that where I am, *there* ye may be also.

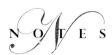

Footnotes:

[1] Dallimore, Arnold. C.H.Spurgeon. Chicago: Moody Press, 1984. Pages 224-225.

Lesson 12

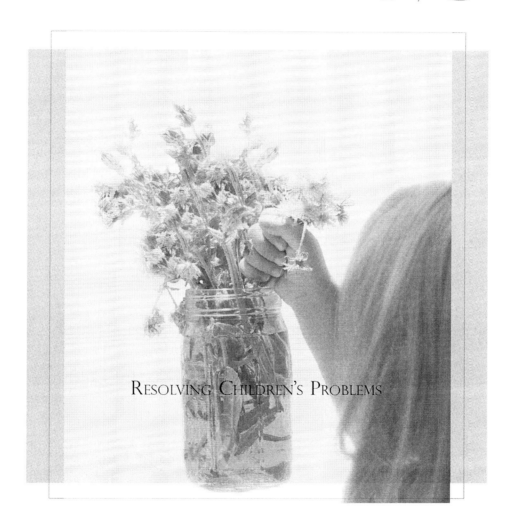

RESOLVING CHILDREN'S PROBLEMS

And call upon me in the day of trouble:
I will deliver thee, and thou shalt glorify me.
Psalm 50:15

Let us therefore come boldly unto the
throne of grace, that we may obtain mercy,
and find grace to help in time of need.
Hebrews 4:16

Key THOUGHTS

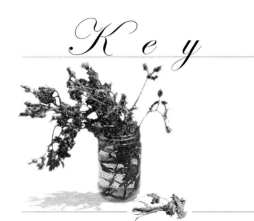

Resolving children's problems Biblically involves first seeking God's wisdom, identifying any possible underlying problems or sins, constructing practical solutions as necessary, and putting off all wrong behavior while at the same time putting on its opposite righteous counterpart. The main objective is to address the underlying motivations of a child's choices and teach him how to understand and apply Biblical principles, not to just blindly do what he is told.

Discussion Problem

Danny's mother caught Danny stealing a small toy from the store. After talking with him and explaining the seriousness of stealing, she immediately spanked him and had him return the toy to the store manager and then ask forgiveness. Danny was repentant and cooperative. Is there anything more Danny's mother can do to help her son keep this from happening again?

Brenda is an outgoing six-year-old. She can't seem to sit still even for a short period of time. She has a hard time finishing anything, especially when it comes to picking up *all* her toys. She's easily distracted and often responds by saying, "I forgot." What can her mom do?

Joey, age eight, and Steven, age ten, are brothers. Their constant fights seem to be getting worse. Usually they have to be forcibly separated when one or the other gets hurt and starts screaming. Joey wants to tag along everywhere with Steven. Mom constantly admonishes Steven to let his brother play with him. What can be done to help the situation?

Fifteen-year-old Cindy never hangs up things such as her clothes, jacket, and towel. Her mom constantly yells at her, but Cindy doesn't seem to get any neater. In fact, Cindy is getting lazier in every area of her life. What can her mother do about this?

Tara, like many other three-year-olds, hates to go to bed at night. Bedtime has become a daily battle. Tara gets up every ten minutes to get a drink, to go to the bathroom, or to complain she's scared of the dark. Often she comes into Mom and Dad's room wanting to crawl into bed with them. How can Mom solve the problem?

Bible Study

1. Ephesians 4:22-24 and Colossians 3:5-15 tell us to "put off the old man" and "put on the new." What does this mean? _____

2. Based on 1 Corinthians 2:14-16, Galatians 2:20, and Philippians 4:13, what makes it possible for a Christian to put off and put on? _____

"A mother is neither cocky nor proud, because she knows the school principal may call at any minute to report that her child has just driven a motorcycle through the gymnasium."
Author Unknown

Will Your Child Sink or Swim?

Suppose a company specializing in building huge ocean liners launched its ships only to have a great many sink shortly afterward? You would think, given the tremendous loss, someone would question why so many sank—but suppose the company president just shook his head in sadness and continued making ships the same way only to have them sink time and time again? It certainly wouldn't take long for stockholders to get involved and changes to be made in upper management. No one with an interest in building seaworthy ships for profit would tolerate such a dismal track record. Yet many in the Christian school movement who claim to value the tremendous worth of a child "launch" graduating seniors into the world only to watch a great many of them sink, few stopping to reevaluate the methods being used to build them. Furthermore, many Christian parents accept failure, supposing it happened by chance, and expend little effort attempting to discover why their grown youngsters left home only to sink spiritually.

No one can presume to know all the many reasons children from Christian homes might grow up and fail to thrive spiritually, but certainly, a great many of them reject the faith and convictions of their parents for reasons that *can* be traced. I believe one major cause of failure is the common practice of solving children's problems in ways that discourage rather than encourage spiritual growth. Quite typically school personnel and parents adopt methods of dealing with problems that focus on stopping outward behavior without changing inward causes. The immensely popular "demerit" system used in many Christian schools tends to encourage such an approach, as do many discipline plans promoted by supposed experts in childrearing. Let's examine the basic structure underlying many of these methods.

In a demerit system children are typically issued a "demerit" slip for offenses they commit in the school environment. Offenses are generally regarded as being more or less serious, and are therefore given demerit values. Forgetting one's book, for example, might result in two demerits while engaging in a playground scuffle might score a whopping twenty five demerits. After students accumulate a certain number of demerits, consequences are issued which vary in severity from after-school detentions to suspension. At the end of each quarter or semester, demerits are usually cancelled so students can start "fresh" at zero. However, if students regularly rack up large amounts of demerits or accumulate an excessive number, students may be asked to leave or be refused admittance to the school the following year. In this way, the fear of detentions, suspensions, or expulsion presumably acts as a deterrent and resolves problems.

What such a plan really does is teach students how to accumulate demerits without actually having to "pay the time" (or change inwardly). Students quickly learn how many demerits they can add up before consequences occur, or how long they have to abstain from getting more demerits before their list is cancelled out at the end of a quarter. Once some students begin accumulating large numbers of demerits and detentions, many give up trying to prevent them and enjoy the process of racking up even more. Other students who possess a high level of self-control learn how to beat

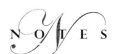

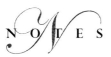

the system by avoiding demerits altogether, earning them the esteem of their parents and teachers alike. These tend to be labeled the "good" students while the others are the "bad" or "rebellious" students. By graduation time, all hopes are pinned on the good students while few expect the bad students to "make it." Predictably, the "bad" students are inclined to live up to their reputation and become as bad as people told them they were. The real surprise is that the "good" students quite often astound school staff by returning to visit with the look of a rock star or worldly fashion icon.

Everyone with a vested interest in these students wonders what happened and are saddened with disappointment. Some question if their sacrifices are worth it. Others aren't fazed in the least and just go on with their work, matriculating youngsters through the system and taking pleasure in the ones that do thrive after graduation—even if they are the minority. Parents, meanwhile, often aren't any more successful with their efforts and are often just as surprised when their children seem to morph overnight into worldly or spiritually apathetic adults. Some had blamed the Christian school and thought home schooling would thwart disaster while others simply never had a clue something less obvious was amiss. Still others followed every suggestion the books had to offer and can't understand why all their rules and restrictions seem to have backfired on them. Could it be that a great many of these parents handled problems with the same focus on outward behavior that some schools adopt?

What happens when Johnny comes home from school with a demerit slip? Is his well-rehearsed defense believed and the teacher's efforts dismissed as unreasonable, or is he spanked or restricted yet further for daring to commit an offense worthy of a demerit slip? Has anyone taken the time to investigate all the details of the offense to determine the underlying cause of the problem? Is it possible the teacher misjudged the situation? Or has it occurred to parent or teacher that Johnny might be learning how to fly below the radar so he can further indulge his selfish desires without getting caught? Doesn't anyone recognize that Johnny is being trained to deal with human weaknesses and sinful desires of the flesh with the weapons of the world, not the weapons of Christian warfare?

Think about it…many children are told to try harder, or pray Jesus helps them be good. The emphasis is invariably on what the child is doing wrong, not what the child could do differently that is right. Of greatest concern is usually the outward unacceptable behavior, not what prompted or contributed to the behavior in the first place. Keeping the letter of the law is acceptable, even when the spirit of the law is ignored. Stopping wrong behavior becomes the primary goal rather than changing the way the child thinks and believes. Compliance toward human authority is valued more than understanding God's authoritative Word. Problems are viewed as a necessary evil to be tolerated or eradicated as quickly as possible rather than an opportunity for growth and understanding. Parents and school personnel see the child's difficulties as wholly the child's responsibility to change rather than a red flag signaling parents and teachers may need to change something as well.

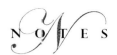

It seems wherever there are children and caretakers, the possibility for misunderstanding and errors in judgment exist. And usually, when the bottom line is reached, it becomes apparent that the greatest obstruction to real resolutions and effectiveness is nothing more than a lack of available time and a lack of priority placed on dealing thoroughly and Biblically with problems. In our instant society we often expect instant change in our children and are satisfied with instant compliance even if there is no inward change whatsoever. Quite simply, we choose methods that save time and get the supposed desired result—acceptable behavior—at the expense of behavior that reflects a true resolution or change of heart. When questioning school administrators and teachers regarding their discipline programs, it becomes immediately apparent that they do not have the time to complete all their duties and carefully work with children's problems as well. The demerit system fits well into a school structure that does not leave a significant allotment of time for problem solving. Likewise, parental discipline plans that highlight controlling behavior rather than changing behavior fits better into a busy parent's schedule than a system that requires them to patiently plod through an investigation and training process.

If there were a new way children could be processed more quickly and with less turmoil, parents and school personnel would tend to enthusiastically welcome it. People tend to show interest in systems that will "fix the problems" more quickly. Beware, parents. Beware teachers and administers, pastors and youth leaders. There are *no* easy short cuts, and anyone who tells you otherwise is horribly betraying you and your children. Problem solving requires an investment of time. Schools who really want to produce top notch Christian leaders can sooner afford to cut out the school janitor or school secretary than someone who can lovingly and effectively work with children's problems. Parents who are serious about raising children and who are confident in their faith and filled with Christian joy can sooner afford to live in a one-bedroom house and do without designer labels or hours of television than live without a parent available to work out children's problems in a patient and systematic manner.

Dealing with problems is not always fun—it is more often painstaking work that is undertaken because it is needful, not because it is enjoyable. Jesus pointedly asked Peter if Peter loved Him. Peter answered, "Yea, Lord; thou knowest that I love thee." Then Jesus replied, "Feed my lambs" *(John 21:15)*. The work of a shepherd is tedious, often lonely, and exhausting because sheep cannot thrive without human intervention and care. The care of human sheep is no less demanding or self-sacrificial. Feeding the Lord's littlest lambs requires quite an investment in time and labor and yet it is, in my opinion, one of the greatest labors of love a parent or church leader will ever engage in. What I am going to suggest in the following pages will not be easier, nor will it require "just a little time." It will however, be an expression of love for God's children, and may very well make the difference between joy and sorrow, success and failure.

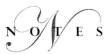

The Perfect Classroom

Problems are a way of life. They are not some kind of freak event of nature. Rather, they are allowed and designed by God for a purpose. Can you say as David said, "Before I was afflicted I went astray: but now have I kept thy word... It is good for me that I have been afflicted; that I might learn thy statutes. Thy hands have made me and fashioned me; give me understanding, that I may learn thy commandments. I know, O Lord, that thy judgments are right, and that thou in faithfulness hast afflicted me" *(Psalm 119:72-73,75)*? Can you say it is good for your children to be "afflicted" so they might learn how to understand and obey God's Word?

Problems and trials are opportunities to learn God's Word, to correct one's thinking, and to compel one to realign himself with what is right. Paul gloried in trials because of the good they produced. Viewed and handled correctly, trials produce patience, humility, obedience, strength, stability, faith in God, joy, and understanding. In the end, these things yield great reward in heaven for all eternity. Trials drive us to the feet of Christ where we find our every need supplied and every desire fulfilled. We learn to pray best in times of trouble, and we learn to love the Word of God when we are driven to search its pages for answers or comfort. Should our children be any different? What an opportunity we have to teach them how to deal with life's disappointments and problems when they squabble with a friend, fail a spelling test, disagree with a teacher, forget their homework, face the ridicule of schoolmates, or choose to be disobedient! How else will we be able to teach children Biblical ways to respond to injustice or injury inflicted by another except we get involved with their childhood problems and walk them through solutions?

When children are told to love their enemy and their enemy suddenly becomes unlovable, we are instantly given the perfect condition in which we can explain that no one can live the life of Christ in their own power or strength for it is impossible without God's enabling grace. When they become angry and retaliate and then believe they are perfectly justified, we are provided with the ideal classroom in which to teach the concept that our reactions to evil reveal our hearts. Another person's sin does not excuse our sinful way of responding to it, and no one makes us angry unless we let them! When children cheat on a test, it provides an excellent opportunity to show them how many sins are involved in one little fateful decision. If we take the time to explain it to them, we have the opportunity to explain how it was dishonest, how it manifested a prideful desire to be thought of more highly than what one deserved, how it reveals laziness, or how a desire becomes so great that we are willing to sin to get it.

It is an opportunity, not an inconvenience, when children call each other names, refuse to allow another child to play, push someone out of line, wear something immodest, write notes in church, or do any number of things sinful human children will do during their childhood. The problem is, we miss our opportunities to teach Biblical principles and instead become annoyed or angry that such childish events throw a monkey wrench into our plans for a smooth and trouble-free day. Better rethink your job description, Mom and Dad! Where there are children, there will be continual opportunities to learn, all cleverly disguised as interruptions to your day.

Change Takes Place on the Inside, Not the Outside

In order to effectively facilitate inward changes or solutions, we need to understand the inner human mechanism and process by which people, including children, make choices and changes. We first *reason* and weigh our understanding and desires. Then we judge which choice we prefer. Finally, we *will* to pursue that which is determined in our heart to be most preferable or valuable. If our own desires are judged preferable, we will choose to embrace our own ways and persist in them. If God's desires are judged preferable, we will choose to embrace His ways and persist in them. When addressing childhood problems, parents are confronted with more than a challenge to change a child's apparent actions or behavior; they are dealing with their child's heart, will, and thoughts as well. Spend some time pondering what the following passages of Scripture say to do and not do and the reasons that are given for the instruction.

- **Heart**—*Keep thy heart with all diligence; for out of it are the issues of life (Proverbs 4:23).*

- **Will**—*Make not provision for the flesh, to fulfill the lusts [desires] thereof (Romans 13:14b).*

- **Thoughts**—*For though we walk in the flesh, we do not war after the flesh; (for the weapons of our warfare are not carnal, but mighty through God to the pulling down of strong holds;) casting down imaginations, and every high thing that exalteth itself against the knowledge of God, and bringing into captivity every thought to the obedience of Christ (2 Corinthians 10:5).*

- **Actions**—*This I say then, Walk in the Spirit, and ye shall not fulfill the lust [desires] of the flesh (Galatians 5:16).*

When we, or our children, are not taught to do right and love God, our sinful hearts will always gravitate towards doing that which is selfish and evil.

A great passage of Scripture that summarizes the way these four areas function together in concert is found in *2 Timothy 3:16*. Paul tells Timothy, "All scripture is given by inspiration of God, and is profitable for **doctrine**, for **reproof**, for **correction**, for **instruction** in righteousness." In a nutshell, God changes our heart, will, thoughts, and actions as we 1) understand *doctrine*, which is truth and understanding through the Word; 2) accept *reproof* which leads to repentance and a change of heart; 3) *correct* or put off, old behavior, thoughts, words, actions; 4) receive *instruction* that disciplines us to put on new habits, thoughts, words, and actions.

The primary activity taking place in this process involves changing one's mind in such a way that we **put off** what is wrong and **put on** what is righteous. Change does not take place simply because we stop sinning in some way. There are many reasons one might stop behaving badly other than a change of heart about the sin or the problem. We are to stop behaving badly, or **put off** sinful behavior, because we come to realize and believe such behavior is a sin that brings sorrow to God. Yet simply **putting off** sinful behavior for the right reasons is not enough either. God tells us the second half of the process is to **put on** right behavior. Again, there are many selfish reasons one might decide to act righteous other than a godly reason. We are to **put on** righteous behavior because we desire to please God. This concept of replacing wrong behavior with its right counterpart operates effectively even when problems do not involve sin.

Blindly ceasing to do wrong and exercising righteousness has its benefits, but apart from engaging the mind in such as way that it is accompanied by understanding, or the heart in such a way that it is accompanied with a desire for what is right, putting on what is right is merely a work of the flesh. It is not an act of faith that is born out of true repentance nor does the Holy Spirit energize it. Parents who are satisfied with right outward behavior and give no thought to the condition of their child's heart make their children like those Jesus condemned, who "make clean the outside of the cup and the platter" while the inward part is "full of ravening and wickedness" *(Luke 11:39)*. Again, majoring on using external pressure to conform behavior produces a form of godliness, while denying the power with which true godliness is produced. (See *2 Timothy 3:5.*)

When a sinner expresses saving faith, the Bible tells us that "with the heart" he believes unto righteousness and with the mouth confession is made unto salvation *(Romans 10:10)*. A sinner is able to pray a prayer and not be saved because faith requires him to engage his heart and mind and *believe*, or rely completely on the Lord Jesus Christ—not just say a "magic" prayer. In a similar way, merely going through the actions of putting off wrong behavior and putting on right behavior does not necessarily mean one has a change of heart or mind about sinful or righteous behavior. We must understand truth; we must accept reproof in such a way that we have a change of heart about the behavior; we must engage our will and reject wrong behavior, choosing its righteous counterpart instead. Then we must willfully choose to practice right behavior, depending on God's Spirit to enable and change our inclinations toward doing wrong.

We will want to teach our children what behavior to put off and what behavior to put on in its place, assuming that we are also teaching our children in such a way that his heart, will, and mind are being renewed and transformed at the same time. *Ephesians 4:22-24* says this, "That ye put off concerning the former conversation [behavior] the old man, which is corrupt according to the deceitful lusts [desires]; and be renewed in the spirit of your mind; and that ye put on the new man, which after God is created in righteousness and true holiness." Putting off wrong behavior and putting on righteous behavior without being "transformed by the renewing of your mind" *(Romans 12:2* and *Ephesians 4:23)* produces Pharisees who proudly follow the letter of the law but know nothing about the spirit of the law. They are as Jesus

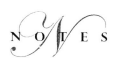

described, "people who draweth nigh unto me with their mouth, and honoureth me with their lips; but their heart is far from me" *(Matthew 15:8)*.

The good actions of Ezra were the outcome of his heartfelt decision to love God and obey Him. "For Ezra had prepared his heart to seek the law of the LORD, and to do it, and to teach in Israel statutes and judgments" *(Ezra 7:10)*. The evil actions of King Rehoboam were the outcome of his heartfelt decision to please himself and ignore God. "And he did evil, because he prepared not his heart to seek the LORD" *(2 Chronicles 12:14)*. When we, or our children, are not taught to do right and love God, our sinful hearts will always gravitate towards doing that which is selfish and evil. The ability to do right is rooted in a heartfelt love for God.

Change Requires Two Basic Actions

Put Off	Put On
Sinful thoughts, words, and actions	Godly thoughts, words, and actions
Sinful habits after judging your life by God's Word	Godly habits by deliberately doing the right behavior
Depending on the power of your flesh to overcome bad habits	Depending on the power found in Christ alone to overcome bad habits
Focusing on yourself and temporal values	Focusing on Christ and eternal values
Focusing on personal failure, sins, personal inadequacy	Focusing on Christ's success, His forgiveness, and His adequacy

Teach your children the wisdom of right behavior. Read through Proverbs with your children, looking for an example in each chapter of behavior to put off and behavior to put on. Read the entire chapter, first summarizing it, then pinpointing at least one thing to put off and put on. For example:

Proverbs	Put Off	Put On
Chapter 1	Hating knowledge and correction	Fearing God and loving instruction
Chapter 2	The neglectful ways of the wicked	Diligently searching God's Word for wisdom

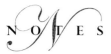

EPHESIANS 4:25-32	PUT OFF	PUT ON
Verse 25	Lying	Speaking truth
Verse 28	Stealing	Working and giving
Verse 29	Destructive speech	Constructive speech
Verses 30-31	Bitterness, anger	Kindness, forgiveness

The following pages describe various problems and possible solutions that are intended to illustrate a basic problem-solving procedure. They are not intended to supply an exhaustive list of possible causes and solutions, but are offered as possibilities for you to consider as you seek God's wisdom in dealing with your own particular child and situation. The principle of engaging your child's heart and mind and leading him to put off wrong behavior and put on its righteous counterpart becomes "second nature" the more you practice it.

You will need to do the work of finding Scripture that applies to what needs to be put off and put on when problems involve sins that need to be dealt with. (The problem of "sassing" is filled out as an example.) Remember that many problems do not involve a sinful choice on the part of parent or child and therefore require a different sort of "put off and put on" application. You will notice that some examples offer very simple solutions, yet still have the element of investigating the precipitating underlying causes, identifying what needs to be eliminated and what needs to be implemented. The way a parent would engage a child's heart and mind as he works through this process varies depending on the problem and the need.

SASSING - NAME CALLING

Possible Underlying Problem
- Resentment of authority
- Rebellion
- Lack of love and respect for others
- Does not know how to make a godly appeal to authority.

Possible Parental Contribution
- Failure to discipline properly
- Failure to admit or correct own wrongs, parental hypocrisy
- Tolerating disrespectful speech or actions

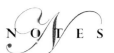

- Does not entreat authority with respect.

Put off—Judging others - *Matthew 7:1-2*

Put on—Examining own faults - *John 8:9*; Bitterness - *Hebrews 12:15*; Tender heart - *Colossians 3:12*; Boasting and conceit - *1 Corinthians 4:7*; Humility - *Proverbs 27:2*; Stubbornness - *1 Samuel 15:23*; Submission - *Romans 6:13*; Disrespect - *2 Timothy 3:6*; Yielded will - *Matthew 6:10*; Sassing - *John 6:43*; Hurtful words - *Ephesians 4:29*; Respect for authority - *Ephesians 5:21*; Words that build up - *1 Timothy 4:12*; Hatred - *Matthew 5:21-22*; Love - *Ephesians 4:32*

Stop your child *immediately* when he engages in unkind or disrespectful speech. Spank him for using disrespectful words to a parent or one in authority. *Do not* try to correct disrespect by lecturing or withholding a privilege. All disrespectful speech must incur an immediate, swift response. If you are in a public place, calmly leave. Go home, correct your child, and return. The inconvenience is worth the results you will achieve if you deal with it decisively, quickly, and seriously.

After you have disciplined your child for disrespect, or stopped him from calling names or using unkind words, have him *replace* his wrong attitude and wrong words with good ones. Demonstrate a way that your child could have said what he wanted to say in a respectful manner. We must put off the sinful speech, and put on kind and loving speech. As you teach children kind and respectful language, they will not have difficulty refraining from using hateful words.

Engage Child's Heart and Mind—A father must not allow his children to talk disrespectfully to their mother. Nor should he ever talk to her disrespectfully. Likewise, mothers must not talk to or about the children's father disrespectfully. When parents tolerate disrespectful speech toward the opposite parent, they encourage their children to disregard the authority of both parents. Model respect for authority; teach your children how to appeal to an authority other than yourself, demonstrating what you are doing and why you are doing it, when possible. Do not ever allow your children to argue with you disrespectfully, or engage in unconstructive, heated discussions. Nevertheless, deliberately teach your children how to express their views and differences with you while at the same time maintaining an attitude of respect.

DAYDREAMING

Possible Underlying Problem

- Too much emotional stimulation that child is not mature enough to handle
- Too much television watching
- Desire to escape discomfort, fears of facing difficulties, or failure
- Means of avoiding or putting off unpleasant tasks, laziness
- Enjoys thinking that is artistic or inventive in nature

- Child is highly distractible, has difficulty staying on task, or keeping focused on uninteresting tasks.

Possible Parental Contribution

- Giving instructions and commands without following through to be sure child responds immediately
- Unresolved difficulties or tension in home
- Lack of encouragement or follow through in requiring child to complete something difficult.
- Leaving child alone for long periods of time.
- Intolerance toward child's differing personality.
- Lack of patience or consistency in helping child develop ability to sustain attention.

It's good to remember that daydreaming is normal, unless it becomes excessive or interferes with your child's routine or ability to concentrate. Some children are more prone to daydreaming than others, although some use it as a means to brood about problems, which is problematic.

Don't stop your child from daydreaming by ordering him to stop. Rather, when it is interfering with his normal routine, interrupt his thoughts by engaging him in conversation. Encourage him to talk with you by asking questions that cannot be answered with a simple yes or no until he begins talking more openly. Then, engage him in a concrete activity that will absorb his thinking in a healthy way.

Deal with possible underlying fears by talking about them and providing information that will better equip him to draw more confident conclusions or to confide in you. Help your child construct and implement solutions to problems that seem to be overwhelming. Become part of his team and work *with* him. Eliminate unnecessary and oppressive pressure on your child in some cases where it is appropriate. Keep your home environment happy. Provide space for the child to fail. Adult intolerance and unrealistic expectations (perfectionism) often fuel a child's desire to escape.

Insist that your child obey immediately without dawdling or arguing. Encourage him when situations or tasks are difficult but do not allow him to quit before he completes them.

Some children respond well to the use of a wind-up timer to help them complete tasks in reasonable amounts of time or a silent egg timer for quiet tasks. Although he may require more time than others to complete a project, do not allow him to spend *excessive* amounts of time doing things that he *can* do much more quickly. Don't allow him to be sidetracked when he's doing a task. Gently keep him focused on what he's to do.

Do not allow excessive television viewing. The rapid pace of changing television scenes condition some children to become intolerant of a normal monotonous pace of life. Television also introduces emotionally stimulating (not intellectually or spiritually stimulating) or confusing subject matter that children often tend to ruminate over. Help your child realize there are more fun things to do besides watching television—then help him do those things.

FEAR

Possible Underlying Problems

- Frightening experiences, television viewing, older playmates who manipulate the younger by such means as fearful storytelling
- General fearfulness, lack of confidence, lack of social confidence.
- Sensitive temperament, perceptions of helplessness
- Too much idle time spent worrying or ruminating real or perceived injustices
- Views failure as unacceptable in any circumstance, fears the outcome of failure.
- Introspective thinking habits, habitual "what if?" type of thinking.

Possible Parental Contribution

- Using ridicule, scorn, or fear as a means of discipline. Over-disciplining or using overly harsh means of instructing children. Perfectionism.
- Forcing child to go through an experience he deeply fears
- Repeated experiences with impatient, intense, and overbearing adults who are in authority over child outside home.
- Failure to communicate adequately with child, explain, or prepare child for changes
- Alienating child, becoming overly occupied in own activities to the excessive exclusion of child
- Parent showing unreasonable fear and lack of control over emotions

Do not use threats of a fearful consequence as a means of controlling or inducing obedience. Do not ridicule or embarrass as a means of discouraging unwanted behavior. Do not administer discipline in anger or use stomach-wrenching lectures as a means of venting your frustration. Do not forcefully compel your child to go through a situation he deeply fears—this will only increase his fear. Do not use bribes and coercion as a means of helping him overcome fears.

Restrain your outward expressions of fear, anxiety, worry, or pessimism. Children cannot adequately discern or objectively handle a parent's problems. They are always exaggerated in a child's mind and interpreted as more severe than they are in actuality. Watch your intensity of emotion when dealing with a sensitive child. Use a soft voice. Slow down. Have a pleasant facial expression as you speak to him. Screaming at a fearful child increases his anxiety.

Help your child gradually gain a sense of control over the thing he fears. He can make a toy dog stop barking or make an obedient dog sit on command while a parent is holding him securely. Let him turn the vacuum cleaner on and off himself to help him overcome a fear of the vacuum cleaner. Many fears are overcome by gradual degrees of controlled exposure to the thing he dreads. At the same time, he needs to be given the opportunity to control the thing he dreads as much as possible. Whenever possible, provide information that will diffuse your child's exaggerated conclusions. As your child becomes familiar or knowledgeable about the thing he excessively fears, his anxiety will usually decrease dramatically.

Talk to your child while you are working. Explain what you are doing. Be predictable. Provide a schedule of your plans for the day. Prepare your child for changes. Speak confidently and quietly. Listen to your child. Provide eye contact. Encourage him to express his feelings. Do not leave your child for excessive amounts of time in the care of others. Don't exclude him from activities that he could be a part of.

A baby needs to form an attachment to his Mom; consequently, he will react more strongly when his Mom leaves. This is normal. Nevertheless, it is good to teach babies and children that Mom needs a break. Short absences are healthy. However, with young children prolonged separations should be avoided, particularly with children who are fearful. Do not sneak out to prevent a baby or child from crying when you leave. While this practice initially makes leaving easier, it only increases insecurity. Say good-bye, hug your baby, smile, tell him when you will return, use a confident voice, then *leave*! Do not express worry, sympathy, distress, or hesitancy for this increased fear; for they will prevent a child from learning to accept Mom's occasional leaving.

Bad Dreams—Ask your child to describe the dream so you can offer appropriate reassurance and also gain an understanding of the possible emotions or fears he's struggling to resolve. Talk about verses of Scripture that assure us of God's loving care. Pray a simple prayer of thanksgiving for God's love. Conclude by talking about things that are of particular delight to your child in order to get his mind engaged in a different direction. Do not ridicule him for his fears or bad dreams.

Fear of the Dark—Night lights are helpful to a child afraid of the dark. Installing a dimmer switch so he can gradually diminish the light needed works particularly well in many cases. This may help produce peace of mind.

JEALOUSY

Possible Underlying Problem

- Resentment over new sibling displacing his one-and-only-status
- Extreme selfishness or self-pity
- Fears of no longer being loved
- Fear of being alone, resentment over younger child interfering with normal activities, preferential treatment of another child

- Evaluating abilities harshly, hearing or engaging in unfavorable comparisons with others
- Too much isolation at home with few opportunities to interact with other children

Possible Parental Contribution

- Forces child to spend too much time playing alone, neglecting to include him in your life and activities whenever possible
- Failure to adequately prepare other children for arrival of a baby or major change in home life
- Overly indulging child's whims and demands
- Lack of warmth, physical contact, expressions of love
- Preferential treatment of a brighter or more talented child
- Family conversation focuses on acquisition of material goods, criticizing others, comparing others, belittling the accomplishments of others

Jealousy primarily stems from a discontent with God's provisions and a lack of thankfulness for what we have or for the limitations God has placed on us. Children must learn that our provisions all come from God and that He works differently in each person's life. We trust that God is good and fair by what we know about Him; therefore, we are able to rest in the knowledge that He knows what He is doing and will bring all things to a fair and just conclusion. The concept "to whom much is given much is required," proportionate giving, etc. all help children gain a proper perspective when tempted to envy others. Show children how things aren't always what they appear to be on the surface by discussing Bible accounts of such errors in judgment.

Because jealousy indicates a lack of love for others and a focus on one's self, make every effort to teach children how to do acts of love and kindness for others. Do not tolerate speech that puts down others such as sarcastic teasing or boastful speech. If children are allowed to practice such behavior repeatedly, it will become habituated into their personality. Teach brothers and sisters to cheer for each other and be happy for each other's accomplishments. Do not allow complaining or encourage comparing of circumstances. Teach your children how to be *thankful* in every situation.

LAZINESS

Possible Underlying Problem

- Resentment of authority
- Poor development of listening habits
- Boredom, self-centered life
- Physical lethargy due to growth spurts, illness, or poor eating habits

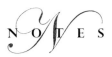

- Lack of physical exercise, stimulation
- Repeated experiences of failure in competitive sports or academic subjects
- Lack of self-discipline

Possible Parental Contribution

- Nagging, irritable parent
- Lack of effort in providing inspiration and motivation
- Lack of discipline and structured activity in parent's lives
- Allowing children to easily manipulate parents
- Allowing children to get by with expending minimum effort
- Failure to recognize limitations of child's ability or learning aptitude
- Allowing child to spend inordinate amounts of time with TV, video games, etc.

Laziness stems primarily from a lack of self-discipline. Therefore, make every effort to structure your child's life and get him in the habit of doing things because it's time to do it, not because he *feels* like doing it. Teach him to use an alarm clock and get himself up at the same time every morning. Do not allow him to stay up so late that he cannot get up properly in the morning.

Make four lists of routine tasks: one to be completed before breakfast, one before lunch, one before dinner, and one before bedtime snack. Keep the lists very short to start with. Your objective is to establish habitual routines by repeatedly doing them in a given time frame. For example, your list before breakfast might include making the bed and brushing teeth; before lunch, washing hands and picking up toys; before dinner, feed dog and clean room; before bedtime snack; brush teeth, lay out clothes for tomorrow. Even after you have established your routine, keep the lists simple and very *limited*. A long list will not work. Do not allow your child to eat *until* the list has been completed at each checkpoint meal, but do not lecture, scold, or show disgust. Simply start the meal without him and allow him to join you or eat his meal when he has completed his tasks. If the child comes to the meal having completed the targeted tasks without having to be prompted, give him points toward a reward at the end of the week or in the very least, commend him warmly.

Lazy children tend to become quite proficient at excuse making and will become indignant if you discover their deception. Be careful not to be easily taken in by clever excuses. Don't allow your child to manipulate you. When children forget, help them remember next time by following through with discipline, even though they forgot.

Do not nag your children. Rather, expect and insist on obedience. Act immediately when they ignore you. Letting them get by with "putting you off" only reinforces their habit of obeying only when they feel like it or when they absolutely have to.

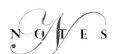

Keep your children involved in structured activities. You don't want them to have so many activities they never have a chance to rest, but neither do you want them to have so little activity they have a surplus of idle time.

Laziness and self-centered thinking go together. Steer your child away from brooding and thinking about himself. Teach him to love God, to serve others, and to enjoy being useful. Show him how to set and achieve goals, both short and long term.

If your child is having difficulty with his social life or is experiencing repeated failures in school, find ways to tutor him as well as build his confidence. Affirm your love for him as you patiently help him through his difficulties.

LYING

Possible Underlying Problems

- Unresolved guilt, which produces a fear of judgment
- Fear of admitting truthful thoughts and feelings
- Desire to avoid disagreeable consequences, accepting personal responsibility, or humbling self to admit wrong
- Fear of making mistakes or failing, or appearing to be a failure
- Fear of losing parent's respect or love, or invoking parent's anger or uncontrolled outburst

Possible Parental Contribution

- Parents indulging in any deceptive behavior and failing to live honestly
- Parents encouraging children to engage in polite lying
- Placing too much importance on what people think, seeking the applause and approval of others rather than of God
- Refusing to model owning up to the truth, accepting blame, or asking forgiveness
- Emotionally charged, intense lectures, or angry outbursts when child's misbehavior or failure is discovered; harsh discipline

Help your child understand that any attempt to deceive is a lie. For example, we are able to lie by being silent when our silence allows someone to believe something that is not true. All deceptive and manipulative behavior must be dealt with thoroughly so a child understands the many ways human beings use deception to avoid discomfort of some kind. Help your child pinpoint the motive he had for being deceptive and the events that preceded or led up to his choice to deceive.

Extol the great benefits of talking truthfully as a desirable virtue that we must always practice. The love of lying is overcome when it is replaced with a love for truth. Explaining God's attribute of truthfulness and the many benefits of God's truth greatly encourages a child to esteem truth and desire it. Express enthusiasm when your child exercises good character traits, rather than putting your major emphasis on child's winning and excelling. For example, commend him for his courage to tell the truth even when it is uncomfortable to do so. Be sure to explain that humility is required in such situations, and this is greatly valued by God, for He promises to give grace to the humble and opposes the proud.

Be sure you are not making too much an ordeal over every little transgression. However, do not make light of lying. Do not spank a child who is repentant and confesses his wrong without being found out. Let him know that if he comes to you on his own, he will not be spanked; though, he still may be required to make his wrong right or to suffer the natural consequences of his sin. Be sure child understands how a Christian resolves guilt and receives assurance of God's forgiveness.

NERVOUS HABITS

Possible Underlying Problems

- Repeated or major frightening experience
- Physical illness or improper rest
- Belief he must conform to adult behavior
- Fear or failure to express feelings, thoughts, or ideas; believes that he must hide them rather than deal with them openly and truthfully
- Underlying tension, tense family relationships; overbearing or bossy older siblings or playmates
- Excessive worry, possible bitterness, blaming others for unhappiness
- Unresolved guilt, inadequate understanding of God's forgiveness
- Lack of thankfulness
- Self-absorbed thinking habits

Possible Parental Contribution

- Perfectionist, critical parents
- Lack of physical outlets provided for tension release
- Using fear (threats) or name calling as a means of controlling behavior
- Inconsistent discipline, poor teamwork between parents
- Loud, angry, intense parents
- Expecting child to maintain too full a schedule
- Disorganized, cluttered environment or home life
- Worry and fretting between parents
- Constant arguing in the home

Simplify your child's daily routines, and do not expect adult behavior of him. Find ways to relieve strains at school or in regard to his social situations. Provide a place

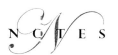

where he can retreat and enjoy quiet time alone when he desires. Be careful he doesn't have too many toys or too many fragile toys. Do not discuss your child's problems openly or within earshot of him. Do not nit-pick, or compare him with siblings or other children. Deal with causes of turmoil in the home.

When giving him choices, limit them between two. "Would you like this or this," not "Which one would you like?" Tone down excitement and activity before bedtime and prior to stressful events. Resting or having quiet time before meals is often helpful. Warm baths before bedtime and before stressful events often help considerably, particularly with small children.

Work at getting your child to associate something good and pleasant with whatever causes him fear or dread. Encourage your child to talk about his concerns and fears, but do not allow prolonged brooding or fretting. Teach him to put yesterday behind him and concern himself only with today. Become aware of what is going on at school even if the child does not complain of problems. Make it your business to know who your child is with and who might be mistreating your child while he is away from home.

QUARRELING

Possible Underlying Problem
- Age and personality differences
- Pride, refusing to yield personal rights
- Selfishness, intolerance
- Jealousy
- Inability to resolve problems or find appropriate solutions
- Immaturity in communication skills

Possible Parental Contribution
- Grudge holding between parents
- Parental fighting, yelling, ungodly communication
- Failure of parents to openly demonstrate Biblical method of repenting, seeking forgiveness, granting forgiveness, and making restitution when applicable
- Failure of parents to teach children how to reasonably resolve difficulties, yield personal rights
- Lack of interaction between parents and children
- Favoritism, expressed or unexpressed

Fighting among Boys—Boys tend to be more physical in their expressions of anger than girls. They are built to withstand active work and play and therefore seek more physical outlets for their energy. If they are not given ways to expend physical energy in a controlled manner, they will tend to misuse it or vent it on others with

Page 253

whom they are unhappy. Boys *need* physical activity! The will to fight is a natural inclination to boys. To a great extent, it is a God-given mechanism that will later prompt them to protect their family, defend their country, and survive in a tough world. Do not shame your son for wanting to wrestle with his brothers or friends, or play war games. However, teach him to control his fighting and playing. Do not ever tolerate bullying or fighting that is vindictive, cruel, or out of control. He must never be allowed to have fun at the expense of others, or tease in ways that are cruel or demeaning.

Do not forbid your son to fight if it is in self-defense; however, do not encourage fighting or allow your son to accept the idea that he can settle his disagreements or anger by fighting. Before he should ever use force, he needs to have done everything possible to stop or resolve problems. Teach your sons that some things are worth fighting for, but other things are not. The values you teach will form your son's opinions as to what and when it is appropriate to fight. Teach your son skills that will help him avoid a fight. Such things include a sense of humor, tolerance, avoidance when possible, negotiation and communication skills, and a willingness to overcome evil with good, according to *Romans 12*. Teach your son how to direct his energy toward constructing solutions to problems rather than venting his anger about his problems.

Fighting among Girls—Girls rarely become physical when they fight amongst themselves. Most often their fights involve words or actions that inflict emotional pain on those they wish to hurt in subtle ways. Rejection, isolation, ridicule, tattling, and teasing are their "weapons of choice" when angry or unhappy with others. Girls have a natural inclination toward honing communication skills that will be a particular asset as a future mother and wife. They need to be taught to control the tongue with the same diligence that boys need to be taught to control their fists. The tongue can be used as a vicious weapon of defense and often leaves many causalities in her wake. Parents need to be aware of the subtle means of provocation that can be utilized by girls in particular, and expend much effort in teaching girls how to use kindness and graciousness in their speech.

Like boys, girls need to learn ways of resolving problems rather than being allowed to resort to hateful means to do so. Girls do tend to use the tongue in situations where they believe they need to defend themselves. Because they generally back away from attempting to use physical means of discouraging abuse, they most often resort to verbal means of defense. You do not want your daughter to become passive toward the abusive behavior of others, but neither do you want her to learn habits of reacting that will only make her interpersonal relationships more complicated and painful. Teach her how to confidently and graciously confront a bully or deflect mistreatment without resorting to retaliation or hurtful speech.

Quarreling among Siblings—Help children learn to understand and appreciate each other's differing personality traits. Provide guidance to help children resolve their own disputes when they cannot do so alone, but avoid always refereeing quarrels. Separate your children and interfere only when they are out of control, or have an unfair advantage over another.

It is important that your children be given opportunities to observe a godly and controlled way of disagreeing and resolving conflicts because children ultimately do whatever they see, either good or bad. To some extent, it is constructive and profitable for children to see Mom and Dad disagree and resolve conflicts Biblically and lovingly. However, it is *not* constructive to openly discuss matters that children are not yet emotionally able to handle or understand. It is also *not* constructive for children to observe Mom and Dad behaving in a disrespectful, petty, selfish, or uncontrolled manner. When this occurs, be sure the children also observe Mom and Dad acknowledging their behavior as sinful and seeking one another's forgiveness.

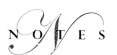

SELFISHNESS

Possible Underlying Problem

Lack of love or regard for others; unaccustomed to putting self in another's place

- Selfishness, greed, covetousness
- Loves to be center of attention, object of other's admiration and devotion.
- Refusal to yield personal rights, expectation that others should yield
- Lack of enjoyment for giving and helping others

Possible Parental Contribution

- Indulgence; unwillingness to refuse child's demands; deny or discipline child appropriately; desire for peace at any cost
- Lack of love for others on part of parent; critical of others, self-righteous
- Covetousness or selfishness on part of parent; refusal to demonstrate yielding his own personal rights
- Child is not made to work or earn privileges or wait for things desired.
- Parent's lack of joy and enthusiasm for giving and helping others

Remember that sharing is gradually learned and does not come naturally to children. Do not just announce, "Share" and demand that children do so. Do not allow your child to bully others or to manipulate you or other children into giving him what he wants.

Help children understand the feelings and wishes of others he is to get along with by describing specifically how his actions affect others. Encourage him to express how he feels when others mistreat him in the manner he is now treating a playmate. Make a game out of taking turns. As much as possible, children should be given the freedom to decide whether or not they will share a toy or object that belongs to them exclusively. In order to help a child learn to give willingly from his heart, he must be allowed to make that decision himself rather than being forced to share something that rightfully belongs to him.

Teach concepts of serving others and sharing by explaining and demonstrating your willingness and enjoyment in sharing with others, including your children. Share with your children when it is clearly your choice to do so, not when your child demands what is yours. Demonstrate the joys of serving and the means by which we serve God.

Do not negotiate your commands with your children or plead with them to obey. Teach your children to immediately respond to a request that is given in a calm, loving, but firm manner. Do not encourage arguments or protest by responding with pleas or threats. Do not allow complaining. Teach your child to be thankful for and content with whatever God has given him. Do not allow your child to have everything he wants. Giving in to a child's demands for instant gratification leads to selfish, indulgent behavior.

STEALING

Possible Underlying Problem

- Selfishness, unwilling to give or share
- Lack of discipline, unwilling to work
- Impatient, unwilling to earn or wait for privileges
- Lack of love for others

Possible Parental Contribution

- Indulging child's whims and demands, failing to teach child concepts of sharing
- Failure to teach child to enjoy work or to discipline him to work and fulfill his responsibilities
- Allowing child to be distracted from tasks, leave work unfinished, giving too many desires without waiting or working for them, giving too much money disproportionate with work expended
- Not providing a means for children to earn money to buy things he desires

Do not allow your child to manipulate you into caving in to his whims and demands for instant gratification. If you have declined a request, do not reward your child's protests, complaining, or arguing by changing your mind. Changing a no answer ought to be a rare occurrence.

Do not force older children to give up toys for a younger child simply because he is whining or crying. This leads the younger to selfish expectations that he should have what he wants. Teach your child to enjoy giving and sharing. Include your child in your projects to give and share with others, and make it fun. Teach your child how to tithe to God.

Give your child a reasonable amount of responsibilities around home, according to his age, time availability, and capacity. Assignments of individual responsibilities should be accepted by all family members and should not be rewarded with money. However, you must also provide work opportunities that children can be paid for, most of which are voluntary. No work, no pay. Do not give automatic weekly allowances if the child does not work for it. Do not give your child a disproportionate amount of money for the work he does.

Work with your child as much as possible. Make work fun by your happy attitude and spirit of cooperation and teamwork. Do not allow him to leave uncompleted tasks or develop a bad habit of not finishing projects. Structure your child's day and encourage routines by doing the same responsibilities at the same time each day as much as possible. This helps your child develop a more disciplined manner of living.

Teach your children how to save and work toward desired goals. Always have both short-term and long-term goals. Encourage him, while he is young, to learn skills that interest him such as sports and hobbies.

Appendix

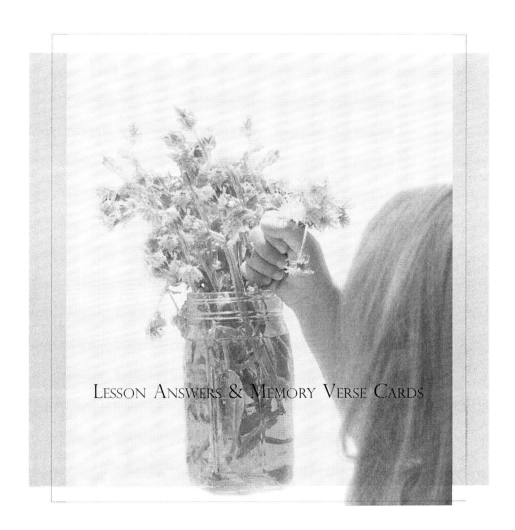

Lesson Answers & Memory Verse Cards

Chapter One: What Makes Christian Parenting Different

Answers:

1. love God and obey Him themselves
2. hear; learn; fear the Lord; observe to do (obey) all God's commandments
3. hear and do them

Chapter Two: The Successful Christian Parent's Secret Ingredient

Answers:

1. fear of the Lord
2. 2:6 – understanding, 2:6 – knowledge of God, 2:12 – discretion, 2:12 – deliverance from evil people
3. a. Where is wisdom found? How does one get understanding?
   b. fear the Lord and depart from evil
4. They were following their own human reasoning and "feelings" rather than conducting themselves according to God's commandments. They did not exercise or discipline themselves to practice godliness.

Chapter Three: How To Really Love Your Child

Answers:

1. joyful parents
2. when the child is young
3. a. rod and reproof
   b. neglecting to discipline
4. parents provoke. *Provoke* means to incite anger by treating child unjustly.

Chapter Four: Understanding Your Child's Unique Personality

Answers:

1. judged
2. cries; father
3. heritage (inheritance, gift, reward)

Chapter Five: Getting Through The Bumpy Stages

Answers:

1. teach; example; ashamed
2. observe; lovingkindess

3. example (ways)
4. godliness; good; evil

Chapter Six: Discipline That Works, Part One

Answers:

1. God chastises us so we can be partakers of His holiness, for our benefit.
2. These passages allude to the fact that children might mistake the purpose of correction and wrongfully believe God (or a parent) doesn't love them or is rejecting them.
3. He doesn't understand that chastisement is a deterrent to sins that destroy him in adulthood. When he is an adult who is suffering the painful consequences of sin, he wishes he had been chastised in childhood so he would not have chosen such a destructive path.

Chapter Seven: Discipline That Works, Part Two

Answers:

Psalm 119:75,67,71

1. He no longer goes astray – he learns God's laws (Word).
2. God cares about him, loves him, knows him.
3. They recognize the loving motives of parents who were willing to discipline righteously.

Psalm 107:10-13

1. They rebelled against His Word.
2. When they cried to Him
3. Trouble and distress

Chapter Eight: Motivating Children to Do What They Don't Want To Do

Answers:

1. hear and be wise
2. observe; ways
3. strong; God's charge, statutes and judgments; prosper
4. wisdom

Chapter Nine: Preventing and Dealing With Rebellion

Answers:

1. He warned but did not restrain them from doing evil.
2. Lot was hypocritical; children did not view him as a godly man.

Chapter Ten: Teaching Precept Upon Precept

Answers:

1. picture/example
2. inspiring/teaching
3. God's Word

Chapter Eleven: Your Child's Future: Disaster or Delight?

Answers:

1. singing
2. praise/thanksgiving
3. prayer
4. comfort
5. instruction
6. exhort/encourage

Chapter Twelve: Resolving Children's Problems

Answers:

1. stop practicing sinful ways of an unbeliever and start deliberately obeying/practicing the right ways of a believer.
2. the Holy Spirit living within him.

Lesson One
What Makes Christian Parenting Different

Lesson Two
The Successful Christian Parent's Secret Ingredient

Lesson Three
How To Really Love Your Child

Lesson Four
Understanding Your Child's Unique Personality

Lesson Five
Getting through the Bumpy Stages

Lesson Six
Discipline That Works, Part One

Lesson Seven
Discipline That Works, Part Two

Lesson Eight
Motivating Children To Do What They Don't Want To Do

And when they shall say unto you, Seek unto them that have familiar spirits, and unto wizards that peep, and that mutter: should not a people seek unto their God? For the living to the dead? To the law and to the testimony: if they speak not according to this word, *it is* because *there is* no light in them.
Isaiah 8:19-20

Wisdom is the principal thing; therefore get wisdom; and with all thy getting get understanding. Exalt her, and she shall promote thee; she shall bring thee to honor, when thou dost embrace her.
Proverbs 4:7-8

Parenting With Wisdom - Memory Verses

But now, O LORD, thou *art* our father; we *are* the clay, and thou our potter; and we all *are* the work of thy hand.
Isaiah 64:8

I will praise thee; for I am fearfully *and* wonderfully made: marvelous *are* thy works; and *that* my soul knoweth right well.
Psalm 139:14

Parenting With Wisdom - Memory Verses

The rod and reproof give wisdom: but a child left to himself bringeth his mother to shame.
Proverbs 29:15

Correct thy son, and he shall give thee rest; yea, he shall give delight unto thy soul.
Proverbs 29:17

Parenting With Wisdom- Memory Verses

Behold, I set before you this day a blessing and a curse; a blessing, if ye obey the commandments of the LORD your God, which I command you this day: and a curse, if ye will not obey the commandments of the LORD your God.
Deuteronomy 11:26-28a

The LORD hath appeared of old unto me, *saying*, Yea, I have loved thee with an everlasting love: therefore with lovingkindness have I drawn thee.
Jeremiah 31:3

Parenting With Wisdom - Memory Verses

The father of the righteous shall greatly rejoice: and he that begetteth a wise child shall have joy of him. Thy father and thy mother shall be glad, and she that bare thee shall rejoice.
Proverbs 23:24-25

Whatsoever ye do, do all to the glory of God.
1 Corinthians 10:31b

Parenting With Wisdom - Memory Verses

This is my commandment, That ye love one another, as I have loved you. Greater love hath no man than this, that a man lay down his life for his friends.
John 15:12-13

With all lowliness and meekness, with longsuffering, forbearing one another in love; be ye kind one to another, tenderhearted, forgiving one another, even as God for Christ's sake hath forgiven you.
Ephesians 4:2, 32

Parenting With Wisdom - Memory Verses

Charity suffereth long, *and* is kind…beareth all things, believeth all things, hopeth all things, endureth all things.
1 Corinthians 13:4a, 7

Being confident of this very thing, that he which hath begun a good work in you will perform it until the day of Jesus Christ.
Philippians 1:6

Parenting With Wisdom- Memory Verses

My son, despise not the chastening of the LORD; neither be weary of his correction: for whom the Lord loveth hecorrecteth; even the son in whom he delighteth.
Proverbs 3:11-12

For I have given you an example, that ye should do as I have done to you.
John 13:15

Parenting With Wisdom - Memory Verses

Lesson Nine
Preventing and Dealing with Rebellion

Lesson Ten
Teaching Precept upon Precept

Lesson Eleven
Your Child's Future: Disaster or Delight?

Lesson Twelve
Resolving Children's Problems

Theme Verse
Precept Upon Precept

Series Verse
Titus 2 Bible Study Series

Whom shall he teach knowledge? And whom shall he make to understand doctrine? Them that are weaned from the milk, and drawn from the breasts. For precept must be upon precept, precept upon precept; line upon line, line upon line; here a little, and there a little.

Isaiah 28:9-10

But continue thou in the things which thou hast learned and hast been assured of, knowing of whom thou hast learned them; and that from a child thou hast known the holy scriptures, which are able to make thee wise unto salvation through faith which is in Christ Jesus.

2 Timothy 3:15

Parenting With Wisdom - Memory Verses

And call upon me in the day of trouble: I will deliver thee, and thou shalt glorify me.

Psalm 50:15

Let us therefore come boldly unto the throne of grace, that we may obtain mercy, and find grace to help in time of need.

Hebrews 4:16

Parenting With Wisdom - Memory Verses

Young men likewise exhort to be sober minded. In all things showing thyself a pattern of good works: in doctrine *showing* uncorruptness, gravity, sincerity, sound speech, that cannot be condemned; that he that is of the contrary part may be ashamed, having no evil thing to say of you.

Titus 2:6-8

Parenting With Wisdom - Memory Verses

Fathers, provoke not your children *to anger*, lest they be discouraged.

Colossians 3:21

And Samuel said, Hath the LORD *as great* delight in burnt offerings and sacrifices, as in obeying the voice of the LORD? Behold, to obey *is* better than sacrifice, *and* to hearken than the fat of rams. For rebellion *is as* the sin of witchcraft, and stubbornness *is as* iniquity and idolatry.

1 Samuel 15:22-23a

Parenting With Wisdom - Memory Verses

But as it is written, Eye hath not seen, nor ear heard, neither have entered into the heart of man, the things which God hath prepared for them that love him.

1 Corinthians 2:9

Thus saith the LORD, Behold, I set before you the way of life, and the way of death.

Jeremiah 21:8

Parenting With Wisdom - Memory Verses

But the word of the LORD was unto them precept upon precept, precept upon precept; line upon line, line upon line; here a little, *and* there a little.

Isaiah 28:13a

Parenting With Wisdom - Memory Verses